The Pocket Pediatrician

An A–Z Guide to Your Child's Health

Dear Paul + Yvonne,
...For our children's future!

David Zigelman

D1316860

The Pocket Pediatrician

An A–Z Guide to Your Child's Health

David Zigelman,
M.D., F.A.A.P.

MAIN STREET BOOKS

Doubleday
New York   London   Toronto
Sydney   Auckland

A Main Street Book
PUBLISHED BY DOUBLEDAY
a division of Bantam Doubleday Dell Publishing Group, Inc.
1540 Broadway, New York, New York 10036

Main Street Books, Doubleday, and the portrayal of a
building with a tree are trademarks of Doubleday, a
division of Bantam Doubleday Dell Publishing Group, Inc.

Library of Congress Cataloging-in-Publication Data
Zigelman, David, 1948–
    The pocket pediatrician: an A–Z guide to your
child's health / David Zigelman.
        p. cm.
    Includes index.
    1. Children—Health and hygiene—Handbooks,
manuals, etc.   2. Children—Diseases—Handbooks,
manuals, etc.   3. Children's accidents—Prevention—
Handbooks, manuals, etc.   I. Title.
RJ61.Z54   1995   94-11969
613'.0432—dc20   CIP

ISBN 0-385-47088-6

THIS BOOK IS DEDICATED TO:

Shaindy

for sharing this adventure.

for creating an environment that helps me learn.

for taking on added responsibilities while I was preoccupied with preparation of the manuscript.

and she does it all with style and with a smile.

Michelle and Moshe

for teaching me the most about children. Due to their patience, understanding, and sacrifice, this book is as much theirs as it is mine.

Abraham and Beatrice Zigelman

for instilling in me the desire to learn.

and to my father's cluttered den, which attests to his love of books, a love he instilled in me.

John Lewy, M.D.

who allowed his fountain of pediatric knowledge to spill a little in my direction.

Charles Kleinman, M.D.

who set the standard on approaching each pediatric challenge in a thorough and organized manner.

George Azzariti, M.D.

who showed me how to incorporate, mold, and adapt "ivory tower" academic medicine into the care of children in the real world.

FINALLY, THIS BOOK IS DEDICATED

to the health of children throughout the world, particularly of those who are victims of disease, abuse, and poverty.

DISCLAIMER

THE INFORMATION contained in this publication should be used in conjunction with ongoing discussions with your pediatrician. There may be variations in treatment that your pediatrician will recommend based on individual facts and circumstances, and this is not a substitution for the advice of your physician about your child.

The pronouns "he" and "she" are used when referring to a baby or child merely for simplicity. The information applies to both boys and girls, except when it is obviously gender-related.

Since medical information constantly changes, this book should be used to encourage frequent discussions between parents, their children, and their pediatricians.

ACKNOWLEDGMENTS

MY HAND HAS BEEN GUIDED by doctors, authors, and teachers who came before me, for this book draws greatly on the knowledge of others. However, as the years accumulate, it becomes difficult to separate my own practical tips from those of others. I have read extensively and listened very well, and would have to list far too many sources to credit all the information and tips I have included in this book.

First and foremost, I thank the children and their parents who have encouraged me to share their advice and experiences with many other families. These children make coming to "work" each day a joyful experience.

My partners and co-workers have given me support and have provided a wonderfully satisfying environment in which to practice medicine. They have enriched my life and helped me grow. My office staff has created a working atmosphere conducive to running a busy pediatric practice as well as writing this book during "spare time." Special thanks go to Terry and Walter Truppe, whose remarkable secretarial and computer skills and infectious enthusiasm make them both very "user friendly." I am grateful to Jo Ann Magnone, who has developed a relationship with the office copy machine.

My sincere thanks go to Michele Martin, who nourished this project in its embryonic stages. I thank my

ACKNOWLEDGMENTS

editors, Lori Lipsky and Frances Jones, for their insight and their comments on the original manuscript, and Frances Apt, whose copy editing made my ideas and thoughts more comprehensible. I am grateful to Dr. Harry Leider, whose clever suggestion for the title, *The Pocket Pediatrician,* came to fruition.

I offer my thanks to all my friends and relatives who have patiently listened to discussions about the book and have offered advice, support, and encouraging words. Another group of people to whom I am indebted are the students, interns, residents, and fellows whom I have taught and learned from through the years. Sometimes, without even realizing it, they have added their own practical tips to my list.

To all these people, my grateful thanks.

David Zigelman, M.D., F.A.A.P.

Contents

Introduction	xv
Acne	1
AIDS	4
Anemias	6
Anorexia and Bulimia	11
Apgar Score	12
Asthma	14
Bad Breath	21
Bed-wetting	22
Birthmarks	25
Bites and Stings	27
Bones	32
Bottle Mouth Syndrome	34
Breast Milk Versus Formula	36
Bronchitis	40
Burns	43
Caregivers and Day Care Centers	46
Carriages and Strollers	49
Chest Pain	50
Chickenpox	54
Child Abuse	58
Choking	64
Cholesterol	66
Cold Sores and Fever Blisters	71
Colic	73
Common Colds	76
Constipation	80
Contact Dermatitis	83

CONTENTS

Cough Medicines 86

Cradle Cap 89

Crib Death 90

Cribs 96

Croup 98

Crying 100

Cystic Fibrosis 102

Developmental Milestones 104

Diabetes 107

Diaper Rash 110

Diarrhea 112

Diphtheria 115

Ears 116

Eating Habits and Picky Eaters 122

Eczema 126

Erythema Toxicum (Newborn Rash) 128

Eyes 129

Feet 132

Fever 134

Fifth Disease 139

Food 141

Food Allergies 147

Frostbite 151

Growing Pains 152

Hair Loss (Alopecia) 153

Head 154

Headaches 157

Head Trauma 161

Heart Murmurs 164

Heat Rash 164

Hemophilia and Other Bleeding Disorders 165

Hepatitis 172

Hiccups 178

High Blood Pressure 179

Highchairs 180

Hips 181

Hives 183

Hospitalizations: Do's and Don'ts 185

Humidifiers 187

Imaginary Friends 188

Immunizations: Parts 1 and 2 189

Impetigo 198

Influenza 199

Jaundice in the Newborn 201

Kawasaki Disease 204

Learning Disabilities, Hyperactivity,
and Attention Deficit Disorder 205

Lice 212

Limping and Joint Problems 213

Lyme Disease 219

Masturbation 222

Measles 223

Measurements and Doses 225

Meningitis 225

Mononucleosis 228

Motion Sickness 230

Mumps 231

Nails 232

Nervous Tics 234

Newborn's Appearance 236

Nosebleeds 244

Osgood-Schlatter Disease 246

Pacifiers 247

Penis 248

Pertussis 255

Phenylketonuria 256

Pinworms 257

Pityriasis Rosea 259

Poisonings 260

Polio 264

CONTENTS

Returning to School and Day Care
  After Respiratory Infections 265
Reye's Syndrome 266
Ringworm 267
Roseola 268
Rubella 269
Scabies 270
Scoliosis 272
Seizures 274
Sensitive Topics 277
Separation Anxiety 279
Sexual Development 281
Sibling Rivalry 284
Sinusitis 287
Sleeping and Bedtime Problems 289
Sore Throat (Pharyngitis) and Tonsillitis 299
Stitches 306
Stomachaches 307
Stool Color 315
Stuttering 316
Teeth 317
Teething 321
Television 323
Temper Tantrums 325
Testes 333
Tetanus 334
Things to Prepare Before the Baby Comes 335
Thumbsucking 339
Thyroid 341
Toilet Training 344
Tongue 346
Tongue-Tie 347
Torticollis (Wryneck) 347
Toys 349
Tuberculosis 352

Twins   355
Umbilicus (Bellybutton)   357
Urinary Problems   359
Vagina   366
Vitamins   369
Walkers   371
Warts   372

SAFETY TIPS:
Airplane Safety   374
Bicycle Safety   375
Calling the Doctor   377
Car Safety   378
Giving and Taking Medications   381
Halloween and Party Precautions   385
Injury Prevention: Six Basic Tips   386
Kitchen Safety   387
Lead Poisoning   390
The Newborn: Crowds and Going
    Outside   395
Playground and Backyard Safety   397
Sunburns and Sunscreens   399
Traveling with Children   403

INDEX   407

INTRODUCTION

MEDICINE IS an art, not a science, possessing few "wrongs" and "rights." In the field of pediatrics especially, there are many ways to achieve the desired goal, whether it's a type of treatment for a specific disease or disciplinary advice for a behavior problem. Five different pediatricians may offer five different ways to deal with the problem at hand, and all may succeed. Some "old wives' tales" are effective, and are based on sound medical facts. Some work well, even though there is no logical or scientific basis for their effectiveness, while others simply don't work at all or are even potentially harmful.

Much of my responsibility as a pediatrician has been to go through the thousands of pieces of information presented to me by my teachers, training, books, journals, parents, old wives, and, yes, even children.

This book represents the culmination of almost twenty-five years of deciphering and collating pediatric and adolescent advice and solutions for the myriad problems I have faced, and still face, each and every day. It relates how I advise my parents to do things, as Sinatra has said, "my way." Experience has taught me that this advice works.

I've written the book at the request of the parents of my patients. The parents, I may add, sometimes require my help more than their children do. My goal has been to present a practical, concise, and easy-to-read format for them, designed as a handy guide for pediatric situations. The topics are listed alphabetically to make each one easier to find, rather than "in order of appearance" in a child's development. When appropriate, I have supplied the logical, medical, and scientific explanations.

Children don't mind one bit that their parents are not experts at child rearing. If parents just relax and display the love and warmth they feel for their children, then the kids will be happy and will develop a positive self-image.

What's the best way to use these pages? By doing the same thing I advise my parents to do with their kids.

ENJOY THEM!

David Zigelman, M.D., F.A.A.P.

Acne

IT IS ONE OF the cruel ironies of adolescence that this is the age group most frequently troubled with acne. Although we adults never enjoy our "zits," teenagers have to deal with enough social adjustments and body image problems without the added pressure of facial and body acne. As if this is not enough, acne is one of those problems associated with many myths and old wives' tales. I will try to separate the facts from fiction.

At the onset of puberty, certain hormones stimulate the oil glands in the skin. Hair and oil glands plug up with a pasty material that traps the oil. Normal skin bacteria combine with this extra oil, resulting in inflammation of the surrounding skin. When these plugs of oil and bacteria become oxidized right at the surface of the open skin, "blackheads" result. When the plugs remain closed over, they are called "whiteheads." Emotional tension and fatigue exacerbate acne in some people. Girls tend to develop the lesions just prior to their menstrual periods. Scars develop only if the acne process is severe and chronic. Areas commonly involved are the face, shoulders, chest, and back. Greasy hair preparations are thought to contribute to the frequent occurrence of pimples on the forehead. Acne usually disappears by the early twenties.

In newborn acne, the baby's glands are stimulated by mother's hormones in utero. An untrue old wives' tale is that newborn acne is caused by the mother's eating chocolate during her pregnancy or while breast feeding. Infantile acne appears in 30 percent of infants after one month of age and can last until eighteen months. It spreads from the scalp and forehead down to the face and shoulders. Other than keeping the face clean, you

1

need administer no specific treatment. Newborn acne usually does not leave scars.

TIPS:

1. Wash the face two to three times a day to decrease the oiliness. Avoid squeezing pimples, as they may rupture under the skin and cause an infection. Use a baby shampoo daily.

2. Avoid oil-based skin preparations. Use water-based makeup products.

3. Try to avoid working around hot areas, such as stoves with heavy grease and oils, which can worsen acne.

4. Avoid having oily hair hang over the forehead and face.

5. Don't let the teenager's face rest on his hands while he is watching television or, with luck, while studying.

6. Topical benzoyl peroxide is available both by prescription and over the counter. It is antibacterial and gets rid of oil. Although it is available in many strengths and preparations, it is best to start with the 5 percent gel, once a day. After two weeks, progress to a twice-a-day regimen if needed. If there still is no improvement, the 10 percent gel can be used, following the same procedure.

7. Retinoic acid (Retin-A) is an effective prescription topical agent that causes peeling of the skin. It too is available in different strengths and preparations, but it is best to start with the cream, since it has few adverse effects. The lower strength and frequency of use can be increased after two months. Retinoic acid causes an increased skin sensitivity to sunlight, so use a sunscreen to prevent burning.

8. Topical prescription antibiotics, such as clindamycin (Cleocin T) and erythromycin (T-Stat), can also be used. Discuss these medicines with your doctor.

9. Oral antibiotics are to be used if topical treatment does not work. Tetracycline or erythromycin is beneficial. Although these medicines are initially taken three to four times a day, they can eventually be lowered to a once-a-day maintenance dose. Be sure the adolescent female is not pregnant when she is taking tetracycline. Remember that taking antibiotics for a long time can cause vaginitis.

10. Accutane is a prescription oral medicine used for severe acne. Certain liver-function blood tests should be monitored while the teenager is on this medicine. Because of teratogenic effects in animal models—that is, malformation of the embryo—it is important to be sure that there is no risk of pregnancy.

11. If these topical and/or oral medications do not help, a consultation with a dermatologist is appropriate. Dermatologists sometimes use ultraviolet light and dermabrasion for severe cases. For older teenage girls, they occasionally recommend low-dose steroids and estrogen hormonal therapy.

Discarding Old Myths:

• The extra oil produced at puberty is not the result of eating french fries or potato chips. Foods do not cause acne.

• The dark centers of blackheads are not due to dirt in the pores.

• Acne has nothing to do with masturbation. Sexual relations will not affect acne one way or the other.

• Neither extra vitamins nor laxatives help acne.

AIDS

FOLLOWING is a list of statistics that illustrate and emphasize the importance of AIDS—acquired immunodeficiency syndrome.

• Only ten years into the epidemic, one million Americans, *1 in every 250 people,* are infected with HIV (the human immunodeficiency virus), the virus that causes AIDS.

• By 1999, every school district in the country will have at least one child or teacher infected with the AIDS virus.

• An American is infected with HIV *every 13 minutes.*

• Since 1989, AIDS has become the sixth leading cause of death in people fifteen to twenty-four years of age.

• More than 160,000 Americans have died of AIDS-related illnesses.

Since national surveys show that 50 percent of girls and 60 percent of boys between the ages of fifteen and nineteen have had sexual intercourse, it is our responsibility as parents to teach our children how to avoid this preventable disease. This includes discussions about reproduction, love, birth control, condoms, homosexuality, abstinence, and illegal drug use. All of these important and sensitive topics cannot be dealt with appropriately in one conversation. TV and radio programs, celebrity involvements, car rides—all can be used as springboards to discuss this multifaceted problem. As with many sensitive subjects, a primary goal is to make it comfortable and easy for your child to approach you, the parent, about these issues, and not to rely upon strangers for potentially false and misleading information. Even three- to four-year-olds can be told that AIDS is a disease, but that it is unlikely that they— or you, their parents—will get it. They can be shown that all sick people, including those with AIDS, deserve compassion and care. Age-appropriate information should be given throughout elementary school. Studies show that kids as young as twelve years of age are having intercourse, so it is not appropriate to wait until high school to discuss AIDS. Prevention is still the only cure for AIDS. No vaccine is available.

Separating Facts from Myths:

• AIDS is a disease that weakens the body's ability to fight off some infections and cancers.

• HIV, the virus that causes AIDS, can be present in the body for ten to fifteen years before it causes any symptoms. Therefore, many people with AIDS continue to lead normal lives for months, even years.

• All kinds of people have AIDS: men, women, teenagers, children, homosexuals, heterosexuals, people of all races in countries all over the world.

• Although there are many studies going on for treatment of AIDS, it is still a fatal disease.

• It is not easy to get AIDS. It is transmitted by blood, semen, cervical secretions, and breast milk. The HIV virus must be introduced into a person's bloodstream. This can be done by sharing dirty needles, such as with illegal drug use. Another way is through sex. Abstinence, condoms, and spermicides are some ways to avoid this pitfall, although only abstinence is foolproof. Some people have contracted AIDS through blood transfusions, but this is increasingly rare, because regulations safeguarding the nation's blood supply have become much stricter since the mid-1980s. Anyone who received blood between 1978 and 1986 should be tested for HIV.

If a mother is infected, there is a 50 percent chance of the baby's contracting HIV while still in utero, or during birth, or while being breast-fed. The blood test for AIDS measures the antibodies against the HIV virus. Some infants obtain these maternal HIV *antibodies* in utero or at birth, without actually contracting the HIV *virus*. Since it can take up to fifteen months for the maternal antibodies to leave the baby's blood, the diagnosis of AIDS can't be determined unless these antibodies are present when the baby is older than fifteen months. That would then mean the antibodies are the baby's own.

• AIDS *cannot* be contracted by hugging, shaking hands, getting a mosquito bite, being sneezed or coughed on, donating blood, drinking from a water fountain, touching a doorknob, sharing a snack, holding hands, sitting on a toilet seat, swimming in a pool, or being in a classroom with someone who has AIDS.

• Children with AIDS may attend day care and schools and may participate in all sports programs. There are no reported cases to date of one classmate acquiring AIDS from another.

For more information about AIDS, call the U.S. Public Health Services AIDS toll-free hotline: 1-800-342-2437.

Anemias

ANEMIA is a condition in which either the total number of red blood cells in the blood is below normal, or the amount of hemoglobin in each red blood cell is below normal. In a normal sample of blood, the red and white blood cells make up slightly less than half the total volume of blood, and plasma, the liquid that transports them, makes up the difference. Hemoglobin is the protein molecule in the red blood cells that picks up oxygen from the lungs and carries oxygen to the cells of the body. It is the pigment that gives red cells their color. The many types of anemia of childhood are generally divided into two large groups:

1. Those in which the normal number of red blood cells or hemoglobin is not made. Such anemias are caused by infection, cancer, kidney disease, and nutritional deficiencies—like low amounts of vitamins and minerals (iron, zinc).

2. Those in which the red blood cells are destroyed after they enter the bloodstream from the bone marrow, where they originate. Examples of this are sickle cell anemia, thalassemia, blood group or blood type incompatibilities (such as A, B, and Rh factors), lupus, as well as toxic poisoning from drugs and chemicals.

Since the list of types of anemias is long, we will focus on two of the more common anemias of childhood—one from each group. Iron deficiency anemia belongs in the first group, and sickle cell anemia is part of the second.

Iron Deficiency Anemia:

Although the prevalence of iron deficiency anemia has decreased over the past thirty years, it remains the leading anemia in infants and children. Iron is absorbed more efficiently from breast milk than from cow's milk, which is one reason that, today, more infants receive breast milk during the first year of life than cow's milk. Another reason to avoid giving whole cow's milk at an early age is that chronic intestinal blood loss caused by the irritating effect of the protein in cow's milk on the baby's gastrointestinal tract results in severe iron deficiency. This has nothing to do with lactase deficiency or typical "milk allergy." Infant cereals have also been fortified with iron, as have many infant formulas. Although government-sponsored programs, such as the WIC program for low-income families, have improved the nutritional status of these children, lower socioeconomic status is still a factor in the development of iron deficiency anemia.

During pregnancy, the mother's dietary iron is absorbed twice as efficiently as it is when she is not pregnant. The normal full-term baby receives enough of his mother's iron during the last month of pregnancy to last him for four to six months of life. Therefore, an iron supplement should be started when the baby is four months of age, in the form of cereal, iron-fortified formula, or iron drops if the infant is solely breast-fed. Many pediatricians recommend using iron-fortified formula as a supplement to breast milk or as the sole source of nutrition (when breast feeding is not an option) as soon as the newborn starts feeding. Since premature babies don't get the iron boost from that final month of pregnancy, their diets need to be supplemented with iron much earlier. Iron deficiency can develop in premature babies by the time they are two months of age.

Symptoms of iron deficiency include pallor, tiredness, irritability, decreased appetite, rapid heart rate, a blue tinge to the whites of the eyes, and a decrease in subsequent cognitive performance. Iron deficiency can affect attention span, alertness, and learning in both infants and adolescents. Iron-deficient adolescents complain of exercise fatigue, impairment of short-term memory, and just not feeling right. Menstruating girls have an additional need for iron supplements. Pediatricians should therefore routinely do finger-stick blood tests for anemia on infants, children, and adolescents.

Treatment consists of the oral administration of iron drops or tablets, which are better absorbed when given between meals. Large amounts of milk may decrease the absorption of iron. Oral iron supplements can make the bowel movements turn black. If a child simply refuses to take the iron orally, an injectable form is available. The family should learn about foods rich in iron, such as meats, leafy green vegetables, whole-grain cereals, peas, beans, egg yolks, raisins, nuts, and peanut butter. Vitamin C (found in orange juice) helps in the absorption of iron. A repeat blood test should show improvement after two to three months of treatment.

Many parents are concerned about their child's

"pale" appearance. It is important not to confuse abnormal pale coloring with normal fair complexion. The normal hereditary fair coloring of skin has nothing to do with anemia. Most children appear fairer in the winter than in the summer. If the child's lips and nail beds are pale, then anemia is usually present.

If poor oral intake is not the cause of the child's iron deficiency, then the child is losing blood from the body —usually into the gastrointestinal tract. Some reasons for this are esophagitis (inflammation of the esophagus), ulcers, Crohn's disease (refer to the section on "Inflammatory Bowel Disease" in the entry on "Stomachaches"), malabsorption problems, food allergies (e.g., an allergy to milk), and infections.

Sickle Cell Anemia:

Whereas normal red blood cells have a flexible, concave shape, those which contain the abnormal "sickle" hemoglobin assume a more rigid curved shape (like the letter *C)*. These inflexible red blood cells clog small capillaries as they try to pass through them. As a result, needed oxygen does not diffuse out to the surrounding tissues. This causes pain in the child's bones and in the muscles of the fingers, toes, and intestines (leading to stomachaches). When the capillaries of the brain are blocked, the person can suffer a stroke. Anemia occurs because these brittle red blood cells easily break up. Blockage of capillaries in the spleen interferes with the spleen's growth and makes it shrink in size until, by the time the child is one year of age, it is useless. Since the spleen normally helps fight infections, bacterial diseases become the leading cause of death in children under five years of age with sickle cell disease. Bilirubin, a yellow pigment, is also released from inside these red blood cells, so jaundice develops in the skin and eyes. First symptoms can develop as early as six months.

Sickle cell anemia does not affect the child's intelligence or academic performance. However, his teachers and school nurse should be informed of the diagnosis, because the child can have an acute attack of pain and swelling of the hands or feet—called a crisis—at any time.

Sickle cell disease and sickle cell trait are hereditary and very common in the black population. Those children who have only one sickle cell gene are considered to have the sickle cell trait. Seven percent of black Americans have that trait. Their red blood cells do not sickle, so they lead normal lives. If each parent has one sickle cell gene, there is a 25 percent chance that the child will inherit both faulty genes, resulting in the full-blown sickle cell disease, with its anemia, infections, and other problems. This occurs in 1 out of 500 black Americans. Any couple with a family history of sickle cell disease or trait on either side should receive genetic counseling. Many people with sickle cell disease have successful pregnancies and deliveries. Every black child should be screened for this disease with a blood test in the hospital after birth or during his first year of life.

There is no cure for sickle cell disease, but bone marrow transplants offer a promising future in severe cases. It is imperative for these children to be fully immunized against such diseases as the flu, hepatitis, and pneumococcal and Hib (haemophilus influenzae type B) infections. Children with full-blown sickle cell disease are kept on penicillin prophylactically until they are six years old. The liberal use of antibiotics is appropriate for those children with early signs of infection. In the natural course of the disease there will be intermittent flare-ups, of varying intensity. Painful crises will require acetaminophen, ibuprofen, or codeine. More severe episodes will require hospitalization for the administration of intravenous fluids and for pain relief with narcotics. Transfusions of normal red blood cells are given to patients with chronic pain or those being prepared for major surgery. With aggressive medical care, many young adults can lead fruitful and productive lives.

Anorexia and Bulimia

PRETEENS and teenagers, especially girls, may eat poorly because of excessive concern about their appearance, or because of a deep emotional need to establish control over some area of their lives. Anorexia nervosa occurs in the extreme case where the adolescent has such a distorted body image that she loses weight because she sees herself as fat, although she is actually dangerously thin. The gradual starvation may lead to hospitalization, and up to 10 percent of these adolescents literally starve to death. One in every hundred females between sixteen and eighteen years of age has some degree of anorexia. The female-to-male ratio is ten to one. Children and teenagers from all socioeconomic levels and all ethnic and racial groups can suffer from this psychological disease. The parents of anorectic teenagers are usually said to be smart, demanding, and controlling. Most of the ill teenagers are described as having been model children and excellent students before the onset of the illness. However, they tend to be very dependent and socially immature. Many families refuse to believe that a serious problem exists, and they may even resist the therapy.

Whereas anorectics restrict their intake of food, those teenagers with bulimia eat in binges and then throw up immediately afterward or take laxatives. Parents are usually not aware of this problem because the purging is done quietly, in private. If allowed to go unstopped, anorexia and bulimia can affect the gastrointestinal tract (constipation, heartburn), kidneys, brain, central nervous system, skin (hair loss), liver, and hormones. As a matter of fact, it is common for a female with one of these eating disorders to miss several peri-

11

ods or to stop having periods completely. She also becomes very sensitive to cold weather.

Anorexia and bulimia commonly begin as innocent dieting behavior. This is one reason why even overweight children should not be placed on an "adult-type" diet. Children have special nutritional needs to maintain their normal growth and development. Any weight-loss program, therefore, should involve a pediatrician, a qualified nutritionist, and an exercise program.

Treatment for these multifaceted illnesses combines psychotherapy for the patient and family, nutritional rehabilitation (sometimes requiring hospitalization), and, occasionally, antidepressant medications. There are special hospitals or floors for adolescents that combine the needed modes of therapy. Out-patients may need to make weekly office visits so that the doctor can monitor weight, blood pressure, and pulse, and watch for any changes in hair, bowel habits, and menstrual periods. Multivitamins, calcium, and iron may be prescribed. Ask your pediatrician or local mental health professional for information about your regional anorexia and bulimia association.

Apgar Score

WE AMERICANS are preoccupied and obsessed with numbers, grades, and scores. Amazingly, this scoring and grading system begins as early as one minute of age.

In the early 1950s, Dr. Virginia Apgar developed a scoring system by which a newborn's condition could be evaluated, based on five signs. Each sign is given 0, 1, or 2 points. Thus, the baby is rated from 1 (bad condition) . . . to 10 (excellent condition). The evaluation is done twice: when the baby is one minute old and again at five minutes. If the Apgar score is less than

The following chart explains the Apgar score.

Condition	Score (in points)		
	0	1	2
A = Appearance (color)	Entire body is blue or pale.	Body is pink, extremities are blue.	Completely pink.
P = Pulse (heart rate)	None.	Below 100 beats per minute.	Over 100 beats per minute.
G = Grimace (from nasal catheter)	No response.	Grimace.	Cough or sneeze.
A = Activity	Limp, flaccid, poor muscle tone.	Some flexion of extremities.	Active motion, good flexion.
R = Respiration	None.	Slow irregular breathing with a weak cry.	Good, regular breathing with a strong cry.

7 at five minutes of age, it may be repeated every five minutes. The five measured indicators are the baby's heart rate, breathing, color, activity, and reflexes. The tester judges the reflexes by looking for a grimace after a catheter is inserted into the baby's nostril. This is normally done, anyway, to suction out some amniotic fluid from the nose and mouth. The Apgar score helps determine which babies need immediate attention and care. It is of minimal benefit in predicting future neurological status and intelligence. Things that adversely influence the Apgar score are prematurity and some drugs (narcotics, sedatives) taken by the mother before delivery. The Apgar score is determined by the doctor, midwife, or nurse present at the time of delivery.

We have taken Dr. Virginia Apgar's last name, and

related to its five letters each of these five conditions. This mnemonic device makes it easy to remember. Thus:

A   Appearance (color)

P   Pulse (heart rate)

G   Grimace (from the nasal catheter)

A   Activity

R   Respiration

Asthma

ASTHMA, also called "reactive airway disease," is a chronic condition in which the bronchi, the tubes leading from the windpipe to the lungs, become swollen and narrowed when exposed to various allergic and/or inflammatory irritants. They also react to changes in weather, certain types of exercise, and to periods of emotional stress. As a result, the air "whistles" or "wheezes" as it flows through these constricted airways. This "bronchospasm" is reversible. The reaction can lie dormant for weeks, months, or even years, only to be triggered by an irritant. Some irritants known to set off an asthma attack are the common cold virus, other viruses and bacteria, pollen, smoke, dust, air pollution, ragweed, perfumes or other strong smells (including, ironically, some powerful disinfectants), animal dander, certain foods (including eggs, wheat, milk, soybeans, peanuts, chocolate, oranges), some drugs, and stress. Wheezing caused by strenuous athletic activity is called exercise-induced bronchospasm. Although stress can occasionally trigger an asthmatic attack, emotional problems are not the cause of asthma.

Approximately 5 to 10 percent of children are diagnosed with asthma and many have a family history of hay fever, eczema, or asthma. Asthma accounts for more missed schooldays than any other chronic health problem. However, asthma is not contagious, and the child may attend classes if her wheezing is mild. She should avoid gym on these days, and her asthma medicines should be available in school. Symptoms in children with asthma include coughing, chest congestion, wheezing, shortness of breath, chest pain, difficulty in breathing, blueness around the mouth, and the sucking in of the skin between the ribs and between the neck muscles, as these muscles work hard to assist in breathing. The feeling of suffocation is so frightening that the resulting panic makes breathing all the more difficult. If the bronchial narrowing is mild, the only symptom may be a persistent cough, with no wheezing or difficulty in breathing. If the constriction is more severe, the other symptoms will develop. In asthma, the wheezing occurs during expiration (breathing out). In unusual circumstances, acute episodes can be fatal. However, when appropriate treatment and preventive measures are followed, there are no permanent lung changes. Over half of the children with asthma outgrow it during adolescence.

If the child has a severe cough but no wheezing, the diagnosis is aided with the use of a peak flow meter. If the child is over five years old, she blows into this hand-held instrument, and the strength of her expiration (peak flow) is measured. If she has asthma, her peak flow will be low. If she is too young to master this technique, a diagnostic trial of medication may be necessary. A bronchodilator can be given orally or through a nebulizer—a machine that puts the medicine into a mist, which is then breathed in through a mask. If the child improves immediately, it is likely she has asthma. Most pediatricians like to wait until the child has had at least two episodes of wheezing before they label her as having asthma.

Many babies under one year of age have one or two wheezing attacks if their small airways become inflamed. These episodes are called bronchiolitis and are not clear-cut harbingers of asthma. Respiratory syncytial virus is the main cause of bronchiolitis. As children with this disorder get older, their airways widen and the wheezing stops. Some babies, though, do respond to medications similar to those used for asthma.

Asthma is not progressive. Unlike some other chronic pulmonary diseases, such as chronic bronchitis or cystic fibrosis, asthma does not progress from mild to severe. Instead, the clinical course is characterized by exacerbations and remissions. It is also important to remember that a sudden onset of wheezing, especially during inspiration (breathing in), could mean that the child has inhaled a foreign object. Peanuts, pieces of hot dogs, hard candies, coins, and small toys are notorious hazards. This situation requires immediate medical evaluation.

Some mild asthmatic episodes can be handled by parents who are experienced and confident in their management at home. The majority of episodes will require an office visit. Sometimes hospitalization will be needed.

TIPS:

1. Refer to the entry on "Cough Medicines" on page 86. Bronchodilators are medications that treat the bronchospasm by widening the narrowed airways, thus helping the child cough up the accumulated mucus. Some medications work by preventing the bronchospasm. Bronchodilators, like albuterol (Proventil, Ventolin) and metaproterenol (Alupent), are available in both an oral form and an inhaled form, and the latter has very few side effects. Some children as young as three can use a small portable inhaler if a "spacer" is attached. The spacer is a plastic reservoir (tube or chamber) into which the inhaler sprays the medicine. The child then merely breathes in the medicine from the spacer. It is imperative to follow carefully the directions on the correct use of an inhaler. Refer to "Giving and Taking Medications" under "Safety Tips" on page 381, for directions on using an inhaler. Have your child's doctor demonstrate its proper use. For children under three years of age, a nebulizer (see above) can administer these medicines through a mask. The medicines are

usually prescribed for one to two weeks after an asthmatic attack or until the child has been completely free of symptoms for three days.

Two medicines used to prevent asthma are cromolyn sodium (Intal) and steroids. Cromolyn has some immediate beneficial effects, but its main use is to prevent attacks by blocking the release of one of the body's chemicals that causes bronchoconstriction. It takes several weeks for its preventive effects to work. Oral and inhaled steroids treat the inflammation of the bronchi so that the airways are not so sensitive. Although long-term effects are not known, early indications are that inhaled steroids (Vanceril, Beconase) in prescribed doses do not cause the serious side effects caused by prolonged use of oral steroids—growth retardation, weight gain, and cataracts. Inhaled steroids can be given safely for weeks and even months to children over six years of age. Oral steroids (Prednisone, Prelone, Pediapred) can be given safely for four to five days at a time, but they should be administered only under the guidance of the child's doctor. Theophylline (Slo-bid, Theo-Dur, etc.) is an oral bronchodilator available in long-acting forms that need to be given only every eight to twelve hours. They are particularly helpful in treating nocturnal episodes. Occasional side effects are hyperactivity and poor concentration. Adjustments of all medications depend on the child's symptoms and the readings of the peak flow meter. If a child has one or more asthmatic attacks each month, she probably needs to be on continuous medication. For more severe episodes, a shot of Adrenalin, intravenous fluids, oxygen, and sometimes antibiotics will be needed. Fever with asthma does not always indicate that a secondary bacterial infection has set in. A moderate fever may occur during the height of an asthmatic attack, but it should subside as the asthma clears.

2. The child will be more comfortable in a sitting or an upright position.

3. Stay calm. Making the child more anxious will

only exacerbate the problem. Distract her with other activities.

4. Encourage the child to drink extra fluids. If she stays well hydrated, the mucus won't thicken, and it can be coughed up more easily.

5. Treat a fever as you would in other illnesses. (Refer to the entry on "Fever" on page 134).

PREVENTION:

1. Keep the child's home (and especially her bedroom) clean and free of dust and mold. Low humidity levels discourage mold growth. A bare wood or tile floor is preferable to carpeting. The greatest dust collector of all is wall-to-wall carpeting, regardless of the material or the frequency with which it is cleaned. A thickly waxed hardwood floor can easily be wiped free of dust.

2. Choose synthetic fibers (polyester, rayon, Dacron) for clothes, drapes, and rugs. Natural fibers (wool, corduroy, cotton) accumulate more dust. Pillows should be stuffed with synthetic fabric. Use only washable blankets and comforters. Mattresses, box springs, and pillows should be placed in airtight, soft vinyl encasings, because even "hypoallergenic" materials can harbor the strongly allergenic dust mites. Dust mites are common to all households and have nothing to do with good or bad housekeeping.

3. The home should be vacuumed and dusted frequently. Sweeping the floors should be avoided, because it merely sends the dust into the air. A vacuum with a water filter helps to prevent recirculation of dust. Some strong cleaning fluids, however, can aggravate asthma.

4. Get rid of stuffed animals, especially the ones that are filled with animal hair. Replace them with toys that do not collect dust. Refer to the entry on "Toys" on page 349.

5. Check your air conditioner, heating system, and humidifier regularly for mold growth. Change filters frequently and spray them with an aerosol mold killer.

Mold from the outdoors varies according to the season, but indoor mold can produce symptoms year-round.

6. Clean the mold from bathroom tiles and grout. Moisture commonly collects behind the toilet and under the sink. Since bathrooms and basements harbor high amounts of mold, the allergic child's bedroom should not be located below ground or have an attached bathroom. Other household items that promote mold growth are carpet padding, fireplace logs, clothes hampers, and certain foods, such as cheeses, mushrooms, melons, dried fruits, and vinegar (in sauerkraut, relish, and pickles).

7. Plants and dried flowers grow mold. Some asthmatic children will do better in homes with hydroponic plants (plants grown in water instead of soil).

8. Avoid hairy or feathered pets. It can take weeks or months for animal dander to disappear after a pet is removed. If the pet is to stay, wash it every other week to remove the dander before it becomes airborne. The pet should not sleep in the same room as the allergic child.

9. Avoid all sorts of smoke—cigarette, industrial, barbecue, etc. Avoid strong perfumes, hair sprays, and paint fumes. Clothes dryers should be vented to the outdoors.

10. The child should stay away from woods and fields during the pollen season. If the pollen count and/or air pollution are high, the child should stay in an air-conditioned room.

11. Some asthmatic children are sensitive to food preservatives called sulfites. They are found in lettuce, precut fruit, maraschino cherries, fresh mushrooms, shrimp, wine, and beer. Monosodium glutamate (MSG), the flavor enhancer, aggravates asthma in some children.

12. Get prompt medical care for any illness, especially of the respiratory tract—sore throat, earache, sinusitis. Be sure immunizations are up-to-date and

that asthmatic children receive the flu vaccine each year.

13. If the asthma is triggered by exercise, ask the pediatrician about the use of inhaled medicine fifteen to twenty minutes before any strenuous athletic activity. Alternatively, oral asthma medicine should be taken one hour before the strenuous exercise.

14. Support groups for asthmatic children offer practical tips and emotional support to the child with asthma and to his family. Contact your local branch of the American Lung Association as well as Mothers of Asthmatics (1-800-878-4403) for further information.

15. Inform your child's school about the possible occurrence of asthma attacks. Make sure his prescribed medicines are available.

16. Don't let your child get overweight, for this puts an extra burden on his lungs.

17. If the child is responding poorly to treatment, a nurse should visit the home to detect irritating fumes (such as from a furnace) or to look for a source of mold (such as a water leak) to which the family has become accustomed. Your pediatrician or local health department can advise you on how to obtain care from a visiting nurse or health professional.

Before leaving this important topic, let's discuss the pros and cons of allergy testing and injections. A person who is allergic to a specific item, like pollen, can be desensitized by weekly, and then monthly, injections of increasing amounts of that item. The substances to which the child has a positive skin test are put into a serum for these injections. Some allergists do blood tests to determine what the child is allergic to, but many allergists do not feel that the blood test is as accurate as skin testing. Only rarely is skin testing done on a child under two years of age.

Should the child undergo allergy testing and desensitization tests, or not? This is a commonly asked question. Here are some guidelines.

DO ALLERGY TESTING:

1. To determine if a child is allergic to a specific pet or food.

2. To help the child who has such severe asthma or allergic symptoms that medicines do not afford complete relief; the child who has four or more asthmatic episodes per year; the child who misses school frequently due to asthma; the child who cannot participate in sports because of his severe allergies; the child who has undergone several hospitalizations for asthma.

3. For those children (they are rare) who prefer allergy shots to taking medication.

Some children improve so much with allergy shots that their personalities and school performance improve dramatically. However, if your child does not experience relief of symptoms after a reasonable period of time (one to two years for seasonal allergies), it is appropriate to re-evaluate the situation.

Bad Breath

CHILDREN over three years of age have bad breath for similar reasons as adults. If it is due to overnight stale breath, frequent brushing of teeth solves the problem. A sore throat or other mouth infections can cause bad breath, and medical attention is needed to help any of these problems.

Some causes of bad breath are unique to children. One is the foreign-body-in-the-nose problem. My five-year-old daughter has yet to figure out how an eraser from a pencil ended up in her nostril, but it did. These retained foreign bodies in the nose can cause a foul-smelling yellow or bloody discharge from the involved nostril. Unless the foreign body is accessible and easily removable, don't try to remove it yourself. Seek medical attention.

Tooth decay and gum infections can also cause bad breath. Regular trips to the dentist are necessary for children over the age of three.

Bed-wetting

BED-WETTING, also called enuresis, is a common but disturbing problem, especially as six- to seven-year-old children become more social. Approximately 15 percent of bed-wetters outgrow the problem each year. This means that at the age of five—10 percent of children bed-wet. By ten years—5 percent of children bed-wet. At eighteen years—1 percent of teenagers still bed-wet. As these children become old enough to start sleeping over at the houses of friends and relatives, or as they begin thinking about sleep-away camp, they may be afraid of being teased about this problem. This contributes to poor self-esteem, which can damage other aspects of their lives.

Many stressful situations can precipitate bed-wetting in a child who was dry, e.g., birth of a sibling, death or illness of a close relative, divorce of parents, the move to a new home and school, etc. This "secondary" enuresis may also be evidence of a medical problem, like a urinary tract infection, vaginitis, pinworms, or diabetes.

In some children bed-wetting occurs because they are such sound sleepers that they simply don't feel their full bladder. The parents commonly say, "He could sleep through an earthquake!" It is important to remember that bed-wetting is not a disease but just a stage in normal development. Bed-wetting tends to run in families, so if one or both parents were bed-wetters, their children are more likely to be the same, and these children may stop bed-wetting at the age that their parents did.

It is appropriate for the child's pediatrician to do a urinalysis and/or urine culture to rule out diabetes or a urinary tract infection, even though it is rare that a true physical abnormality causes the bed-wetting. Most physicians agree that radiological studies are not routinely needed.

Following is a list of therapeutic measures as well as a philosophical approach to help these kids. Since the main goal is to improve their self-esteem, best results are obtained by seriously starting these measures when the child is six years old. This is when social issues become important.

TIPS:

1. Don't punish or berate your child after a "wet" night. He is not bed-wetting on purpose and usually can't control the problem. Punitive measures merely contribute to his lack of self-confidence.

2. Protect the mattress with a heavy plastic cover. Large diapers should be used until the child is dry at night. Going to "pull-ups" is a reward for success. If these are used too early, they will only compound the frustration level. Be practical.

3. Decrease fluid intake after supper. It's not reasonable to stop all of his drinking, but the amount drunk after supper should be half the previously acceptable amount.

4. Starting four hours before bedtime, avoid any foods that have caffeine and diuretic properties, like colas, chocolate, etc. A nutritionist or dietitian can advise you on whether your child's favorite nighttime snack contains chemicals with these properties.

5. Reward the child for dry nights, both verbally and physically. A calendar with stickers representing dry nights is something the child can look at, feel proud of, and use to show off his accomplishments. Sometimes accidents occur even after several weeks of success. Be patient.

6. Every child should be encouraged to urinate before he goes to bed. Some children are helped further if the parents wake them up when the parents go to sleep. However, if the child is carried or dragged to the bath-

room and placed in front of or on the toilet, the parents are actually encouraging the child to "let go" and urinate in a groggy and sleepy state. This could actually *promote* bed-wetting. Therefore, the child should first be fully awakened, should walk to the bathroom on his own, and then urinate in a more awakened state.

7. If the child agrees, leave a potty or portable toilet in his bedroom so that he doesn't have to go far in the middle of the night to urinate. Keep a night light on in his bedroom and in the bathroom so that he won't be afraid to get out of bed.

8. Some children have been aided by low doses of imipramine (Tofranil), an antidepressant that enables them to "feel" the full bladder. They can either hold their urine in better or get up to go to the bathroom. One hour before bedtime, one 25 mg tablet is given. If no response is achieved after one month, one 50 mg tablet nightly can be tried. Once dry nights are achieved, the child should be tapered off the medicine slowly. The medicine should not be given to children less than six years old and should be used only under the direction of your pediatrician. Imipramine can be given again for a few days or weeks for various social overnights, camps, or other activities.

9. Some children have good results with an alarm that rings and awakens them as they are urinating onto a moisture detector in the underpants or diaper. The child can then go to the toilet to finish urinating. This type of behavior modification requires that the child cooperate and that the alarm actually wakes him. Sometimes the alarm works better on the rest of the family than on the child, who may be a very sound sleeper.

10. DDAVP (Desmopressin) is a nasal spray that has recently become popular in helping these kids. It is an antidiuretic hormone that reduces urinary output. Combining DDAVP Nasal Spray with behavior-conditioning techniques like the one mentioned above has helped many children.

11. If your child has *only* daytime wetting, he may have an emotional or neurological problem. Discuss this with your pediatrician.

Birthmarks

THERE ARE many types of birthmarks, also called nevi. Some develop before and shortly after birth, and many are still forming years after. Any concern about a given lesion should be discussed with your pediatrician. However, the following ABC rules can act as a guide for such discussions:

A stands for **Asymmetry.** Benign birthmarks are generally symmetrical in color and texture. If a birthmark changes, becoming asymmetrical (e.g., if it becomes rough in one area and smooth in another, or darker in one area than another), bring it to your pediatrician's attention.

B stands for **Border.** If the border of the nevus (birthmark) is sharp, with a clear delineation between birthmark and the surrounding skin, this is usually not a medical problem. If the border gradually fades into the neighboring skin, thus enlarging the size of the entire lesion, bring it to your doctor's attention.

C stands for **Color.** If there is a dramatic change in the color, for instance, from light brown to black, over a period of a month or two, advise your pediatrician. In addition, have the birthmark checked if the different shades of tan, brown, and black produce a mottled appearance.

Some additional warning signs are scaliness, oozing, bleeding, the appearance of a bump near the birthmark, and a change in sensation, including itchiness, tenderness, or pain.

There is such a variety of birthmarks that it is difficult to pinpoint any one characteristic that should alert you to potential problems. One rule, though, is always in effect. Never hesitate to ask!

Some of the more common birthmarks of the newborn period include:

"Storkbites" (salmon patches): Some of these pink, flat birthmarks most commonly appear on the back of the neck, just above the nose, and on the eyelids (where it is called nevus flammeus because it resembles a flame). Forty percent of all babies have one. When the child cries or gets upset, the salmon patch tends to get redder and more obvious. It usually disappears within a few years.

"Strawberry nevi": These are red, raised, bumpy birthmarks that grow larger in the first year or two. They occur in 10 percent of babies under one year of age. Blood vessels actually supply the birthmark with oxygen and nutrients. As the nevus outgrows its own blood supply, the center turns grayish. It may occur anywhere on the body, and it usually disappears by five years. If it bleeds, gets infected, or is very unsightly, it might be advisable to consult with a dermatologist or a plastic surgeon to consider surgery, steroid injections, or laser therapy. Some parents apply camouflage hypoallergenic makeup from the mother's own makeup kit.

"Mongolian spots": These brownish or bluish-black flat birthmarks are present in 90 percent of dark-skinned children. They commonly occur on the buttocks and lower back, and range in diameter from 1 to 6 inches. They are harmless and fade into the surrounding skin during early childhood.

None of the birthmarks is the result of anything a mother did during her pregnancy. These distinctive skin markings are merely part of a baby's unique and individual features.

Bites and Stings

BASIC FIRST-AID rules apply to all types of bites, cuts, scrapes, scratches, puncture wounds, and claw injuries. Refer to the section below for discussion of specific bites and stings; for all wounds, though, try to identify the source. If it is an animal, see whether you can determine its location and a description of its behavior. Elevate the injured part of the body to slow the blood flow. Apply a cold compress or run cold water over it immediately to relieve the pain. Wash the wound well with antibacterial soap and water; apply a bandage. A deep wound may become infected with the bacteria that cause tetanus (also called lockjaw), resulting in muscle pain, difficulty in swallowing, fever, and breathing problems. If your child's immunizations are up-to-date, he is probably well protected. If not, your doctor will recommend a tetanus booster shot and/or human tetanus immune globulin. If your child has a bite that itches, cut his fingernails so that he won't scratch the bite and possibly cause an infection. Call your pediatrician if any of the following signs of infection develop: increasing pain, swelling and redness, a discharge from the wound, fever, or a red streak leading from the bite area.

Human:

Aside from the above first-aid measures, aggressive scrubbing—rather than mere washing—is necessary because of the high incidence of infection. Human bites transmit more germs than do animal bites. Your doctor may prescribe an antibiotic to help prevent infection.

Insects:

Bees, wasps, yellow jackets, and *hornets* usually inflict a single sting. Bees commonly leave their stinger

27

behind, but wasps rarely do. *Fire ants* may leave several stingers. Carefully remove stingers with a clean tweezers or gently scrape out stingers with a clean knife blade, plastic credit card, or fingernail. If you are using tweezers, try to grasp one end of the stinger, being careful not to squeeze it, because venom could be released into the wound. Aside from taking the usual first-aid measures, watch for local and systemic allergic reactions. If the skin around the bite swells quickly and itches, apply a cold compress, elevate the swollen part, apply calamine lotion, and give Benadryl or another antihistamine orally. The skin around the eyes is prone to swell a lot because it is flaccid and offers very little resistance. Acetaminophen or ibuprofen can be given for pain. Call the doctor immediately if any of the following develop: wheezing, facial swelling, difficulty in breathing, faintness, pale color in the face, or joint swelling. If a child is known to have severe allergic reactions to stings by these insects, he should wear an identification tag or Medic Alert bracelet describing his problem and the need for immediate medical treatment. He can be given allergy injections to prevent future reactions to bee stings and other animal bites. He may need to carry an Epi-Pen—which can administer epinephrine quickly in emergencies. Epinephrine counteracts the life-threatening swelling of the airway and lungs. Don't let your child play outside in clothing with bright colors that resemble flowers. Don't let him wash with perfumed soaps that could attract insects. Be sure he wears shoes, even on grass. Keep all garbage cans covered.

Spider bites tend to be particularly painful, but should be treated the same way.

Flea bites leave a flock of itchy welts in one area. Clean the carpet, curtains, and furniture by applying a special flea powder obtained from your veterinarian. Have your pet checked thoroughly.

Lice. Refer to the entry on "Lice" on page 212.

Bedbugs may attack one person but not another in the same bed. They tend to leave a series of three bites in a straight line. Clean the sheets and pillowcases, and beat the mattress outside with a tennis racket. Bedbugs do not hide on the body or in clothes, so use an insecticide spray on the bed (mattress, baseboard, sides of crib) and in theroom.

Mosquito bites are very itchy. Use insect repellent on the child and spray his room.

Ticks. See "Lyme Disease" on page 219. There are several other rare diseases that can be transmitted by ticks, including Rocky Mountain spotted fever and Colorado tick fever.

Animals:

Bats, skunks, raccoons, and **foxes** are among the wild animals that can carry rabies, which means "rage" or "madness" in Latin. In the United States, the disease is rarely carried by cattle, dogs, and cats. Squirrels, hamsters, gerbils, chipmunks, rats, and mice carry the virus so rarely that no such animal has been implicated in human rabies in the United States. Unless the animal is obviously rabid, rabies treatment is not recommended. Whereas in the United States dogs account for less than 5 percent of cases of rabies in animals, in developing countries worldwide, dogs account for 90 percent of rabid animals. This is why the majority of U.S. cases are in immigrants or travelers who were infected in another country.

Raccoons and animals infected by raccoons (such as groundhogs) account for more than 60 percent of all cases of rabid animals in the United States. Although 4000 animals with rabies are found each year in this country, only one or two humans get the disease each year. Actually, since 1980, only eight people have acquired rabies in the United States.

The animal's saliva can transmit the rabies virus. If the animal is rabid, wounds to the child's head are more dangerous than wounds to the body, because the virus travels retrograde (backward) along the nerves near the bite to the central nervous system at a rate of 1 to 2 cm per day. Since the head is closer to the brain and spinal cord than the extremities, head bites produce earlier symptoms. The incubation period, therefore, can be from one week to several months after the bite, after which the child would develop flu-like symptoms of fever and fatigue, as well as throat spasms. Within one to two weeks, these symptoms progress to coma. A series of shots can prevent these complications, even if they are started five days after the bite. The police should be notified to arrange for the animal's capture. Medical experts will observe the animal for two weeks, and, if appropriate, will analyze the brain for the rabies virus. Rush your child to the hospital if the bite was inflicted by an animal that was foaming at the mouth and that attacked unprovoked.

All patients with rabies who recall their contact with the animal report that they were bitten. Cases of rabies after scratching or licking open wounds are extremely rare. Petting a rabid animal or coming in contact with its urine, stool, or blood is not considered an exposure and does not need vaccine prophylaxis. Nevertheless, vaccination of all dogs and cats is still recommended.

Emergency care is needed for any deep, crushing bite with resultant mangling of tissue. Immediate and thorough washing of all bite wounds with soap and water greatly reduces the chance of rabies. Even in the absence of obvious bacterial infection, your doctor may prescribe an antibiotic on a preventive basis. Since the tetanus bacteria can be introduced into a wound by an animal bite, be sure all immunizations are up-to-date.

Cat-scratch disease:

This self-limiting illness causes swelling of the lymph glands in the area near a bite or scratch from a cat. Half of the infected children also complain of being tired, and they have a low-grade fever. This illness can also occur after bites or scratches from dogs and monkeys. It is caused by a bacterium that is sensitive to several antibiotics. Cat-scratch disease is limited to humans; the infecting animals themselves are not sick. Cat-scratch disease is not contagious to others. A pimple develops at the wound site within ten days, and nearby swollen glands appear two weeks later. These usually disappear without medicine in two months. If antibiotics are used, the glands disappear sooner.

Jellyfish stings:

Jellyfish stings should be treated like insect stings (see above). However, treat them as an emergency if the jellyfish could be a Portuguese man-of-war. Do not use dry sand to rub away bits of remaining jellyfish, because this procedure could release more venom into the child. Jellyfish washed ashore (perhaps after a storm) may appear dead but are still able to inflict stings.

Rat-bite fever:

Rat-bite fever follows the bite by a rat and requires antibiotic treatment.

Snakes:

There are four poisonous snakes in the United States: coral, moccasin, rattlesnake, and copperhead. Clean and dress the wound. Keep the involved areas below the heart to decrease spread of the venom while you seek medical treatment. Unless you have been taught the correct way, do not apply a tourniquet, because gangrene and nerve injury can result if the tourniquet is applied too tightly. Likewise, do not suck out the poison, because this can introduce further infection into the wound. Follow the usual first-aid measures. Try to identify the snake, or kill it and take it with you to the emergency room. If the snake is thought to be poisonous, your child will receive an antivenom injection. Bites by nonpoisonous snakes don't have distinct fang marks and don't cause much surrounding pain or redness.

Bones

Broken Bones:

SINCE CHILDREN'S BONES are more flexible than adult bones, they bend in response to trauma and don't always break. This produces a "greenstick" fracture. Whether the break is of the greenstick variety or a true break, medical treatment is needed. If the involved area is cold, blue, or numb, nerves and major blood vessels could be involved. It is not true that if you can move the involved area (finger, toe, hand, etc.) the bones are intact. If the muscles over the involved fracture are intact, it is still possible to move the broken bone.

The growth plates in children are at the ends of the bones. Injuries to these bone ends are serious because they could interfere with the normal growth of the bone.

Occasionally, the fracture does not show up on an x-ray until a few days after the injury, so your doctor may treat the injury as a fracture even if the initial x-rays are normal. If the involved area is not broken, it may be sprained, which means the underlying muscles or ligaments are stretched or torn. The sprain should be treated with rest, cold compresses initially but warm compresses after the swelling goes down, and elevation.

TIPS:

1. If the involved area appears bent, don't try to straighten it out yourself.

2. Stabilize fingers or toes by taping them to nearby digits until help is obtained.

3. If the arm is involved, grab the nearest magazine or rolled newspaper and tape it around the tender area as a temporary splint. Rest the arm on a pillow or blanket.

4. Immobilize the joints above and below the break.

5. Don't give the child anything to eat or drink. He may vomit from the pain or the excitement of the event. In addition, if immediate surgery is needed, he may need general anesthesia, which must be administered on an empty stomach. Later on, ibuprofen will help alleviate any musculoskeletal pain.

6. Never move the child if the injury involves the neck or spine. Call an ambulance or await trained medical personnel.

7. Ear, nose, and throat doctors usually wait two or three days to evaluate a swollen, injured nose. This gives the swelling a chance to recede.

8. Skull fractures are either depressed or nondepressed. A depressed (pushed-down) skull fracture can be associated with underlying bleeding, with resultant pressure on the brain. This can cause life-threatening neurological problems. Hospitalization will be needed for observation, with the possibility of surgery. A nondepressed, straight crack of the skull, if not associated with neurological problems, requires no surgical treatment, but the child should still be examined by a physician. Refer to the entry on "Head Trauma" on page 161. Many doctors recommend repeating the skull x-ray four to six months after the injury to make sure that a cyst did not develop between the healing bones.

9. Newborns and children frequently fracture their collarbones (clavicles). These bones, just in front of the shoulders, heal very well with either no treatment or merely with the application of an Ace bandage to support the shoulder.

Dislocated Elbow:

A young child can sustain an injury when an adult or older child pulls on the younger one's wrists or hands. One of the forearm bones (the radius) may separate from the elbow. The child will be unable to lift the forearm and will be in pain. He should be seen immediately, because your doctor, with a simple manipulation, can slip the radius back into place. If the bone has been dislocated for a short time (less than an hour), the improvement will be immediate and dramatic. If it has been dislocated for several hours, there may be soreness even after the elbow is reduced (put back in place). In this case, the child may still favor the arm and prefer not to move it for a few hours.

High school athletes sometimes experience a similar dislocation, which involves the shoulder. The area at the end of the collarbone appears deformed and is very tender. This usually requires care from an orthopedist or a sports medicine specialist.

Bottle Mouth Syndrome

"BOTTLE MOUTH" syndrome is a condition of severe decay, cavities, and malocclusion of the primary (baby) teeth. It is thought to be due to:

- Prolonged bottle feeding (beyond fifteen months).
- Use of sugar-containing liquids in the bottle.
- Allowing the baby to fall asleep with the bottle in his mouth.
- Child's genetic predisposition to tooth decay.
- Unrestricted use of a pacifier.
- Inappropriate fluoride supplement.

Bottle mouth syndrome is an entirely preventable disease, yet it occurs in 5 percent of American children. It initially shows up as dental cavities in some toddlers who are not yet weaned off a bottle by fifteen months of age and are allowed to sleep with a bottle. Too often, the bottle is misused as a pacifier for comforting the infant or for controlling his behavior. Use of the bottle is often prolonged due to parental frustration or convenience.

Bottle mouth syndrome does not occur in breast-fed babies who are weaned directly to a cup, bypassing the bottle. Pacifiers should be discontinued when the first teeth erupt, around six months of age. Bottles should be discontinued between twelve and fifteen months of age, before the child becomes more "attached" to them. The length of time per bottle feeding as well as the number of bottle feedings per day can influence the extent of decay of the teeth.

Early enamel demineralization and cavity development parallel the gum lining. The white areas of the teeth cavitate and become yellow, brown, or black. Total destruction occurs if the disease is not treated. This is a serious problem, because if primary teeth are lost too early, the incoming permanent teeth may be crowded or crooked. The decay and loss of primary teeth can also cause speech problems, a poor self-image, and a sensitivity to cold, hot, or hard foods. A consultation with a pediatric dentist is appropriate.

TIPS:

1. Fluoride should be provided daily if it is not in the local water supply.

2. Parents should introduce the cup by the second half of the infant's first year.

3. The parents' reaction to this problem is often one of anxiety and guilt, and they ask why they weren't told early in the infant's life that such a thing might happen. A pediatrician performs an important service by informing the parents how to avoid bottle mouth syndrome.

Breast Milk Versus Formula

I HAVE a stack of journal articles, twelve inches tall, that clearly demonstrate that breast feeding is better than formula feeding. I have another stack of articles, one foot tall, that make absolutely clear that formula feeding is as beneficial as breast feeding. The answer, in a nutshell, is that both work!

Despite everything that has been written about the antibodies, allergies, and immunological benefits of breast feeding, if you were to spend a week in a busy pediatrician's office, you would notice that breast-fed babies catch colds and illnesses just as formula-fed babies do, and that the latter group grow and develop just as well as the former.

Having determined that babies will do fine on either breast or formula from a health standpoint, let's explore the real-world advantages of breast feeding.

• Breast feeding is convenient in that you don't even have to get out of bed to go to the refrigerator for the milk. You also don't have to fuss with cold bottles. Breast milk is already warm, and it is cheaper than formula.

• It supplies the bonding advantages of closeness and skin contact, and provides the mother with the warm and protective feeling of being the baby's main source of nourishment. Although the feedings may take longer at first and the baby may have only one breast per feeding, eventually the baby will nurse ten to fifteen minutes at each breast for each feeding. Alternate breasts to start each feeding.

• Breast feeding can help, to a slight extent, to

36

shrink the postpartum uterus, because it stimulates the hormone responsible for uterine contraction.

• You can breast feed, changing to formula, if and when you choose. However, you can't feed first with formula and then decide to breast feed, since the breast milk will have dried up.

The success and enjoyment of breast feeding have nothing to do with breast size. Large breasts merely contain more fatty tissue, which is not involved in the production of milk.

If you decide not to breast feed, or if you've tried and want to stop, it's perfectly all right. Too many women get depressed and feel they have failed as mothers, women, or wives if they choose to stop breast feeding. This is simply not the case. Other than the inconvenience and expense of buying formula, getting up at night to go to the fridge, and warming the bottle, you and your baby will do just fine with the commercially prepared formulas, which have vitamins and minerals added to closely approximate your breast milk. In addition, the baby's father or other caregiver can share in your baby's feeding time. Bottle feeding, too, can provide the rewarding and enjoyable feeling that accompanies cuddling with close contact. Bottle feeding also allows the mother to be more mobile and makes it easier for her to pursue a job away from home.

Although most "pro-breast" organizations have excellent ideas and suggestions for some of the problems of breast feeding, they may not adequately prepare mothers for the unnecessary feelings of inadequacy and guilt if breast feeding fails. Sometimes the reasons women stop breast feeding are not just physical, such as cracked nipples or infections. Some find it inconvenient as they resume their careers, and some worry that the baby is not drinking enough, because you can't measure how much breast milk the baby gets, as you can when using formula. The point here is that whether you breast or bottle feed, the baby will do well *as long as you enjoy yourself too*. Always remember, **never allow** the baby to tell you what to do. You tell the baby! The baby will adapt to your schedule sooner than you will adapt to the baby's.

You might want to compromise, as many of my mothers have done, especially those who work. These mothers breast feed in the morning and at night, and the fathers or other caregivers formula feed the rest of the day. After a while, your breasts should adapt to this schedule, and there will be little or no leaking during the day.

One note of caution. *Never prop the bottle and leave the baby alone to feed!* If the baby should cough, sneeze, or hiccup while the milk continues to drip down, he could choke on the milk, aspirate it, and develop "milk pneumonia," a stubborn and difficult problem to treat. Even if you leave for only a short period of time, stop the feeding.

Be sure to burp the baby after every five minutes of breast feeding or after every ounce of formula feeding. Hold the baby upright, gently pat the back, and rock back and forth or go for a short walk. If the baby doesn't burp within two to three minutes, resume feedings and try again five minutes (or one ounce) later.

Milk, whether it is formula or breast milk, can stay in a closed bottle in the refrigerator for two to three days. Either form of milk will last for two to three weeks if it is stored in a freezer. Label the containers with the date, and use the older milk first. When the container is being filled, leave about a half-inch at the top to allow for the expansion that occurs during freezing.

To warm up frozen or refrigerated milk, it is best to set the container in a bowl of warm water or hold it under lukewarm water from a faucet. This should be done only for the few minutes required to take the chill out of the milk. It is preferable not to use a microwave, because microwave heating is uneven. The milk in the center could get scaldingly hot even though the outside of the container may feel fine, and the baby might get burned. Always test a few drops on your wrist to be sure the milk is lukewarm. By the time babies are six months old, they can drink milk just as it comes from the refrigerator.

It is best to stop using a bottle when your child is twelve to fifteen months of age. This helps to prevent bottle mouth syndrome. Refer to the entry on "Bottle Mouth Syndrome" on page 34 for details. The baby's sucking reflex is gone, and he has not yet become "attached" to the bottle by one year of age. Thus, by not creating a habit, you don't have to break one. When weaning from the breast at any age (bottle mouth syndrome does not occur with breast feeding), pick one feeding time and switch to a bottle or cup every day for that feeding. After four or five days, do the same for a second breast feeding time. Continue with other feeding times thereafter. Within two weeks, your child will have weaned from the breast painlessly.

Finally, it simply is not necessary to "sterilize" a baby's bottle. The bottles and nipples should be carefully and thoroughly cleaned by hand, with soap and water, or by dishwasher. A baby sucks many things that are not sterile—his thumb, pacifier, the sheet he sleeps on, the cloth diaper or clothes he leans on while being burped, etc. Even his own mouth is not sterile. Just as breast-feeding mothers must keep their nipples clean, so must bottles be kept clean but not sterile.

TIPS:

1. Whether breast or bottle feeding, sit in a comfortable chair with cushioned arms to help support the baby's weight. Approach the period of feeding as a time of physical rest and relaxation.

2. When breast feeding, keep undergarments, sheets, and blankets out of the way. This will make it easier for the baby to feel and smell the breast.

3. Be sure to have the baby weighed and examined within two weeks of birth. This helps to determine how well the breast or bottle feedings are going.

4. In bottle feeding, a clean nipple should drip at a rate of one drop per second when the bottle is turned upside down.

5. Don't allow yourself to be pressured into choosing breast feeding or bottle feeding. Breast feeding is better for some mothers and bottle feeding is better for others. Don't feel guilty! Your baby will be happier when you are happy.

Bronchitis

BRONCHITIS is an infection of the larger airways that lead to the lungs. The insides of these tubes swell, produce extra mucus, and make breathing difficult. This causes a productive cough, and the child brings up phlegm. When the swelling in the air passages is extreme, air whistles through the narrowed openings. This is called wheezing, usually due to asthmatic bronchitis. Refer to the entry on "Asthma" on page 14. A foreign body stuck in the bronchus can cause the same wheezing sounds.

When a child swallows the extra mucus produced by bronchitis, it can upset his stomach, making him vomit. It is good to encourage him to cough up this infected mucus so that it does not settle lower into the lungs, causing pneumonia. Some children spit out the mucus; others swallow it. Either way, it doesn't go back into the lungs. If it is swallowed, it works its way through the child's stomach and intestines, and can sometimes be seen in his stools.

Bronchitis is often secondary to a common cold or sore throat, and, like them, can be caused by viruses or bacteria. It is difficult to distinguish between viral and bacterial bronchitis, although usually the children are sicker with the bacterial variety. Even though viral bronchitis will clear up by itself, most pediatricians treat all bronchitis infections with antibiotics (unless they are confident that the infection is caused by a virus). Unlike sore throats, in which a throat culture easily distinguishes viral from bacterial infections, there are no "lung cultures" to help distinguish viral from bacterial causes in an office setting. Most children will not provide a specimen of phlegm to culture. That is why antibiotics are empirically used. As mentioned above, another cause of bronchitis is aspiration of a foreign body into an airway. In this case, even antibiotics will not help until the foreign body is removed.

Fever commonly, but not always, accompanies bronchitis. Occasionally, fever will be the only symptom, and the physical exam will not reveal its source. If the fever persists, a chest x-ray may show the bronchitis.

Many people wonder what it means when they feel vibrations as they place their hands on their child's chest or back. Although this can be a sign of bronchitis, it certainly is not definitive or diagnostic. Sometimes the vibrations merely reflect the upper respiratory sounds transmitted through a clear chest. One way to understand this is to picture a drum. Place your right hand on one side of a drum and hit the other side. You will feel the vibrations with your right hand even though the drum is clear inside. The same vibrations can be felt on the child's chest or back even when there is no bronchitis. You are feeling the vibrations transmitted from the upper airway.

Bronchiolitis is a form of bronchitis, but the smaller airways (bronchioles) are infected. As a result, coughing, wheezing, and rapid breathing develop. Respiratory syncytial virus (RSV) is the main cause of bronchiolitis, which usually attacks infants and toddlers, most often during the winter months. The virus is found in the nasal secretions of infected individuals, and therefore is spread by coughing and sneezing. Permanent immunity does not develop after one bout of RSV bronchiolitis, so a child can suffer through several bouts, each lasting one to two weeks. Aerosol bronchodilators can be useful in treating these children. RSV can leave the lungs in a sensitive state (called a reactive airway) for several months afterward.

TIPS:

1. Refer to the entry on "Fever" on page 134, for treatment.

2. Encourage the child to drink extra fluids to prevent dehydration and to keep the mucus loose. Some pediatricians advocate stopping milk and dairy products, because they feel that these increase mucus production in the chest. However, breast feeding does not have to be stopped.

3. Avoid cough suppressants. Some children may need the opposite—cough expectorants—to help them bring up the phlegm. Refer to the entry on "Cough Medicines" on page 86.

4. Sometimes a child may be more comfortable sleeping with her head in an elevated position.

5. Don't smoke around your children. Coughing and wheezing are far more frequent in children exposed to passive smoking. Similarly, bronchitis will take weeks longer to heal in the teenager who smokes.

6. A cool-mist humidifier will make some children more comfortable. Refer to the entry on "Humidifiers" on page 187.

7. Consult with your pediatrician about the need for antibiotics.

8. Severe cases may need hospitalization so that oxygen, intravenous fluids, and medications can be administered.

9. Getting chilled (as when going out in the rain) does not cause bronchitis.

10. It is not true that if your child has had bronchitis or pneumonia once, he will be prone to recurrences. If episodes do occur frequently, there may be several reasons, such as asthma, tobacco smoke, allergies, chemical or paint fumes, cystic fibrosis, tuberculosis, or the

presence of a foreign body. These children should undergo lab tests to help determine whether there is an
underlying problem.

Burns

CHILDREN are like some stubborn adults we all
know, in one important and unfortunate way. The experience of others means nothing to them. They have to
learn for themselves. So it is that too many children
have to learn through hands-on experience about the
dangers of fire, wires, hot utensils, chemicals, and the
sun.

With a first-degree burn, the outer layer of skin reddens and is painful to the touch, but no blisters form,
and it does not scar. Most sunburns cause first-degree
burns. With a second-degree burn, the skin reddens,
blisters, swells, and is tender to touch. It is more serious, more prone to infection, and takes longer to heal.
Scarring is usually minimal. With a third-degree burn,
the skin turns red, white, or black. The burn is so deep
that even nerves are destroyed. As a result, the skin is
not painful to the touch. When this serious burn heals,
the skin loses its elasticity, usually scars, and may require skin grafts. However, most burn cases that can be
managed outside the hospital will heal well if infection
is not allowed to settle in.

Sunburn: Refer to "Sunburns and Sunscreens" in
"Safety Tips" on page 399.

Fire: Burns from a fire may be first, second, or
third degree. If the child's clothing is on fire, stop him
from running around, because the activity will increase
the flames. Lay him down, douse him with water, or, if
no water is available, cover him with a blanket or coat.
Roll him over to smother the flames.

Chemicals: Acids, drain cleaners, and other caustic chemicals may cause first-, second-, or third-degree burns when they come in contact with skin. Remove any clothing that has touched the chemicals. Wash the affected area of the body with large amounts of cool water. Wash the eyes continuously until medical attention is obtained.

Heat: Boiling water, hot coffee or other drinks (including hot milk or formula in a bottle), hot surfaces (stove, iron) may produce first-, second-, or third-degree burns. The affected area should be rinsed with cold water, and cool compresses should be applied. Do not apply fats, oils, or homemade ointments.

Electric Current: Electrical burns (from chewing on wires, sticking fingers into sockets) are tricky and misleading because they are often more severe (second or third degree) than they first seem. If the child is still in contact with the electrical source, push him away from it with something that does not conduct electricity (like wood), or you could electrocute yourself. Look for burns on the skin where the electricity enters as well as leaves the body.

TIPS:

1. Small areas of first-degree burns can be treated at home with cold compresses (washcloths, clean handkerchiefs, etc.). If possible, hold the affected area under a cold faucet for ten minutes. Topical antibiotic ointments (such as Neosporin) and bandages can then be applied. If no bandages are readily available, a clean plastic bag will do temporarily. Notify your doctor if large areas of the body are involved, even with first-degree burns, or if the eyes, face, or genitals are involved. Whenever large blisters develop, seek medical attention.

2. A blister is "nature's Band-Aid," protecting the raw, underlying skin from the outside world. When this new skin is "epithelialized" and ready to be exposed,

the outer thin layer of tissue will burst and peel away. If the blister is broken too early, there is a risk of infection. If it does burst, apply an antibiotic ointment and cover it with a bandage. If the blister becomes filled with pus, or if a red streak extends from it, notify your doctor.

3. Be sure tetanus immunizations are up-to-date, because burned skin is an invitation for infection by the tetanus bacteria.

4. Give acetaminophen and/or ibuprofen for pain relief.

5. Encourage the child to drink extra liquids to prevent dehydration from loss of fluids at the burn sites.

6. The child should wear loose-fitting cotton clothing to promote "breathing" of the skin and to minimize skin irritation.

7. Try to make the bed without wrinkles in the sheets, because they may irritate the skin.

8. Apply lubricating skin lotion when the burn peels in five to ten days.

9. For extensive second- and third-degree burns, lay the child down, with his legs elevated, until medical attention is obtained. Burns on the hands and face require special care. A team of specialists in a burn trauma center will coordinate the various treatments needed for severe burns.

10. When dealing with chemical burns, put rubber gloves on your own hands to protect yourself.

11. Safeguard your home. Refer to "Safety Tips."

12. Use clothing made of fabric that is nonflammable.

13. Home hot water burners should be set so that the water at the faucet never exceeds 120° F (48° C).

14. Be sure to have safety guards on all electrical outlets.

15. Teach your older child these tips in case he or a younger sibling gets burned.

Caregivers and Day Care Centers

IN TODAY'S society, it is common for both parents to pursue careers, with the mother resuming hers following a short maternity leave. One of the most gut-wrenching decisions parents have to make regards the type of child care (nanny or au pair, baby sitter, day care center) most appropriate for their way of life. Even if one parent remains home as the primary caregiver, sooner or later the need will arise for a baby sitter. What are the pros and cons of the alternatives available?

Baby Sitter:

There are several advantages to relying on a home-based sitter rather than a day care center.

• Your child will stay in his own or the baby sitter's home and play with his own toys.

• He is not directly exposed to the colds, viruses, and illnesses of other children.

• His schedule can vary and be more flexible when you have the one-on-one attention of a baby sitter.

Interviewing and Choosing a Baby Sitter:

• It is most important to meet each candidate in your own home, with your child present, so that you can observe their interaction.

• Ascertain whether each candidate's values and moral standards are similar to yours. You can ask appropriate questions without "tipping your hand" to what you would like to hear. Try to find out, for exam-

46

ple, whether the baby sitter smokes or drinks or uses drugs.

• Ask for references from people with whom the candidates have had past experience. Call and speak to these people.

• Inquire about the candidates' opinions regarding discipline (including spanking), displaying affection, and use of television. Do they mind taking the baby outside or playing outside with an older child?

• Discuss the hours of availability and anticipated duration of availability. Discuss pay scales, and whether or not a candidate is willing or able to do additional chores, like laundry, ironing, cooking, housekeeping, or other tasks you may request.

• Present a potential emergency, such as a fire or a fall, to get a feeling for how calm a candidate would be and how appropriate her actions seem.

TRUST YOUR GUT REACTION!

Day Care Center:

A day care center supplies stability and reliability for the parents as well as the stimulation and interaction with other children that a baby sitter cannot offer. Here are some points to consider and some questions to ask.

• Always ask for references, and speak to some of the other parents who send their children to the center.

• Inquire about how many children are cared for by the same person or people. What is the caregiver-to-child ratio? Infants and toddlers require much attention, so there should be at least one caregiver for every four children. Children over three years of age require fewer staff members.

• Is first aid available? Is there a doctor available as back-up? Are the supervisors certified for CPR?

• What activities and hobbies are routine? Are the kids taken outside? Do the caregivers allow television to act as a baby sitter? Do the children nap?

• Does the group take occasional organized trips?

• How does the staff deal with discipline? What if a child blatantly misbehaves, gets into fights, or bites or kicks other children?

• Do the children have to be toilet trained? If the child is in the process of being toilet trained, does the staff have the time and patience to help?

• Discuss the types of food served. When babies are fed a bottle, is the bottle propped or will your baby be held?

• While visiting the center, notice whether the other children are happily interacting with one another as well as with their supervisor. Is the center clean? Are there protective door and cabinet locks, outdoor fences, indoor gates, appropriately placed locks, and outlet protection devices? Are the toys in good condition? Is there lead paint in the rooms?

• **MOST IMPORTANT,** is any parent welcome to stop in and visit *at any time?*

It is normal and healthy for one or both parents to feel nervous, guilty, and even jealous when a child is first left with a caregiver. Share these feelings with your friends and relatives. You'll be amazed at how common these feelings are. With time, and a competent caregiver, the concerns will pass.

Whether you choose a nanny, au pair, or a day care center, don't be surprised, hurt, or worried if, at the end of her day with the caregiver, your child is not bursting with as much excitement to tell you about her day as you are to hear about it. She may simply be too tired to rehash the day's activities or she may be so excited to be back with her parents that she wants to talk about other things first. If you change the subject temporarily or wait for the special half-hour before bedtime (see "Bedtime Routine" in the entry on "Sleeping and Bedtime Problems" on page 289), you will get an earful of her thoughts and feelings.

Carriages and Strollers

IF YOU ARE lucky enough to have inherited a baby carriage that still works, enjoy it! However, it is not necessary to mortgage your house to buy an expensive carriage or stroller. Many are bulky, cumbersome, and difficult to use on stairs. Remember that a lightweight version will do just fine, especially since you can use the more practical stroller when the baby is as young as four or five months old. As a matter of fact, a more recent model of strollers supplies a horizontal surface that can be used for infants as well. They are light and collapsible, which make it easier for you to get in and out of the car or bus. In addition, your baby will be able to sit up and look ahead, where all the action is. Some babies may need to be propped up with a blanket or diaper to help them sit securely.

TIPS:

There are many features of strollers, but these five in particular will help the younger child:

1. The straight, hard back is preferable to a curved, soft back, since it will supply the necessary support that the younger child requires.

2. The stroller must have a safety strap. Infant swings, which can be used for six-week-old babies if they have good head control, must also have a secure safety strap.

3. Be sure the stroller has brakes that lock all four wheels, and use them regularly.

4. The stroller should have a basket underneath it. If it doesn't, bear in mind that putting heavy shopping bags on the handles could tip the stroller over.

5. If you need a twin stroller, be sure the footrest extends all the way across both sitting areas. Otherwise, a child's foot might get trapped between the separate footrests.

Chest Pain

ALTHOUGH adolescents frequently go to the doctor's office with the complaint of chest pain, rarely is it serious and even more rarely is the heart involved. The general term "chest pain" includes pain caused by coughing, "heartburn" (see below), pain caused by turning or taking a deep breath, and pain felt when any part of the chest is touched. It is helpful to determine how and when the pain begins, where it occurs, and how long it lasts, as well as any pattern it follows (day or night, relation to physical activity, stress, or eating). If the pain is muscular in origin, the doctor may learn about it while watching the patient remove his shirt and hop onto an examining table; these movements sometimes elicit the pain. It is also important for the doctor to know if there is a past history of surgery, asthma, or other illnesses, such as sickle cell disease. Sometimes x-rays, blood tests, and electrocardiograms or echocardiograms are needed to sift through the list of possible causes of chest pain.

Irritation of the Musculoskeletal Chest Wall: All the ribs are connected by the intercostal muscles. These muscles are frequently strained or "pulled" during the physical activity of sports or work or merely by a sudden, fast turn of the body. The resulting pains and aches will come and go with certain movements and deep breaths. If a sharp blow to the chest injures or fractures a rib, the pain over the involved bone will be severe. Finally, there is a frequent cause of chest pain called "Tsetse syndrome" (unrelated to the African fly). This is a costochondritis, or inflammation of the cartilage, at the junction of the ribs and the sternum (breast-bone). Once again, strenuous exercise is usually the cause. Pressure on the area will induce the pain. For most of these musculoskeletal injuries, rest, heat, and ibuprofen usually do the trick. An Ace bandage wrapped around the entire chest will help to limit the movements of a tender chest wall. As important as a cure is the reassurance to the adolescent and his parents that the chest pain is not due to a heart attack and does not involve the heart at all.

Functional Chest Pain: The word *functional* means that no physical cause for the problem is found. Some headaches and even some heart murmurs are called functional (and therefore less serious) because there is no underlying pathology. Some children with functional chest pain may imitate an adult with angina (heart pains) to get attention. Emotional problems, school phobias, and peer pressure may manifest themselves as chest pains. This pain is real to the child or the adolescent even though the ribs, muscles, lungs, and heart are normal. There is no association of functional chest pain with exercise or trauma. As a matter of fact, this type of chest pain usually does not interrupt a favorite physical activity or sleep. In these cases, reassurance that there is nothing wrong with the heart is the main treatment. Of course, the underlying emotional problem must be addressed.

Heartburn: When the acid contents of the stomach back up into the esophagus (food pipe), esophagitis results. This causes indigestion and sharp, burning pains in the chest, referred to as "heartburn." The condition has nothing whatever to do with the patient's heart. Irritation of the lining of the esophagus and resulting chest pain can also occur if a swallowed foreign body lodges itself in the esophagus. Both esophageal conditions require medical attention.

Enlarging Breasts at Puberty for Girls and Boys: Refer to the entry on "Sexual Development" on page 281.

Lung and Heart Infections: Children with serious lung infections will have a cough and usually a fever. If the lining of the lungs becomes infected, the child will take short, shallow breaths to avoid the stabbing pain associated with the rubbing of the tender lung lining against the chest wall that takes place during a deep breath. An infection of the lining of the heart and of the heart muscle itself can also cause chest pain. Finally, Coxsackie virus can infect the muscles of the chest wall. This condition, called pleurodynia, causes spasms of pain lasting fifteen to thirty minutes. This problem is self-limiting and leaves after three to five days. Again, these children will look ill and will need medical attention.

Asthma: Children who are wheezing and coughing forcefully may irritate the chest muscles and feel chest pain.

Pneumothorax: If a small piece of lung tissue tears or ruptures, air from in the lung leaks into the space between the lung and chest wall. This condition, called a pneumothorax, is associated with severe chest pain. A pneumothorax often occurs in children or teenagers with asthma, but it can also arise spontaneously in children with no history of lung problems. If only a small amount of air leaks out, pain may be the single symptom. If a lot of air leaks out, the lung may collapse, causing respiratory distress. Although mild cases stop on their own, and need only bed rest as treatment, severe cases may call for the air to be removed through a suction tube placed into the chest wall for a few days.

Pulmonary embolism: A blood clot in the lung, called an embolism, is a rare complication for female adolescents on birth control pills. When blood clots are present, they cause chest pains.

Sickle cell disease: This condition can cause pains in the chest muscles and ribs. Refer to the section on

"Sickle Cell Anemia" in the entry on "Anemias," on page 6.

Heart problems: Rarely, the cause of chest pain does involve the heart. Here are a few of these problems.

• Irregular Heart Beats (Arrhythmias): A very rare cause of chest pain is an abnormal heart rhythm, which results in a decreased flow of blood to the heart muscle itself. The child may feel his heart racing or pounding, and the pain will last for the several minutes it takes for the palpitations to revert to normal. An electrocardiogram, sometimes taped to the chest for twenty-four hours (allowing mobility and normal activity), is used to detect the intermittent nature of this abnormal rhythm. A cardiologist will usually be consulted.

• Heart Attack: A true heart attack, with interruption of the blood flow to the heart itself, is very rare in children. Severe cases of hyperlipidemia (refer to the entry on "Cholesterol" on page 66) and Kawasaki disease (refer to the entry on "Kawasaki Disease" on page 204) can predispose a child to heart attacks.

• Congenital Heart Problems: Another rare cause of chest pain is a congenital narrowing of the aorta, the blood vessel through which the blood leaves the heart. Since the coronary arteries, which supply blood to the heart muscle, originate just beyond this narrowed opening of the aorta, the resulting decrease in blood flow to the heart muscle causes chest pain. Another congenital condition, called mitral valve prolapse, only rarely causes chest pain even though the valve between the left atrium and left ventricle balloons and stretches back into the atrium. Most children with mitral valve prolapse have no symptoms. Other than prophylactic antibiotics before dental work or urological surgery, no specific treatment is needed.

Rheumatic fever is another disease that can cause inflammation of the heart. Refer to the section on "Rheumatic Fever" in the entry on "Sore Throat (Pharyngitis) and Tonsillitis" on page 299.

Juvenile Rheumatoid Arthritis, Lupus, Dermatomyositis: In these diseases, the body makes antibodies against its own organs, including its joints. Since the connections between the ribs and breastbone are also a type of joint, this area can become inflamed, swollen, tender, and painful. This type of pain is chronic and does not go away with rest. Refer to the entry on "Limping and Joint Problems" on page 213 for a discussion of these disorders.

Precordial Catch Syndrome: A sudden, sharp, frightening chest pain, in the front or on the side of the chest, may last just a few seconds or up to a minute. This "stitch" of pain is self-limiting and is not related to activity. Once again, reassurance is the only needed therapy.

Chickenpox

CHICKENPOX (also known as Varicella) is a common childhood viral illness. It usually occurs during late winter and early spring, but can develop year-round, and is spread by direct contact, coughing, or sneezing. In addition, exposure to someone with shingles can trigger chickenpox (see below). The incubation period is twenty-one days. Chickenpox is contagious from one day before the rash appears (so the contact is known only in retrospect) until all the lesions are crusted over. The virus is present in fresh blisters but not in dry scabs. Your child may go back to school once there are no new blisters and all the lesions have become dried scabs. He does not have to stay home until all the scabs fall off, which could take an additional two weeks. Mild cases take approximately five days to form scabs, but more severe cases may take ten days. The average case of chickenpox has about five hundred sores.

A mild upper respiratory infection can precede and accompany the rash. The rash usually begins as a group of small, clear, oval "tear drop" blisters with some surrounding red pimples. Within one or two days, some of these progress to pustules and then crusted scabs, even as new lesions are cropping up. One of the hallmarks of chickenpox is the appearance of several of these different stages of lesions, all near one another, at the same time. They start somewhere on the trunk (abdomen, chest, or back) and then spread peripherally to the extremities and head. The rash is itchy, but the lesions on sensitive areas (mouth, genitalia, eyes) actually burn. The temperature can be normal or as high as 105° F. Although the scabs from the lesions are gone within one month, it can take up to two years for the last discolorations to fully disappear. Chickenpox leaves scars only if the lesions become badly infected.

There are several things to be done to make these children more comfortable:

TIPS:

1. Cut all fingernails to prevent even inadvertent scratching, which may cause scarring. Some children may need mittens and some babies may need cotton socks on their hands to stop their scratching. Wash the child's hands frequently with an antibacterial soap like Dial or Safeguard.

2. Antihistamines (Benadryl, Tavist, etc.) may help the itching. Some topical lotions, creams, and sprays contain antihistamines, but these should not be used if oral antihistamines are being given. Calamine lotion is helpful in particularly itchy areas.

3. Acetaminophen (Tylenol, Panadol, etc.) can be used for fever reduction or for pain. *Avoid aspirin because of its association with Reye's syndrome when given to someone with chickenpox or influenza.* Reye's syndrome is a serious neurological condition marked by vomiting, lethargy, delirium, and even coma. Ibuprofen (Advil, Motrin, etc.) is an anti-inflammatory agent available in pediatric doses for control of fever and pain. Check with your pediatrician for its use together with acetaminophen. People allergic to aspirin should not use ibuprofen. However, ibuprofen has not been associated with the development of Reye's syndrome, so it may be used for chickenpox and influenza.

4. A sponge bath can reduce a high temperature. A mild soap with gentle washing can help prevent the lesions from getting infected. Aveeno bath treatments can be used to help the itching.

5. The child should drink extra liquids to help the body keep up with the increased metabolic demands caused by the fever.

6. Light cotton clothes are less irritating than heavy woolen clothes or nonporous synthetic materials.

Rare complications include pneumonia, bleeding tendencies, heart problems, and encephalitis, which is marked by a loss of balance, convulsions, and coma. Infants of mothers who had chickenpox during the first 3 months of their pregnancy tend to be smaller than average and are prone to seizures, eye problems, scarring of the skin, and mental retardation.

One old wives' tale that seems to be true is that a more severe case of chickenpox is usual in the sibling who contracted the virus from another member of his family. Perhaps this is because the first family member transmitted a higher dose of the virus during his sibling's prolonged exposure.

A chickenpox vaccine is currently being studied for release in the United States. A type of gamma globulin shot (called V-ZIG) is available for people who are at high risk of developing complications from exposure to chickenpox. This includes people with cancer, immunodeficiency diseases, and newborns whose mothers develop chickenpox within five days after delivery.

Once he has had chickenpox, the child theoretically has lifelong immunity and should not get chickenpox again. However, I have seen mild cases of clinically diagnosed chickenpox followed, years later, by another true case. The initial cases were probably so mild that the child developed only partial immunity. Regardless, after a person gets chickenpox, the virus lies dormant in his spinal cord without causing any problem at all. Years later, this virus can be reactivated by stress, steroids, or immunosuppressive medicines, such as chemotherapy for cancer, and other still unknown factors. The virus then tracks its way back to the skin, resulting in shingles (herpes zoster), but *not* in chickenpox. If a grandparent has had chickenpox, he need not worry that he'll acquire shingles by being in the presence of a grandchild with chickenpox.

The Committee on Infectious Diseases of the American Academy of Pediatrics recently made the following observations after the Food and Drug Administration approved the use of oral acyclovir to treat chickenpox infections in otherwise healthy children. Immunocompromised children, babies less than one year old, and patients receiving systemic steroids may experience severe disease or a higher rate of complications from chickenpox. However, no data currently exist that delineate the benefits of oral acyclovir for these high-risk patients. Although acyclovir will result in a one-day reduction of fever, and a 15 to 30 percent reduction of symptoms with no significant adverse effects, it has not been shown to reduce the rate of complications, itching, spread of infection, or the length of the child's absence from school.

RECOMMENDATIONS:

1. Oral acyclovir therapy is not recommended routinely for chickenpox in healthy children.

2. For certain groups at increased risk of severe chickenpox or its complications, oral acyclovir should be considered if it can be started within twenty-four hours of the onset of the rash. These groups include:

- Teenagers, but not pregnant adolescents, because the risk to the fetus is unknown.

- Children over one year of age with a chronic skin or pulmonary disorder (asthma, cystic fibrosis, etc.).

- Children receiving long-term aspirin therapy.

- Children receiving steroids. These children should stop the steroids, if possible, after known chicken-pox exposure.

3. Not enough data exist to make a recommendation for children under one year of age.

4. Oral acyclovir should not be used prophylactically in the otherwise normal child exposed to chicken-pox as a means to prevent infection or illness.

Child Abuse

MOST parents engage in some form of mild disciplinary action at one time or another during their parenting years. This does not mean that they are child abusers, but rather that they are normal, concerned parents. However, when such action in any form becomes repetitive behavior, it is child abuse. If physical discipline is severe, and results in bruises, cuts, burns, or bites, it is child abuse. If discipline is not designed to educate, but is arbitrary and inconsistent, it is child abuse.

More than a million children are abused each year in the United States. Approximately four thousand children die each year of child abuse and neglect. The six recognized forms of abuse are physical abuse, physical neglect, emotional abuse, emotional deprivation, verbal assault, and sexual abuse. Abused children often grow up to abuse their own children. Parents who abuse their children belong to all ethnic, religious, educational, geographic, occupational, and socioeconomic groups. The suspected abuser may be a relative other than a parent, a baby sitter, or a teacher. The presence of spouse abuse doubles the likelihood of child abuse. Where there is marital discord, unemployment, or drug abuse, parental stress heightens the likelihood of child abuse.

Abusive parents share the following characteristics which form a pattern of child abuse. They are immature; they see themselves as inadequate and worthless; and they are unwilling to perceive the child as dependent on them. Because of their low self-esteem, they are easily shattered by criticism. They view the child as a small adult and turn to the child for reassurance. Since the small child cannot meet their needs, and the parents have a low frustration level, they act out their frustrations through violence against the child.

A parent who abuses his child usually feels guilty about his behavior. People often mistakenly think that when a parent has abuse problems, his entire relationship with the child is abusive. This is not so. The same parent can relate to his child in healthy, loving ways. Ironically, most abused children are as closely attached to their parents as are nonabused children.

Bruises in varying stages of healing are often the result of repeated beatings. These bruises sometimes display the imprint of the offending object—a belt, rope, or doubled-over electrical cord. The imprints of a hand or fingers may be seen where the child was grabbed and squeezed. Rope burns on the arms, neck, and ankles may mean that a child has been tied to a stationary object. Symmetrical burn injuries on the buttocks, genitals, legs, or hands may mean that these body parts were forcibly held in hot water. Cigarette burns resemble impetigo, except that they leave craters in the flesh. Human bite marks have deep crushing characteristics, whereas dog bites rip and tear the skin. Traumatic hair loss occurs when the abuser pulls the child's hair. Physical neglect includes failure of the caretaker to provide adequate food, clothing, shelter, or medical and dental attention.

With emotional and verbal abuse, the child is ridiculed, threatened, rejected, and discouraged. Emotional deprivation results in the child being ignored and upset by other negative relationships in the home.

CHILD ABUSE

Although sexual abuse is certainly a type of physical abuse, it merits special attention. Child sexual abuse is much more common than most people realize. One out of every six adult women was sexually abused as a child. One out of every ten adult men was sexually abused. Unlike physical abuse, which is dealt with by the civil court, sexual abuse is a criminal offense and is investigated by the police. The young victim commonly keeps the abuse secret at the urging of the offender, who is seeking a continuing relationship with the child. The victim usually depends on the larger and older offender for food and shelter. Those who abuse children sexually have low self-esteem and feel safer relating to children than to adults. These acts usually do not involve force or violence. Less than 10 percent of sexual abuse is violent, forced intercourse (rape).

The more common forms of sexual abuse are molestation and unforced intercourse. Child molestation involves fondling the child's genitals or asking the child to fondle the adult's genitals. Forcibly exposing the child to sexual acts or pornography falls in this category. Sexual intercourse includes attempted or actual oral and/or rectal penetration.

The strong preponderance of victims of sexual abuse are female, and children of all ages are at risk. At least 80 percent of the cases of sexual abuse happen between a child and an adult the child knows. Incest is commonly repeated by one father with successive daughters. The offenders are almost all male. Females are the occasional offenders in a child care setting. Stepfathers are abusers five times more often than are natural fathers. In the rare cases of violent family-related rape, the father's sexual abuse usually extends outside the family circle.

Children who are sexually abused tend to suffer sexually transmitted infections, genital or anal bruises and abrasions, and urinary tract infections. Complaints relating to sexual abuse can masquerade as stomachaches. The child may revert to bed-wetting or lose bowel control. In extreme cases, sexual abuse may show up in the child as a sore throat, which tests show to be due to gonorrhea. Most vaginal injuries are found on the lower half of the vagina when the child is examined on her back by her pediatrician.

Every child suspected of being abused must be reported immediately, by anybody, to a local child protective service, even by phone. Caseworkers are on call twenty-four hours a day. Some people hesitate to report suspected abuse because they do not want to get involved. This is unwarranted, because it is the caseworkers and assigned physicians who will appear in court. The initial caller can remain anonymous.

The first recorded intervention in a child abuse case was dealt with by the Society for the Prevention of Cruelty to *Animals,* because in 1874 there were no laws to protect children. In 1974, the Federal Child Abuse Prevention and Treatment Act allocated federal money to states to "develop, strengthen, and carry out child abuse prevention and treatment programs." The child welfare agencies make home visits to determine and evaluate the therapy for the entire family. Since no single agency can provide all the needed services, self-help parent groups (Parent Aides, Homemakers, Parents Anonymous) have also emerged. They provide telephone hotlines, emergency crisis therapy, and child-rearing counseling. Untreated families tend to produce juvenile delinquents and the next generation of child abusers. The victims of repeated sexual abuse almost always need long-term psychotherapy.

TIPS:

1. Encourage your child to "say no" and to "tell someone." Since, in most cases, the child already knows the offender, warning her to beware of strangers is not enough.

2. When teaching your child about safety, provide specific definitions of what sexual abuse is. She should be taught that "private parts" are the parts of the body that a bathing suit covers.

3. Support your child, after she tells you about a potential episode of abuse, with praise, belief, sympathy, and lack of blame. Many professionals feel that a child does not make up stories of sexual abuse. If she can describe sexual activity, she has experienced or watched it. She should be told that this is *not* a secret to keep, even if the offending adult told her to keep it a secret.

4. Playing "what if" games can help to make your point. Ask: "What if someone you didn't know asked you to go with him into his basement to play a game? What if someone offered you a quarter to work alone with him, but told you not to tell anyone? What if the baby sitter said you could stay up late if the two of you played 'funny' games with each other's private parts?"

5. Take a course in your community to increase your awareness of the signs and symptoms of abuse.

6. High school parenting classes promote bonding between parent and child and teach parenting skills. Some examples of these skills are learning to distract your child from misbehavior (especially when in a store); ignoring unacceptable behavior (such as tantrums, whining, and interrupting); expressing disapproval by getting close to your child, making eye contact, and simply saying *no* or *stop;* using time-out when she misbehaves (for about one minute per year of age, up to five minutes); stopping any physical punishment, which only teaches that it's okay to be aggressive; avoiding any yelling; and rewarding desired behavior.

7. Remember, there are no "bad children." Sometimes good and caring children make mistakes and do bad things. Another example of verbal abuse is: "You never do anything right."

8. Refer to the section on "Spanking" in Tip 5 of "Temper Tantrums" on page 325. Even those pediatricians who feel that an occasional isolated spanking is acceptable agree that:

• A spanking is inappropriate for a child less than one year old and unnecessary after five or six years.

• No one should ever shake a baby or child, because that could cause blood clots in the brain.

• A parent should spank rarely, or the action will have no effect.

• A parent should never spank when he or she is drinking or out of control.

• A parent should never allow baby sitters or teachers to spank the child.

9. Expect your child to cry. The younger the child, the harder it is for you to distinguish between cries for needs and cries for wants. But soon you will learn the difference in your child's cry. When she cries from pain or fear or hunger, respond immediately. If she cries as part of a tantrum, it is harmless and should not be punished. Don't let this upset you. Refer to the entry on "Temper Tantrums" on page 325.

10. Teach your child to occupy herself. You too need some time off, even if it's just a few minutes. You should supply toys, books, or other distractions for your child while you cool off. Don't merely send her away to "go do something." However, even three-year-olds can be expected to entertain themselves for short periods.

11. Teach your child, even at a young age, to respect her parents' rights and their time together. Your child's needs (love, food, shelter, safety) should always come first. Your needs, though, should come next. Scheduled nights out with your spouse will help every marriage and thus improve parenting skills.

Choking

APPROXIMATELY three thousand deaths occur annually in the United States due to inhaled foreign bodies. Children under four years of age account for 20 percent of these cases. Common objects aspirated by children are safety pins, coins, peanuts, uninflated balloons, torn-off pieces of plastic-lined disposable diapers, beverage can pop tops, paper clips, eggshells, marbles, "button" batteries, whole grapes, and baby powder. If a toy or toy part can fit through the center of a roll of toilet paper, your baby could choke on it. Pacifiers, teething rings, and rubber toys in their most compressed state should still be too large to fit through the cardboard tube in a roll of toilet paper.

TIPS:

   1. Avoid toys with small parts, including stuffed animals with eyes or noses that could be pulled off and swallowed.

   2. Cut food into bite-size pieces. Hard, smooth vegetables, hot dog chunks, popcorn, nuts, and adult-type pills should not be given to children until they are six or seven years old. These foods require a grinding, chewing motion, which is not well established until five years of age. Chewable pills for children can be given to two- or three-year-olds.

   3. Do not allow uninflated balloons or plastic bags to be around small children.

   4. Never prop a baby's bottle in his mouth and leave him unattended.

   5. A doorstop with a small rubber or plastic tip that can be pulled off is a particular choking danger because

it is at ground level, easily within a child's reach. Use a doorstop that is one solid piece instead.

6. If an infant or child starts to choke:

• Turn the infant upside down on his stomach and hit him several times rapidly, high on his back between the shoulder blades. An older child can be placed across your lap with his face down, lower than his trunk. (However, if he is coughing, speaking, and breathing on his own, none of these measures is necessary, as it may make the foreign body move farther down.)

• If this does not work, turn the child over with his face up. Push on his chest four times with your fingertips just below an imaginary line between the nipples.

• The use of the Heimlich maneuver on children is controversial, but there are many reports of its successful use for those over one year of age. Put your arms around the child's stomach while standing behind him. Place your fist, with thumb toward the child, between the child's bellybutton and sternum (breastbone). Squeeze quickly four or five times by pulling your fist inward and upward.

• If this does not work, open the mouth wide and try to see the foreign body. If you see it, remove it. Do not, though, thrust a groping finger blindly into the throat, because that could push the object farther down.

• If the above moves are unsuccessful, give mouth-to-mouth breathing. If the chest does not move, repeat the above four steps. Call for emergency assistance.

Every parent should enroll in a local CPR course to receive instruction on the proper management of a choking child.

Cholesterol

OUR AMERICAN nutritional vocabularies have been bombarded with such terms and phrases as monounsaturated fats, low-density lipoproteins, peanut oil, diet therapy, fully saturated fats, "good" and "bad" cholesterol, fish oil, cholesterol lowered with drugs, olive oil, fatty meat, coronary artery disease, high-density lipoproteins, triglycerides, cholestyramine, atherosclerosis, and familial hypercholesterolemia . . . wow!

The coronary arteries supply blood and nutrients to the heart muscle itself. When these arteries become narrowed and eventually blocked by the build-up of fat (called atherosclerotic plaque) along their inner lining, the condition is called coronary artery disease. The earliest fatty streaks can be seen in the coronary arteries of ten-year-old American children. As the atherosclerotic plaque grows and causes the coronary arteries of adults to narrow, the result is chest pain, heart attacks, and sudden death.

Low-density lipoprotein is the name of the molecule that carries cholesterol around the blood. Therefore, an excessive amount of low-density lipoproteins in the blood contributes to the formation of atherosclerotic plaque, thus increasing the risk of coronary artery disease. This is why low-density lipoprotein cholesterol is called the "bad" cholesterol. In contrast, high-density lipoprotein is the molecule that carries cholesterol away from the arteries and to the liver, where the cholesterol is eliminated. So high-density lipoprotein cholesterol is the "good" cholesterol and high levels of it are healthy. Finally, triglycerides are the major source of fats in our diets. Although triglycerides are not an important part of the atherosclerotic plaque itself, an elevation of triglycerides reflects the high level of fats in the blood in general, a factor contributing to coronary artery disease.

Because of its association with heart disease, cholesterol has acquired only negative connotations. Actually, cholesterol also has good and even necessary functions in our bodies. It is an important component of cell membranes, of bile salts (which help digestion), and of steroid hormones. What is harmful is the excess cholesterol. Two thirds of our cholesterol is made by the body; only one third of our cholesterol comes from our diet. Even if we eliminate all cholesterol from our diets, there still will be some cholesterol, made by the body, in our blood. Doctors agree that the best advice is to eat fat in moderation, not to eliminate it totally. Foods that come from animals (milk, other dairy products, eggs, meats) do contain cholesterol. Foods that come from plants (fruits, vegetables, grains) have no cholesterol.

Most American children eat too much saturated fat and cholesterol. Unless diet and exercise intervene, the elevated levels of cholesterol and low-density lipoproteins are relatively constant in the first two decades of life. In half of these children, the elevated cholesterol and low-density lipoprotein levels persist into adulthood. All American children over two years of age should be on a low-cholesterol and low-saturated-fat diet. Not only does the child benefit from the lowered fat content of the blood, but obese kids benefit because fat has twice as many calories as the same amount of protein and carbohydrates. By substituting protein or carbohydrates for fatty foods, they will consume fewer calories. Children under two years of age need the extra fat in their diets for normal growth and neurological development. (Fat is an important component of the nerves of the brain and is needed for the brain's rapid growth in a child's early years. The head circumference, which reflects brain growth, expands rapidly during these first two years and approaches adult size when the child is around two.)

Although universal screening was initially controversial, most pediatricians now agree that there should be cholesterol screening of all children and adolescents. If nothing else, it acts as a stimulus for education and discussions about correct eating habits and appropriate exercise patterns that children can follow through adulthood. If one or both of a child's parents have markedly elevated cholesterols (called familial hyper-cholesterolemia), a sample of the baby's umbilical cord blood can be sent for a cholesterol test. Otherwise, cholesterol screening should begin once the child is two years old. Ideally, though it is not always practical, this blood test should be done after an overnight fast, before the child eats any breakfast. If the test is done after breakfast, lunch, or supper, and if the cholesterol is elevated, then a repeat test within the next month should be done after a twelve-hour overnight fast. It can be done with a finger-stick. If the cholesterol is still elevated, then blood should be drawn from an arm vein for a full lipid profile, which measures low-density and high-density lipoproteins as well as triglycerides. The blood tests should be repeated three months after dietary treatment is started, and carried out yearly from then on. (The measurement of cholesterol, and not a full lipid profile, is used as a universal screening test because it is less expensive, and it is easier to do a finger-stick than to draw blood from the arm.)

The upper acceptable limit for blood cholesterol is 200 (mg/dl, or milligram per deciliter), for low-density lipoprotein it is 130 (mg/dl), and for triglycerides it is 130 (mg/dl). The lower acceptable limit for high-density lipoprotein is 30 (mg/dl). Each 1 percent decrease in blood cholesterol results in a 2 percent decrease in risk of coronary artery disease. Each 1 percent rise in high-density lipoprotein results in a 3 percent decrease in risk of coronary artery disease. Obesity enters into this equation as well, because for every pound greater than ten that an adult is over his or her ideal weight, life will be one month shorter.

Occasionally, a family history will reveal the presence of familial hypercholesterolemia. Twenty percent of children with a fasting cholesterol above 200 have familial hypercholesterolemia. If only one parent has an elevated cholesterol level, the child's cholesterol could be in the 300-to-500 range. If both parents have elevated levels, their children may have cholesterol levels as high as 600 to 1000. These families develop xanthomas, which are flat, orange, fatty skin lesions. Chest pain and even heart attacks may occur in a child as young as six. Since few of the children with the hereditary trait will be able significantly to lower their cholesterols with diet and exercise alone, most of them will need drug therapy. Cholestyramine (Questran, Cholybar) and colestipol (Colestid) are the drugs used to lower cholesterol by binding it in the intestinal tract. Both total and low-density lipoprotein cholesterol have been lowered to the normal range with these drugs.

Other risk factors for coronary artery disease are diabetes, hypertension, obesity, inactivity, smoking, and a history of coronary artery disease in parents, grandparents, uncles, and aunts. Some medicines that may increase cholesterol are oral contraceptives, prednisone, and Accutane.

TIPS:

1. If a child's cholesterol is elevated, there is an 80 percent likelihood that his parents and siblings also have high cholesterol. The entire immediate family should therefore be tested.

2. Stopping smoking raises the high-density lipoprotein cholesterol (the "good" cholesterol) level. Avoid exposing your child to passive smoking.

3. Exercise also raises the high-density lipoprotein cholesterol level. My suggestion, a practical and realistic one, is that the child and at least one other family member do five minutes of exercise each day, above and beyond normal bike riding, participating in gym in school, and playing with friends. The goal is for this to become part of the child's daily or nightly routine, just like getting dressed and undressed, going to the bathroom, and brushing teeth. I have found that five minutes seems to be acceptable to all families. If I ask for ten to fifteen minutes each day, enthusiasm may last for

a week or a month, but then fizzles out. I suggest combinations of different types of exercise to avoid boredom and to involve all muscle groups. Sit-ups, push-ups, jumping jacks, running in place, and other activities can be done in any order and in any amount, for a total of five minutes. The program is most likely to succeed if at least one parent joins the child in exercising daily.

4. We can actually *use* television to increase the amount of time spent exercising. Instead of fighting your child's need to watch television, let him watch if he exercises five minutes during each half-hour of viewing time. Using exercise bikes and running in place are types of activities that can be done while watching television (with its cholesterol-packed commercials).

5. Although children under two years of age need extra fat in their diets, those with familial hypercholesterolemia should consult a pediatrician, dietitian, or nutritionist for formulas lower in cholesterol than breast milk or cow's milk and for age-appropriate low-fat baby and junior foods.

6. Fish, chicken, and turkey have less fat than red meats. When buying ground beef, be sure it is lean. Trim the fat from meats and remove the skin from the chicken and turkey.

7. The egg, a highly nourishing food, need not be completely avoided. Instead, limit the use to a maximum of three eggs per week. After all, eggs are in many foods that children eat, such as breads, pastries, and desserts.

8. Use low-fat (1 percent) milk instead of whole (4 percent) milk for children over two. Skim milk is only 0.5 percent fat. Use margarine instead of butter.

9. Encourage your child to eat fruits, vegetables, and grains.

Cold Sores and Fever Blisters

FEW THINGS in life are as irritating and bothersome as the cold sore. One of the quirks of medical and lay terminology is that "cold sores" are also called "fever blisters." When clusters of clear blisters occur on the lips and around the skin of the mouth and nose, they are referred to as cold sores, fever blisters, mouth sores, or herpetic sores, because they are caused by the herpes simplex type 1 virus. (This is a cousin to the herpes simplex type 2 virus, which causes genital lesions.) Dermatologists describe these thin-walled blisters on a red irritated base as "drops of dew on a rose petal." They are spread by contact (kissing, touching, and sharing towels, toys, and eating utensils) with another infected person. Blisters occurring inside the mouth, on the tongue or gums, and in the throat are called aphthous ulcers, or canker sores. These are not caused by the herpes virus, and they tend to appear around times of stress and fatigue or with exposure to the sun. Burning and tenderness at the site sometimes precede the appearance of the sore by twenty-four hours. The general term "cold sores" applies to these mouth lesions, too.

When the lesions are confined to the soft palate and back of the throat, the condition is called "herpangina." If, at the same time, the white blisters appear on the palms of the hands and the fingertips and on the soles of the feet, the syndrome is referred to as "hand, foot, and mouth" disease (not to be confused with hoof-and-mouth disease of cattle). Herpangina and hand, foot, and mouth disease are caused by a common virus called Coxsackie. It belongs to a different class of viruses from herpes, although it produces similar skin lesions that usually appear in the summer and fall. Fever, sore throats, and stomachaches may accompany all of these rashes.

When herpes blisters occur in newborns, a severe and sometimes fatal systemic reaction can develop. Although older children tend to get clusters of blisters at one time, rather than individual lesions, antibodies build up after each episode so that, as adults, we have only one or two blisters at a time. The blisters are painful, but they are not serious. The incubation periods are two to twelve days for the herpes virus and four to six days for the Coxsackie virus. The blisters will disappear in one to two weeks. If the herpes virus affects the cornea of the eye, a serious infection could result, requiring care by an ophthalmologist.

TIPS:

1. Topical preparations that contain hydrogen peroxide can be used to clean lesions in the mouth. (They "fizz" when applied.) They help the blisters heal sooner but do not take away the pain. For pain relief, follow these preparations with topical analgesics, like viscous Xylocaine, Anbesol, etc. Topical steroids for oral use also supply symptomatic relief from canker sores.

2. Acetaminophen and/or ibuprofen should be used for pain and fever. Refer to the entry on "Fever" on page 134. The sooner the medicine is started, the more likely it is to help.

3. This is a good time for cold foods, like ice cream, milk, Jell-O, yogurt, and ice pops. Avoid hard, spicy, and salty foods. Even citrus fruits will hurt the blisters, but clear juices, like apple juice, are fine.

4. Gargling and swishing half-strength mouthwash (diluted with water) around the mouth will help. Do this a few times each day.

5. Mashing, blending, and pureeing foods make eating easier. Drinking with a straw helps to bypass the blisters on the gums and inner lining of the mouth.

6. When the blisters are on the outside of the mouth or near the nose, an antibiotic cream (e.g., Neosporin) and/or Vaseline can be applied four times a day.

7. Some pediatricians advocate the use of an antiviral oral medicine called acyclovir, also available as an ointment. Its use is still controversial.

8. Be sure the child practices good hygiene by using separate glasses, utensils, and towels. Avoid kissing until the lesions are gone.

9. Apply sunblock to your child's lips, nose, and surrounding skin before she goes out in the sun.

10. Since these lesions are caused by viruses and other external factors, oral antibiotics do not help.

Colic

COLIC is a description, not a diagnosis. It occurs in a healthy, normal infant, who, for unknown reasons during certain periods of the day, will suddenly cry, become irritable, bring his knees up to his stomach, and appear inconsolable. Also for unknown reasons, it is more common in the first-born child. It is not the result of bad parenting, so don't feel guilty. We don't know what causes it, but:

- It sometimes occurs shortly after feeding has begun.
- It is more common in the late afternoon or evening.
- Only rarely does a formula change help, since colic is not an indication of formula intolerance, which is manifested by diarrhea, vomiting, or weight loss.
- There is no identifiable pathological gastrointestinal problem associated with colic. Babies who suffer from colic are healthy, growing babies.

COLIC

One pediatrician stated that parents know their child has colic if they have an irresistible urge to get him his own apartment. Parents don't cure colic; they endure it. Old wives' tales abound when it comes to "treating" colic, but I will offer you several time-proven tips to help you get through these rough and tough periods.

TIPS:

1. The most important point is that, in the vast majority of cases, colic stops when the baby is three months old. It helps to keep this in mind during those periods when frustration causes you to cry even louder than your baby.

2. Create a calm and relaxed environment and mood, especially during feedings. Take the phone off the hook; play some soft, relaxing music, and smile at the baby. There are cassette tapes that combine vocal and instrumental harmonies with womb sounds. The atmosphere will relax you and the baby and prevent him from swallowing a lot of air. Our personalities are the result of two factors: heredity (our genes) and the environment. We can take an inherently happy baby and make him unhappy, and we can change the unhappy, cranky, and colicky infant into a happier and more relaxed child. It requires patience and understanding.

3. Breast-feeding mothers should try to note any association between the baby's colicky period and the mother's intake of large amounts of caffeine (coffee, colas), spicy foods, nuts, shellfish, or raw vegetables in the previous twenty-four hours. Ironically, some babies have problems if their mothers drink too much milk. Trial and error is the operative rule in these cases.

4. Holding the baby in a more vertical position, even during feedings, helps the air bubble to come up easier. Burp the baby after every ounce of formula or after every five minutes of breast feeding. Do not insert a thermometer into the rectum to "release gas." All it does is irritate the anus.

5. Offering chamomile or fennel or other herbal teas seems to have a calming effect on some babies. Make the tea half-strength, adding 2 tablespoons of sugar or Karo syrup into a quart of the half-strength tea. It can be given between milk feedings or during colicky periods. If the quart is not used up over a three- to four-day period, throw it out, make up a new quart and keep it refrigerated.

6. A warm bath, or even a lukewarm heating pad on the abdomen, seems to help some babies.

7. Some babies are soothed by noises and vibrations. A turned-on vacuum cleaner or a clothes dryer provides calming noises and vibrations, as does your wheeling the baby in the stroller. One observant parent noticed that rides in the car calmed his colicky baby, and he developed Sleep-Tight, a device that attaches to the springs of a crib and mimics the noises and vibrations produced by a moving car. Some parents have found this useful for their colicky babies. This Sleep-Tight Infant Soother is federally classified as a medical device, so the cost (up to $100) is sometimes covered by insurance. For more information, call 1-800-662-6542.

8. One school of thought claims that colicky babies can be soothed with a program of infant massage and touch. Your local library or bookstore has books that provide details of these programs.

9. Some colicky babies are comforted with different types of movement: rocking, walking, riding in an infant swing, a stroller, or a carriage, or being carried in a parent's front pack or pouch.

10. A few colicky babies benefit from some medications your pediatrician may prescribe. Simethicone liquids help to break up swallowed air in the stomach. Antispasmodic agents calm down the stomach cramps.

It is understandable that an exhausted and frustrated parent, following nights of unsuccessful attempts to calm a colicky baby, may have temporary, short-lived violent feelings of anger toward the baby and/or his or her spouse. These feelings are common, crossing all socioeconomic boundaries. However, feelings are not actions. Thoughts are not child abuse, and many people feel guilty for simply having these feelings. Talk with your friends, family, and doctors. They, too, have experienced similar feelings. Remember, there is light at the end of your three-month-long tunnel.

Common Colds

THE MOST common disease of the world is the common cold. Ninety percent of Americans have a cold every year, and over half of us have several. It is the most frequent medical problem seen in pediatric practice. Most healthy children get about six colds each year. Since it is caused by more than two hundred different viruses, let's discuss what bacteria and viruses are. Bacteria are very tiny life forms, visible only under a microscope. If the eight million people of New York City were reduced to the size of bacteria, they would fit very comfortably into a drop of water. Most bacteria are more beneficial than harmful to humankind. In fact, life without bacteria would not be possible. Yet there are many bacteria that cause diseases like tuberculosis, pneumonia, diphtheria, etc. Thank goodness many of these bacteria are susceptible to drugs, such as antibiotics.

Viruses are much smaller than bacteria. A special apparatus, the electron microscope, is needed to see them. If our eight million New Yorkers were shrunk to the size of viruses, they would easily fit on the head of a pin, with room to spare. Viruses, unlike bacteria, are extremely fussy about where they live. It is only with the greatest of difficulty that scientists have been able to grow viruses outside an animal body. Nevertheless, they are highly potent and cause a great many diseases, including polio, influenza, hepatitis, rabies, chickenpox, measles, and mumps. Antibiotics that harm or kill bacteria are useless against viruses. The relationship between the two is that viruses can pave the way for bacteria to infect the host. Viruses impair the body's defense mechanisms so that bacteria can invade and cause complications in the ears, sinuses, lymph nodes, and lungs.

A typical cold may start with a brief "dry" stage, during which the nose feels "prickly." The child will complain of a tickling feeling in the throat. This is followed by watery eyes, sneezing, a runny nose, coughing, a sore throat, irritability, loss of appetite, headache, and occasionally a fever. Then the secretions become thick and the cold begins to dry up. "Three days coming, three days with you, three days going" is a time-honored and still fairly accurate description of the course of a cold. However, the younger the child, the longer it may take for her to fight off the cold.

Among different members of the same family, a given virus may simultaneously produce different illnesses and symptoms. For example, it may cause typical colds in the parents, bronchiolitis in the infant, croup in an older child, pharyngitis (sore throat) in another, and a subclinical infection (i.e., no symptoms) in yet another member. A cold is potentially serious, because it may be accompanied by complications like ear infections and pneumonia. A cold can pose an important threat to children with chronic bronchitis, asthma, kidney or liver disease, diabetes, congenital heart disease, and recurrent sinusitis.

Medical science has not yet discovered an exact method for preventing or curing colds. No vaccine or vitamin is available to prevent them. A person with a cold, especially in its early stages, transmits it to children by close contact, kissing, coughing, sneezing, and by handling contaminated handkerchiefs. Every baby less than one month old should be kept away from crowds. If Aunt Matilda has a cold, she will get over her hurt feelings a lot faster than the baby will get over the cold she may give him. However, the baby need not stay indoors. As a matter of fact, some daily fresh air is a good idea at any age, but public indoor areas like stores, shopping centers, malls, and restaurants should be avoided until the baby is a month old.

It is an old wives' tale that chilling, dampness, drafts, air conditioning, wet feet, and letting a baby go outside without a hat increase susceptibility to infection. These events do reduce the temperature of the inner lining of the nose, causing shrinkage of the blood vessels, which is followed by a reflex opening of these blood vessels, producing nasal irritation and a discharge. These worsen an already existing infection, but they don't cause a cold.

Newborns breathe mainly through their noses rather than through their mouths. Therefore, even a tiny amount of mucus, foreign body (e.g., lint), or swelling of the nasal lining causes snorting, gurgling, and other noisy breathing sounds. New parents think this means that their baby has a cold, but this usually is not the case. As long as the baby is sucking and eating well, is not irritable, and has no fever, there is no need to worry. As a matter of fact, sneezing is the way healthy newborns clear their throats and noses of mucus and tiny foreign objects.

Allergies cause sneezing, coughing, and nasal discharges, just as colds do. A few ways to distinguish between allergies and colds are:

• Colds may cause a fever, but allergies usually do not.

• Allergy symptoms last much longer than cold symptoms.

• Allergies cause itchy noses, bringing on the characteristic "allergic salute"—wiping the nose upward, with the heel of the hand, even when it is not running. "Allergic shiners" are dark circles under the eyes caused by chronic rubbing of the itchy eyes.

• Colds produce thick green mucus, but allergies cause thin, clear, watery, nasal discharges. A green nasal discharge occurs in viral and bacterial infections, but it alone is not an indication that an antibiotic is needed.

TIPS:

1. Dehydration lowers a child's ability to fight germs, so encourage him to drink small amounts of clear liquids frequently. Ice pops are a good means of getting in extra fluid. Milk increases mucus production in some children, so clear liquids are preferable.

2. Acetaminophen and/or ibuprofen should be used for fever or discomfort. They do not help to get rid of congestion or a cough. Avoid aspirin. Refer to the entry on "Fever" on page 134.

3. Nosedrops and cough medicines suppress the symptoms. They do not cure colds. Antihistamines are more effective against allergies, and expectorants do not help head colds. Refer to the entry on "Cough Medicines" on page 86. If a baby's nose is so stuffed that he has a difficult time sucking (because he needs to keep his mouth open to breathe), then he may benefit from medicated nosedrops (e.g., Neosynephrine) or salt water nosedrops. Nonmedicated salt water nosedrops can be made at home by adding 1 teaspoon of salt to a pint of boiled water. Let it cool to room temperature, and make a fresh solution every few days. Two drops can be placed in each nostril four times a day. Nosedrops should never be used for more than four days in a row. Refer to the entry on "Giving and Taking Medications" on page 381.

An older child will help to clear the secretions by gently blowing his nose. However, blowing too hard can force the secretions back into the ears or sinuses. For children prone to ear infections or sinusitis, nosedrops, decongestants, gentle nose blowing, or sniffing backward and swallowing the secretions are better than blowing too hard.

4. Very dry rooms are more conducive to colds than more humid ones. A cool-mist humidifier or vaporizer will make a child breathe more easily, especially when his nose is stuffed and his throat is dry. Humidifiers must be cleaned regularly.

5. Your child may be more comfortable with his head elevated in bed. You can place a blanket under the mattress or raise the legs of the crib.

6. Avoid tobacco smoke or industrial smoke. They further irritate the already compromised lining of the respiratory tree.

7. Teach your child to cover his nose and mouth when sneezing and coughing, and to wash his hands well.

8. Although there is no "proof" that vitamin C prevents or shortens the duration of the common cold, there are many who advocate it and have anecdotes about its benefits. Daily doses of 500 to 1000 mg are safe, but doses of 2000 mg or higher can cause diarrhea.

9. Antibiotics should not be taken for the common cold, because they do not cure viral illnesses.

10. Your child may return to day care or school once the fever is gone for twenty-four hours. It is unnecessary and impractical to keep a child who just has a runny nose out of school, because colds are more contagious one to two days *before* the symptoms appear. His classmates have already been exposed.

11. All immunizations can be given to the child who has an uncomplicated common cold without fever.

Constipation

IF A BABY stools daily, even if the stool is harder in consistency than usual, this is not constipation. Some babies stool every other day, but as long as they are not unduly straining or passing blood, their pattern is normal. True constipation occurs if a baby or child has no bowel movement for three days or more.

Constipation is common among two- to three-year-olds as they become toilet trained. If a child passes an occasional large, hard, and painful stool, he is a "stool holder," with the characteristic scissoring of his legs to hold back the stool. Another reason a child holds back is to express rebellion against parents who are too aggressive and obsessed with the importance of toilet training. Some children are just too busy to take the time to go to the bathroom, or they prefer to use only their home toilets. In general, if your child is free of pain, cramps, and rectal bleeding, no treatment is necessary if he has a bowel movement every other day or even every third day.

Chronic constipation sometimes results in partial blockage of the colon by a large, hard stool. Ironically, only loose, watery stools leak around this partial obstruction, resulting in "paradoxical diarrhea." This is called encopresis, a condition that will require a treatment plan set out by your doctor.

Other causes of constipation are:

- High iron content of various formulas.

- Tight anal ring in an infant.

- Anal fissures—small, painful cuts in the skin of the anus.

- Too few liquids in the diet and foods with too little fiber.

- Reaction to medications (codeine, antihistamines, antacids).

- Emotional disorders.

- Appendicitis.

- Irritable bowel syndrome.

- Hypothyroidism (thyroid deficiency).

- Congenital colon disorders (e.g., Hirschprung's disease). All newborns should have a bowel movement within the first thirty-six hours. Some congenital problems are not discovered until the baby is several days, weeks, or even months old, when solid foods are first introduced.

CONSTIPATION

TIPS:

1. It is essential to have a relaxed attitude toward toilet training.

2. Encourage foods high in fiber, such as whole wheat bread and whole rye bread, as well as fruit juices. Encourage the child to drink extra fluids and to eat prunes, dates, figs, and vegetables.

3. Occasionally, a mild laxative like Karo corn syrup or Maltsupex is helpful, but only when prescribed by your doctor.

4. Apply lubricating ointments, such as Vaseline or Neosporin, to anal fissures.

5. Don't force your child to defecate when he is in the bathroom. Try to allot enough time for your child to relax while sitting on the toilet. Most children prefer to have their feet planted on the floor or on a stool. Refer to the entry on "Toilet Training" on page 344.

6. Be aware that common causes of stress, such as a new baby, a new home, or a new school, can wreak havoc on a child's gastrointestinal tract.

7. Don't punish your child for soiling his pants.

8. In extreme cases a doctor may suggest that you stimulate the rectum with a thermometer, as if you are taking your child's temperature. Another suggestion, reserved only for extreme cases, is to use a pediatric glycerine suppository or a pediatric Fleet enema for temporary relief. It should never be used regularly and never without the approval of your pediatrician. Likewise, it is sometimes necessary to offer a prolonged course of mineral oil for chronic constipation to help the child relearn to have a bowel movement without pain.

9. Encourage regular physical activity and participation in sports.

10. An infant with a tight anal ring will benefit from having the pediatrician stretch the ring by gently inserting his finger (in a lubricated finger cot) into the anus. Parents should not perform this procedure.

Contact Dermatitis

THERE ARE two basic types of contact dermatitis:

Irritation:

Rashes can develop from contact with irritants that damage the skin. Some chemical irritants may be acids, alkalis, soaps, or solvents. Common culprits are lye, paint remover, gasoline, kerosene, turpentine, varnish, lacquer, mineral oil, glue, acetone, floor wax, furniture polish, laundry bleach, window cleaner, metal cleaner, and drain cleaner. Contact dermatitis from jewelry is sometimes caused by nickel. Sweat facilitates the release of nickel from the metal. Precious metals such as gold and platinum rarely cause dermatitis. Sunburn is a type of contact dermatitis. (Refer to the entry on "Sunburn and Sunscreens" on page 399.) There is no practical value, and therefore no clinical use, in patch testing (see below) for irritant contact dermatitis.

Allergy:

Allergic contact dermatitis is caused by an induced, delayed allergic reaction. The rashes of contact dermatitis are the same whether they are caused by irritations or by allergic reactions. The allergic response can frequently be demonstrated by patch testing, which can be thought of as creating the disease in miniature. The suspected allergen is applied to the skin to see whether it produces a small area of dermatitis within two to three days.

Poison ivy is one of the most common causes of rashes due to contact with sensitizing agents. As is the case with many allergies, the very first contact may not produce problems, but it sensitizes the child to future contacts. Blisters and itchy patches of redness develop twelve to forty-eight hours after contact with the plant. The most characteristic feature of the rash, aside from the intense itching, is that the red bumps and the blisters tend to appear in lines. The contact does not have to be direct. Contact with contaminated clothing, with fur from an animal that has recently been in the woods, or with smoke from a burning poison ivy plant can produce the rash. The leaves are hazardous even after they fall off the plant. Poison oak and poison sumac plants cause similar problems. More than 50 percent of Americans are sensitive to poison ivy, oak, or sumac. Jewelry, adhesives, eye makeup, insecticides, animals, rug shampoos, bubble baths, and perfumes are other causes of allergic contact dermatitis.

Since exposed parts of the body are most likely to come in contact with these allergens, the face, arms, and legs are most often involved. The rash may also appear on areas of the body covered by clothing because sap under the fingernails is spread by scratching or rubbing the unexposed areas. Be sure to scrub and clean under the nails. The fluid in the blisters, however, does not contain the antigen, so it does not spread the rash. Likewise, a contact dermatitis rash due to irritation or allergy is not contagious to others. Although most cases of contact dermatitis disappear a few days after the offending agent is removed, poison ivy is stubborn and tends to linger for up to two weeks. There are at present no effective immunization methods to prevent poison ivy dermatitis. Poison ivy dermatitis and other types of allergic dermatitis are not hereditary conditions.

TIPS:

1. Prevention is the best treatment. Wear long pants, shirts with long sleeves, and thick socks when walking through wooded areas. Plastic or vinyl gloves are safer than rubber because rubber itself is very sensitizing. In addition, rubber does not protect the hands against poi-

son ivy, but heavy-duty vinyl does. The best advice is "Leaves of three . . . let them be!"

2. If the plant is in your backyard or nearby, try to get rid of it with leaf spray herbicide. The plants can be dug up, but protective clothing must be worn and later discarded or decontaminated.

3. If you think your child has been in contact with poison ivy, wash off the oil from the plant with soap or alcohol within one hour after exposure to minimize any chance of reaction. Clothes and shoes should also be washed.

4. Cool compresses and baths with Aveeno relieve itching.

5. Calamine lotion can be applied topically to relieve the itching of a particularly bothersome area.

6. One percent hydrocortisone cream helps to stop the itching and allows for prompt healing. Occasionally, a stronger topical steroid is needed. When a steroid ointment is applied under cool compresses, it is absorbed more readily. Reapply the ointment if the lesions ooze or if a dressing change is necessary. As a rule, 3 to 4 daily applications are needed. A child with a severe case may benefit from injected or oral steroids. Your doctor will help you assess the severity of the rash and guide you in the mode of therapy. The damaged skin will require time to heal; the rash won't disappear overnight.

7. If, through scratching, secondary bacterial skin infections occur, healing will be delayed. Topical and/or oral antibiotics may then be necessary.

8. Cut the child's fingernails to prevent even inadvertent scratching and breaking of the skin.

9. An oral antihistamine, such as Benadryl, also helps to relieve itching.

10. Teach your child to recognize the plants. Poison ivy is a vine growing on trees, fences, walls, telephone poles, and other vines. It also can grow as ground shrubs of varying sizes. Poison ivy and poison oak gen-

erally have 3 leaves arising from a short stem; poison sumac has 7 to 13 leaves. The entire 3-leaf cluster is only 3 to 4 inches long. The young leaves are green in spring and summer but change color earlier than most other plants and become yellow or reddish in autumn. They have no odor. The plants have black dots on their leaves, stems, roots, berries, or flowers. These are composed of the sap, which contains the chemical sensitizer. The chemical turns black when the plant is damaged and the chemical is exposed to air.

11. An old wives' tale about the benefit of crushed leaves of plantain (the common lawn weed) is not supported.

Cough Medicines

A PET PEEVE of mine is the misunderstanding and misuse of "cough medicines." The misunderstanding part applies both to parents and to doctors. When we say cough medicines, are we referring to medicines that *stop* the child from coughing, or to medicines that *make* the child cough? As if this problem is not complicated enough, many cough medicines that contain more than one ingredient do *both,* and clearly state so on the label. The label says that the medicine contains an expectorant (to encourage the child to cough) as well as an antitussive (to stop the child from coughing). What is the right approach and the best medicine for your child's cough?

When I examine a child with a cough, I try to determine whether the problem is upper respiratory—such as a common cold, postnasal drip, ear infection, sinusitis, etc.—or lower respiratory—such as bronchitis, asthma, or pneumonia. When the cough originates "upstairs," I prescribe a cough medicine that dries up the mucus and stops the child from coughing. When the cough originates "downstairs," I rely on an expectorant or bronchodilator to loosen up the mucus in the chest and stimulate a more productive cough to eliminate this mucus. Although it is sometimes difficult, parents should try to determine whether the child has a head cold or allergy, which would respond to an antitussive (like a decongestant and/or an antihistamine), or is wheezing or seems to have a chest cold, which would call for an expectorant or a bronchodilator (see examples below). If it is hard or tricky to determine where the cough is coming from, see your pediatrician. With time you will feel more comfortable in choosing the right medicine. If your child has asthma or recurrent bronchitis, it is best to consult with your doctor about all medicines.

Since I prefer to give children less medicine rather than more, I discourage the use of those "combination" medicines described earlier. However, medicines that have similar actions can be combined successfully: decongestants with antihistamines, or expectorants with bronchodilators. It should be clear why it is not advisable to give a drying agent, like a decongestant or an antihistamine, to a child having an asthmatic attack or to a child with bronchitis. Not only will the medicine dry the mucus in the child's head, but it will also dry the mucus in his lungs. The thicker mucus is harder for the child to cough up. Conversely, it is unnecessary to give an expectorant to a child with a head cold when all he needs is something to dry up his postnasal drip.

Below is a list of commonly used drugs—all called "cough medicines." They can be found on the labels of over-the-counter and prescription medicines. For practical purposes, I have separated them into (1) medicines that stop coughing, and (2) medicines that encourage coughing or "open" the bronchi to help coughing.

1. MEDICINES (GENERIC NAMES) THAT STOP COUGHING:

     Astemizole - antihistamine
     Atropine - cough suppressant
     Azatadine - antihistamine

Brompheniramine - antihistamine
Caramiphen - cough suppressant
Carbinoxamine - antihistamine
Carbon - cough suppressant
Chlorpheniramine - antihistamine
Clemastine - antihistamine
Codeine - cough suppressant
Cyproheptadine - antihistamine
Dextromethorphan - cough suppressant
Diphenhydramine - antihistamine
Hydrocodone - cough suppressant
Hydroxyzine - antihistamine
Hyoscyamine - cough suppressant
Oxymetazoline - decongestant
Pheniramine - antihistamine
Phenylephrine - decongestant
Phenylpropanolamine - decongestant
Promethazine - antihistamine
Pseudoephedrine - decongestant
Pyrilamine - antihistamine
Scopolamine - cough suppressant
Terfenadine - antihistamine
Triprolidine - antihistamine

2. MEDICINES THAT ENCOURAGE COUGHING OR "OPEN" THE BRONCHI FOR MORE PRODUCTIVE COUGHING:

Albuterol - bronchodilator
Cromolyn sodium - antiasthmatic
Dyphylline - bronchodilator
Ephedrine - bronchodilator
Guaiacolsulfonate - expectorant
Guaifenesin - expectorant
Iodinated glycerol - expectorant
Isoethamine - bronchodilator
Isoproterenol - bronchodilator
Metaproterenol - bronchodilator
Oxtriphylline - bronchodilator
Terbutaline - bronchodilator
Theophylline - bronchodilator

Cradle Cap

CRADLE CAP, like dandruff, is a type of seborrheic dermatitis—an irritation of the baby's scalp. His natural oil has dried, resulting in yellow scales and patches, which are not itchy or painful. Occasionally, the neck and areas behind the ears may be involved. It occurs most frequently during the baby's first year. The scalp over the "soft spot" tends to be more frequently involved simply because many parents are afraid to clean vigorously in that area.

Most cases of cradle cap will respond to daily washes with baby shampoo. A clean soft toothbrush can be used to scrub particularly stubborn areas. In severe cases, an antidandruff shampoo can be used once a week while the baby shampoo is used on the other days. If the patches become red or inflamed, or if eczema develops, the pediatrician may prescribe a topical steroid.

One of the most common old wives' tales calls for the application of baby oil on cradle cap. I strongly discourage that. One is adding more oil to the baby's own natural oil. Although initially this appears to dissolve the crusty flakes of dried oil, eventually the newly applied oil also dries on the scalp, frequently complicating the problem. The daily thorough use of a shampoo will do the trick.

Crib Death

CRIB DEATH (sudden infant death syndrome, or SIDS) is the sudden death of an infant under one year of age which is unexpected by history and remains unexplained after a case investigation, including performance of an autopsy. The peak incidence of SIDS occurs between two and three months of age. SIDS is as old as the Old Testament and occurred as frequently in the eighteenth and nineteenth centuries as it does now.

In spite of the large number of crib deaths each year —over six thousand in the United States alone—the cause of death remains unknown. Death occurs very rapidly, usually during sleep, and there appears to be no suffering. In about 10 percent of crib deaths, careful examination or autopsy does demonstrate a previously unsuspected abnormality or a rapidly fatal infectious disease, such as meningitis or pneumonia. These children are not considered victims of SIDS.

Many scientific approaches and hypotheses have been pursued, but no one single theory is accepted. Following is a list of potential risk factors and preventive measures.

Low birth weight: SIDS infants are frequently premature and have a low birth weight (less than 5 pounds). There is an increased risk of crib death with decreasing birth weight and with decreasing gestational age, but the reasons for these correlations remain a puzzle.

Gender: Males have a 50 percent larger risk of crib death over females.

Race: American Indians and blacks have a higher risk than whites, Asians, and Hispanics. These racial differences have nothing to do with, and are not explained by, other risk factors, such as cigarette smoking during pregnancy, young maternal age, lower socioeconomic status, or different cultural practices of child care.

Seasonal factors: The incidence of crib death is twice as high in the cold winter months as in the hot summer months. This is not explained by accidental smothering with heavier blankets, because, as stated, autopsies do not show evidence of suffocation as a cause of crib death.

Pregnancy complications: Maternal anemia and infection during pregnancy are risk factors in SIDS.

Smoking: Cigarette smoking during pregnancy has repeatedly been identified as a major risk factor for crib death.

Drug abuse: Maternal abuse of marijuana, cocaine, or heroin during pregnancy may increase the chance of crib death. However, use of analgesic or anesthetic drugs for delivery is not associated with an increased risk.

Maternal profile: Young maternal age, lower socioeconomic status, lower education level, and lack of prenatal care are all risk factors. Seventy-five percent of SIDS mothers are teenagers at the time of their first birth.

Marital status: Fifty-nine percent of SIDS mothers are unmarried.

Sibling order: SIDS infants are often not the first-born.

Intervals between pregnancies: An intriguing observation is that the risk of crib death is increased when there is a shorter interval between pregnancies. This phenomenon is particularly evident if the mother becomes pregnant less than seven months after her previous delivery. Once again, we don't know why.

Previous sibling who dies of SIDS: The risk of having a baby die of crib death in a family where one baby already died of SIDS is increased approximately fivefold. The risk is still very small, less than 1 percent. This means that the incidence increases from 2 per 1000 to 10 per 1000, but the figures need explanation, because they can be misleading. The most likely reason for an increased incidence in "subsequent siblings" is that some crib deaths result from a mixed group of genetic diseases that recur in families. If you eliminate these diseases, the incidence for true SIDS in siblings is essentially unchanged, at 2 per 1000. This justifies the statement that SIDS is not hereditary. The occurrence of crib death in a twin increases the risk for the other twin only during the first twenty-four hours after the first twin's death. Reports of later SIDS in a surviving twin are so rare that after twenty-four hours the risk is the same as that for any sibling.

Breath-holding spells and home monitors: Literature refers to the baby born to a family following a death due to SIDS as the "subsequent child." After the subsequent child is born, the parent's natural tendency is to hover over the crib twenty-four hours a day. Eventually, you will get tired, learn to relax, and trust yourself, though there will be uneasy moments. Whereas all parents check to see if the babies are covered, parents of subsequent babies check their respirations. Babies normally pause in their breathing periodically and sometimes pant for a breath or two. Remembering this will save some anxious moments. Most infants who die of SIDS do not have more breath-holding spells in their newborn period than other babies.

Home monitors are electric or battery-powered machines with wires that are attached to a baby as part of a wraparound belt or with small adhesive patches. An alarm goes off if the baby doesn't breathe for a set period of time or if the heart rate drops too low. The justification for the use of home monitors for siblings of SIDS victims and for infants with breath-holding spells is as follows. Although most SIDS infants were not noted to have breath-holding spells before their death, SIDS can be a rare cause of death in those few babies who are breath holders. Parents and caregivers must be taught about monitor use and cardiopulmonary resuscitation (CPR). Selected home monitoring of SIDS siblings with some risk factors has almost certainly prevented recurrences. However, the use of home monitors for all SIDS siblings would mean that thousands of normal infants would be subjected to the monitoring. This approach is hard to justify medically or economically, though it may be of psychological benefit to some parents.

Home monitoring is usually discontinued if there is no problem for four to six months or for one month past the age of the child who previously died of SIDS.

Breast feeding: Some experts feel that breast feeding can protect against crib death, although this remains controversial. We know that crib death occurred in previous centuries, when nearly all babies were breast-fed. Bottle feeding is not a cause of SIDS.

Sleep position: There are studies under way to determine whether there is an increased risk if the baby sleeps on his stomach. There is no conclusive proof that this is a problem, but the rate of SIDS has declined in several communities where the prone position (on the stomach) for infants has been avoided. The American Academy of Pediatrics has recently recommended that a healthy infant should be put to sleep on her side or back. There are many pediatricians who feel that this is an overreaction to some recent data, and they suggest that the baby sleep in the position she finds most comfortable. The prone position doesn't explain the occurrence of SIDS in babies with some of the other variables mentioned, such as higher frequency in the winter, or the baby's sex and race. In addition, the association of SIDS and the prone position varies in different communities. For example, in Sweden the rate of SIDS is low, even though the prone sleeping position is *advised* for babies. However, in New Zealand, sleeping prone has a strong relation to the rate of SIDS. In the United States, as in Sweden, the rate of SIDS is low even though the proportion of babies sleeping prone is almost twice that of New Zealand. Even in the United States, there are certain pediatric conditions, such as vomiting due to gastroesophageal reflux, for which the prone position is an accepted type of treatment.

All these data do not explain why thousands of babies sleep face down and do not die, whereas some who sleep on their backs do die. In summary, I would certainly encourage a baby to sleep on his side or back, but if the baby prefers to sleep on his stomach, it's all right. We hope that current research will soon help to clarify the importance of sleep position as it relates to crib death.

Bedding: Some experts feel that heavy bedding and pillows contribute to sudden death, but this too has not been proven. SIDS is not caused by external suffocation, as evidenced by the lack of typical suffocation findings in autopsies. Nevertheless, common sense dictates that a child does not need a pillow until he moves from crib to bed.

Vomiting: Available data indicate that a baby's vomiting, with its potential for causing choking, has no causal role in SIDS. Autopsies confirm that crib death is not caused by vomiting and choking or other forms of suffocation.

Immunizations: No association has been found between the timing of immunizations, such as DPT, and the occurrence of SIDS. In fact, SIDS infants have been found to be much less likely to have been immunized than were control infants. If anything, there may be a small protective effect from DPT immunization.

Contagion: Since SIDS is not contagious, there is no reason for concern if an infant has been exposed to a SIDS case.

The Sudden Infant Death Syndrome Act of 1974 authorized the Department of Health and Human Services to award grants for counseling to families affected by SIDS. The support for these families is crucial to their recuperation. Since all parents believe that healthy infants do not die without a cause, they feel guilty and responsible for the death. The guilt can be devastating, leading to marital problems and to strained relationships with other children. It is important to assuage those feelings. Parents will be unhappy, but they should not feel responsible.

Before leaving this sensitive topic, I'll say a word about how SIDS affects some older siblings. Young children may infantilize their behavior by clinging to their parents and by misbehaving to get the attention they crave. Older children may feel their own thoughts toward the baby could have caused his death. Also, they can have enormous guilt feelings about having caught a cold and passed it on to the baby. The best way to deal with this is discussed in the entry on "Sensitive Topics" on page 277. The main objective is to discuss the simple truth in a manner that makes it easy and comfortable for the older child to ask any question at all. He should be reassured that he, like all children over one year of age, is not at risk from SIDS.

Since no symptoms precede crib death and there is no known way to prevent it, a parent's extreme anxiety before or after the baby's birth will serve no useful purpose. The last decade has seen a remarkable explosion of concepts and theories regarding crib death. We can only hope that the next decade will answer more questions about this perplexing problem. For more information on SIDS, contact the following organizations:

The National SIDS Resource Center
8201 Greenboro Drive, Suite 600
McLean, VA 22102
1-703-821-8955

The Sudden Infant Death Alliance
10500 Little Patuxent Parkway, Suite 420
Columbia, MD 21044
1-800-221-7437

Cribs

SINCE a crib is made for a child to be left unattended, all measures must be taken to ensure that it is as safe as possible. Most of the problems that have occurred with cribs are now solved by federal government regulations. For example, only lead-free paint can be used on cribs, and the distance between the vertical slats (2⅜ inches) is federally controlled to minimize the chance of babies and toddlers hurting themselves by sticking their heads or extremities between them. However, the potential for newly discovered harm always exists.

TIPS:

1. Most important, think like your child: try to discover what mischief you can get into.

2. Never leave down the side of the crib when the baby is unattended. The top of the side panel, when raised, should be at least 21 inches higher than the top of the mattress. When lowered, the top of the side panel should be at least 4 inches above the mattress.

3. Although most mobiles that attach to only one side of a crib are safe, those which hang across the crib, from one side to the other, can act as a source of strangulation when the child is able to sit and stand. As soon as your child can sit or stand, remove the mobile.

4. The mattress should be firm and flat and should fit snugly. Cover it with a quilted pad and a sheet. Do not use plastic materials to cover mattresses, because a child can suffocate when the plastic sticks to her face. You should have to lift up the mattress to tuck in the sheet. The fit should be that tight! If there is a space between the mattress and the sides of the crib, little things—coins, pieces of toys, "fluffballs," threads—will

accumulate, and sooner or later will make their way into the baby's mouth.

5. Use of a pillow is not advisable throughout the first year of life. After one year, a toddler pillow, not a full-sized pillow, is recommended.

6. Keep the crib away from draperies and blinds so that the baby will not get tangled in the cords. The crib should not be placed near windows, lamps, fans, or heaters.

7. Don't buy a crib with corner posts that extend beyond the end panels. A few years ago, an already approved crib was implicated in the strangulation of some children who could stand in the crib. They trapped their necks between the finials (vertical cornered bedposts) and the blanket rolls (horizontal tops of the end panels of certain types of cribs). Aside from the danger of strangulation, clothing can catch on these posts.

8. Avoid cribs with decorative cutouts in the headboard or footboard that could entrap a child's head, arm, or leg. Similarly, be sure that no slats are missing. Children squeeze their feet into and out of these openings, but their heads get caught, resulting in strangulation.

9. An older crib should be stripped of paint and be repainted with high-quality, nontoxic lead-free paint. All wood surfaces should be free of splinters and cracks.

10. Bumpers should be tied securely, and any excess length of bumper ties should be cut off. When your child can stand, remove bumpers and large toys, which could become steps to help the child climb out of the crib. When the child is at this age, lower the mattress to the lowest position.

11. The tops of the side panels and end panels should be covered with plastic teething guards.

A common question is "How old should my child be when he leaves the crib?" *I can't stress enough that once your child can climb out of the crib after the mattress has been lowered to its bottom rung, it is time to move him to a bed.* The important thing is that your baby never fall from the height of the crib, with the potential for banging his head or an extremity on the sides or legs of the crib, and/or on the floor.

Rarely is a significant trauma sustained by falling off a bed. Some beds come with bed rails, but they are not necessary. Until he gets used to the bed, either keep pillows on the floor for protection, or use a highrise, which opens up on the bottom into another bed and mattress that he can use for climbing into and out of his bed. Refer to the section on "Bedtime Routine" in the entry on "Sleeping and Bedtime Problems," on page 289.

Croup

CROUP is a respiratory illness characterized by a hoarse, barking cough followed by inspiratory stridor —the noise made by air being sucked back into the windpipe. As a matter of fact, "croup" comes from the Scottish word "croak," an appropriate description of the stridorous cough. Croup is usually a viral illness seen in children from three months to five years of age, and it commonly occurs during the change from warm to cold weather. It can come on acutely or be preceded by a cold for one to two days. It usually lasts for seventy-two hours, but is worse at night and better during the day. The first night tends to be the worst. There is a low-grade fever or none at all. The violent nature of the cough and the fact that it occurs at night contribute to the frightening feelings it arouses.

Treatment consists of keeping the child comfortable and relaxed in a suitably humid room. A cool-mist humidifier or vaporizer soothes the throat and windpipe. Just as ice or a cold compress decreases the swelling and soothes an injured ankle, so too does cold steam soothe an irritated and inflamed throat. Create your own "croup tent" by placing three or four sheets around the child's crib or bed to concentrate the humidity from the vaporizer. If you turn on the cold water in a bathroom shower, no steam develops. Therefore, you settle for the next-best humidity, the warm steam from a hot shower. This, too, can be comforting and therapeutic. Since steam rises, do not sit on the floor with your child. Hold the child in your arms in the bathroom to bring him closer to the steam (but not close enough to touch the hot water) and provide the comfort and relaxation that help to relieve the airway spasm. Another source of cold humidity is the outside air, so opening the child's window may help. Although my grandmother would hate to hear me suggest taking a "sick" child outside, the truth is that a twenty-minute drive in a car with a window open helps calm down many children with croup. Speaking of grandmothers—one creative grandmother gave me an interesting suggestion. When her grandson had croup, she opened the freezer door and had him breathe in the cool moist air from the freezer! It worked. I don't approve of teaching children to open the freezer or refrigerator door and stick their heads in, but in an emergency it can help the croupy child.

Sometimes a decongestant will help by shrinking the inflamed tissues of the upper respiratory tract. Acetaminophen can be used if the child has a fever. He may be more comfortable if kept upright. Encourage the child to drink clear liquids in order to soothe the throat and keep any secretions liquefied and thin instead of thick and tenacious. Try to keep the child calm and relaxed and away from any passive smoking, which can further irritate the child's windpipe. Set up a comfortable sleeping area for yourself to spend the night in your child's room. If a fever is gone for twenty-four hours and the child feels better, he may return to school.

Keep in contact with your pediatrician, who may prescribe other medications, like steroids or racemic epinephrine. He may also want to rule out serious conditions that resemble croup, like diphtheria, epiglottitis (see below), measles, throat abscesses, tumors, or aspiration of a foreign body. In rare instances, croup can be psychogenic in origin; that is, there is no identifiable physical problem with the windpipe.

Epiglottitis is a more serious illness, which can mimic croup. This bacterial infection inflames and swells the epiglottis—the small piece of tissue overlying the windpipe. It covers the windpipe when we eat so that food does not go down the "wrong pipe," but it opens when we breathe. In epiglottitis, the tissue may swell to the point of serious compromise or actual obstruction of the windpipe. Children with epiglottitis have serious difficulty in breathing, and assume a characteristic position, with neck extended, to gasp for air. Since it is hard for them to swallow, they will drool profusely. This rare condition requires immediate medical attention and intravenous antibiotics. The Hib (haemophilus influenzae type B) vaccine protects against a bacterium that is a common culprit in epiglottitis.

Crying

THERE ARE as many opinions on how to deal with a crying baby as there are experts. New parents are torn between two divergent philosophies, which can be summarized as follows:

• Let the child cry so as not to spoil him by holding, carrying, or rocking him twenty-four hours a day.

• Never let him cry, because he is, after all, helpless and has no other means of expressing his needs.

Through the years, I have tried to incorporate both ideas into a usable guide for dealing with a crying baby —a compromise that has been successful for most parents. Once we become parents, we temporarily forget that we still serve other roles and have functions in society aside from being the baby's caregiver. For example, we need time for ourselves, spouses, other children and family, and our careers. When we are confronted, then, with a crying baby, it is important to ask ourselves: "Is there something else I should be doing at this time?" I'll explain by discussing daytime and nighttime separately.

Daytime:

When a baby cries after a period of contentment or sleep, it is always appropriate to evaluate her for any obvious needs. Is she hungry or thirsty? Does she require a diaper change? Is she warm? Did a mobile or stuffed animal fall on her? Make a cursory examination to see that everything is all right. Once you've evaluated and taken care of these things, it is time to ask yourself that question: "Is there something else I should be doing now?" If there is, you can put the baby down and deal with those other parts of your life. If there is nothing important to do, this is where the compromise comes in to play. Hold, cuddle, carry, and play with that gorgeous baby! Remember that persistent crying should prompt an evaluation by the pediatrician.

Nighttime:

This is slightly different, because the answer to that question: "Is there something else I should be doing now?" is always yes. You should be sleeping. If the baby has been asleep for a period of time and then cries, you shouldn't ignore that cry. This could be the one time something new and important has developed. Check her out for the obvious and routine problems, such as hunger and need for a diaper change, and, if necessary, try to console her for one or two minutes. Don't turn on bright lights; use a night light. Feed her quietly. Change the diaper without providing any entertainment or stimulation. The middle of the night is not the time to play and carry her around. Put her down, leave the door open, and go back to sleep yourself. As time goes on, she will learn that there's no point in carrying on if, after you've checked her, she is left to her own resources. All children have four or five partial awakenings each night. They must learn to fall back to sleep on their own. Too many parents regret, six months later, that every time their baby cried, they carried her around until she fell asleep in their arms. If she cries continuously, you can check after every twenty minutes, but only for one minute, without taking her out of the crib. If crying continues, as a last resort consider sleeping in her room in a bed or a sleeping bag. When she is six months old, a stuffed animal or a favorite blanket can be comforting.

On the other hand, the baby's cry is the only way she has of telling us she wants something. The compromise allows us both to cater to our nurturing juices and to function in our other roles in society.

Cystic Fibrosis

CYSTIC FIBROSIS is the most common fatal genetic disease in Caucasian Americans, affecting approximately 30,000 children and young adults. It occurs in 1 out of 2500 white children and in 1 out of 17,000 black children. If both normal parents have the defective gene for this disease, each of their children has a 25 percent chance of having cystic fibrosis. Genetic research has disclosed a lot about this disease, so we will soon be able to screen couples to see whether they have this faulty gene.

Cystic fibrosis does not impair intellectual ability. It affects several glands of the body, especially those lining the bronchial tubes and the ducts of the pancreas. The normally thin, slippery secretions of the body (such as sweat, mucus, tears, saliva, and digestive juices) become thick, sticky secretions that develop into plugs in the lungs, sinuses, and intestines. These plugs result in infection and interfere with vital body functions. When the pancreas becomes plugged up, important digestive enzymes are prevented from reaching the intestines. Necessary nutrients cannot be absorbed from the intestine into the body. This leads to diarrhea and foul-smelling, bulky stools. The child will be underweight and may fail to thrive. Occasionally, constipation occurs because the intestines are blocked. As a matter of fact, a newborn's failure to pass meconium (the first stool) for twenty-four to forty-eight hours can be an early warning sign of cystic fibrosis. When the bronchial airways are plugged up, pneumonia can result, with coughing and wheezing. Since sweat is affected, the skin tastes salty.

The sweat test, a reliable diagnostic tool, is painless. A chemical that induces sweat is put on the child's skin, and the sweat is then absorbed onto a filter paper and the salt is measured. A high content of salt in sweat is diagnostic of cystic fibrosis.

Treatment involves a multidisciplined approach, including education of the patient and parents. It calls for a highly enriched diet, vitamin and enzyme replacements, breathing exercises to loosen and drain thick mucus from the lungs ("postural drainage"), antibiotics, bronchodilator drugs, salt replacement, and, when appropriate, steroids. Genetic counseling is strongly recommended for people with a family history of cystic fibrosis.

With good medical care, children with cystic fibrosis generally have good school attendance records and do not, as a rule, need specific activity restrictions.

Developmental Milestones

WHEN Ed Koch was mayor of New York City, he would walk through the streets and ask his fellow New Yorkers, "How am I doin'?" Every newborn, young infant, and toddler being examined by a pediatrician seems to look up with inquisitive eyes and ask the same thing: "How am I doin'?" There are many ways to find an answer. How is the child's growth: length, weight, and head circumference? How is the child's appetite? How are his bowel patterns? Is he sleeping well? One of the best ways to determine how a child is doing is to evaluate his developmental milestones.

All parents worry about whether their child's development is "normal." Early childhood development is a series of transformations—some dramatic, and some barely noticeable even to the parents. Milestones like rolling from stomach to back or back to stomach, and transferring objects from one hand to another may not stand out in a parent's mind as major accomplishments . . . but ask the baby. He's proud of them!

The Denver Developmental Screening Test is one of several "homeowner guides" for making helpful assessments of the child's developmental levels. Parents should not panic about every deviation from "normal." If a developmental problem is evident, it can be investigated to see whether it is specific or generalized. Some developmental disorders are first picked up when the child starts school. A teacher may notice delayed language skills, a short attention span, aggression, or withdrawal. Parents need not be experts; they should be caring, observant, and loving and should rely on both common sense and appropriate professional guidance.

Speech and language problems are particularly subtle

and difficult to pick up in the young child. Before worrying that a child is late in talking, you should know what is within the normal or expected range. The following is a very general list of normal age-to-activity correlations for speech and motor development.

Birth to 1 month	Crying; lifting head
1 month to 4 months	Cooing; laughing; lifting chest while on stomach
6 months to 9 months	Uttering one-syllable sounds (ba-ba, na-na-na, ma, da, di); rolling over, at least from stomach to back; sitting alone; crawling
10 months to 11 months	Saying several syllables; responding appropriately to word cues for familiar things; pulling to stand; standing while holding on
14 months to 15 months	Using "Mama" or "Dada" correctly; walking while holding on; standing alone
16 months to 18 months	Speaking with three- to fifty-word vocabulary; walking
2 years	Using two-word combinations (50 percent of words should be fully intelligible); walking up steps; kicking a ball
3 years	Saying what he thinks and making his intentions clear; riding a tricycle

DEVELOPMENTAL MILESTONES

3 years to 4 years	Being completely intelligible; balancing on one foot for five seconds; toilet training

A sign in my office says, *If your child is not talking by two years of age, ask questions.* Delayed speech sometimes runs in families. It may also signal a hearing loss. Your child can't learn to speak if he can't hear the sounds. Unfortunately, a severe hearing loss may be present for two years before anyone notices, because children learn to respond "appropriately" to visual stimuli around them. A partial hearing loss may go undetected until age four or five. It will affect the way a child says words rather than preventing him from speaking at all. A hearing test is painless, and even newborns can be tested. Hearing tests should be done on babies who were sick as newborns, children with deformities of the ears or neck, children with kidney problems (because the kidneys and ears are formed at the same time in utero), children with deaf relatives, children with delayed milestones, children with repeated ear infections, and children with delayed speech.

The firstborn tends to speak earlier than siblings. There are several theories about this. One is that parents have more time to spend with their first child and therefore can offer more verbal stimulation. Another points out that subsequent children have their parents plus the older sibling(s) to run and do and get for them, so they don't have a "need" to speak at a younger age.

TIPS:

1. Read books with your child, even when she is young. Name objects and ask her to point to them on the page. Let your child see you read so that she can tell how important reading is to you.

2. Sing songs and recite nursery rhymes.

3. Don't use baby talk. Look at your child, talk slowly, and repeat key phrases.

4. Describe what your child is seeing, hearing, and doing.

5. Play games with simple, one-step instructions, like "Kick the ball" or "Throw the ball."

6. Stimulate your child's imagination by letting her tell you stories she has made up or finishing stories you start.

Diabetes

GLUCOSE is a sugar that is the major source of energy for the body. Insulin is a hormone made by the pancreas, an organ inside the abdomen. Insulin removes the glucose from the blood and incorporates it into various muscles and organs for the body to use and into the liver for storage. Diabetes mellitus is a disease caused by the lack of or malfunction of insulin. The glucose, which we ingest in the form of carbohydrates, builds up in the blood and does not get to the important tissues of the body. The body soon looks for other sources of energy, like fat and protein. When these are digested for energy on a regular basis, toxic byproducts are formed, such as acetone and ketones, and these contribute to the problems of diabetes.

When the amount of glucose in the blood surpasses the normal threshold, it spills into the urine. Just as salt soaks up and absorbs ice and snow from sidewalks, so too does this extra sugar in the urine soak up and draw water from the body. This increase in urine volume, if untreated, leads to dehydration.

We still do not know exactly why the pancreas stops making insulin, but most endocrinologists believe that in juvenile-onset diabetes the body starts making antibodies that attack its own pancreas. These, then, interfere with the production of insulin. Heredity, environment, and infection are all thought to be involved in the production of these antibodies. Adult-onset diabetes is different; insulin is made, but it doesn't work right.

Since urinary frequency is one of the symptoms of diabetes, bed-wetting is common, as is the need to urinate many times a day. As a result, the child becomes thirsty and drinks a lot. However, many *normal* children also like to drink a lot, especially if they are very active. A simple urine test will answer whether or not sugar is present. In a normal urine sample, there is none. Other symptoms of diabetes are weight loss, loss of appetite, lethargy, a fruity smell on the breath, and the feeling of being sick.

There are many ways that children with newly developed diabetes first exhibit the problem. On one extreme, some children feel fine, come for their annual check-up, but are diagnosed with diabetes on the basis of urine and blood tests. On the other extreme, a new diabetic can be so sick as to arrive in the emergency room in a comatose state.

Treatment calls for insulin injections, usually twice a day, into the arms, thighs, buttocks, or abdomen to maintain a normal blood glucose. Insulin can't be given by mouth, because the stomach juices destroy the oral form. Giving the right amount of insulin is tricky and should be done initially under a doctor's supervision. Too much insulin will lower the blood sugar too rapidly, causing confusion and even coma. As a child grows and gains weight, his daily insulin requirement increases. In addition, an infectious illness or traumatic event may require a temporary adjustment of the insulin dose. Good nutrition, with well-balanced meals and appropriate between-meal snacks, are outlined and supervised by a nutritionist. For the newly diagnosed diabetic and his family, the initial stabilization of blood sugar, determination of appropriate insulin dose, and intensive daily education are best accomplished in the hospital under the supervision of physicians, nurses, and nutritionists.

As adolescents go through their growth spurt, they require an increase in insulin. Since most adolescents have illusions of invulnerability, they are a particularly tough bunch to convince to maintain good health, nutrition, and medical and dental care. Patient education programs, support groups, and diabetic summer camps are helpful. Immunizations should be kept up-to-date, including a yearly flu vaccine. There should be annual visits to the ophthalmologist and dentist. The goal is to have the youngster lead a completely normal life, with full participation in sports, academics, and social activities.

If diabetes is left untreated or inadequately treated, the high blood sugar will damage blood vessels and nerves. Kidney failure, heart failure, and blindness can follow. Legs and feet can develop life-threatening infections. These long-term complications can be minimized by good blood sugar control. The child should always wear a Medic Alert bracelet with *Diabetes mellitus* engraved on it.

An important problem that all diabetics must know about is the "vicious cycle," known as the Somogyi phenomenon. The patient takes larger doses of insulin in response to an increasing blood sugar. This elevated blood sugar, however, is not from food. It is brought about by counterregulatory hormones, such as epinephrine, cortisol, growth hormone, and glucagon, which raise the body's blood sugar in response to the dramatic decrease in blood sugar caused by insulin. This is why the Somogyi phenomenon is described as "low blood sugar begetting high blood sugar." The symptoms are night sweats, night tremors, bad dreams, seizures, and coma. The diagnosis is suggested by rapid swings in the blood sugar level. Treatment consists of the appropriate regulation of insulin dose under a doctor's supervision.

There is some good news about the future development of an insulin infusion device that can be surgically implanted in the patient's abdomen. This "artificial pancreas" would maintain better control of blood sugar by administering amounts of insulin appropriate to the body's normal variations in blood sugar.

There is one other type of diabetes, which is only

rarely encountered in pediatrics. In diabetes insipidis, large amounts of urine are produced, but not because of problems with sugar. These children have normal amounts of the hormone insulin but insufficient amounts of vasopressin, the antidiuretic hormone. When normal people do not drink enough or lose water through diarrhea, they produce vasopressin, which directs the kidneys to preserve water for the body by not making too much urine. The urine that comes out is therefore more concentrated. People with diabetes insipidis either do not make vasopressin or have kidneys that do not respond to it. Their kidneys cannot decrease urine output by preserving water, so they urinate a lot. These children compensate by drinking a lot. Vasopressin is produced by the pituitary gland, a small but important gland in the head, immediately under the brain, that can be impaired by injury, infection, or tumor of the brain. As a result, the pituitary may fail to produce vasopressin. Treatment involves replacing the vasopressin as well as treating the underlying disease.

Diaper Rash

MANY PARENTS believe that the development of disposable diapers is the breakthrough that will simplify their lives. One of the disposable diaper's few disadvantages is the outer plastic lining, which, being watertight, does not allow the skin to "breathe" and makes the diaper area more susceptible to irritation and infection. It is advisable to put a thin layer of Desitin or A and D Ointment on the diaper area every time you change the baby to protect the skin from urine, stool, sweat, and heat. This will also help to reduce friction in areas of rubbing, like the creases of the hips and thighs. Be sure to wash the ointment off completely at each diaper change so that it doesn't cake and itself cause irritation. You can use lukewarm water and a mild soap. A soft washcloth, cotton balls, or wipes are fine as long as they do not cause an irritation rash. All diapers should be changed every two or three hours or as soon as the baby urinates or defecates.

TIPS:

1. Make two or three small holes in the outer plastic cover of the disposable diaper to allow some air in without letting anything leak out. Keep the diaper slightly loose-fitting. It is a good idea to have cloth diapers available for use for a few days if your baby has a diaper rash. If used without outer plastic panties, they will allow air in to help your other remedies. Some children are sensitive to the perfumes or chemicals in some disposable diapers. Switching to cloth diapers or simply changing brands of disposable diapers may help. When you wash your baby's cloth diapers, use a mild detergent but avoid fabric softeners or other irritating chemicals.

2. The moist, closed, and dark environment of a wet diaper makes the underlying skin prone to a second type of rash—that caused by bacterial and fungal infections. The common yeast (fungal) infection, due to *Monilia* or *Candida albicans,* usually has small red pimples, called "satellite" lesions, surrounding a larger red rash anywhere in the diaper area. Your pediatrician will prescribe a specific topical antifungal medicine for this problem. A source of this yeast infection might be white patches of the same fungus that can infect the inside of a baby's mouth, called "thrush." Sometimes milk or formula leaves a similar white patch inside the mouth, but if gentle wiping leaves a raw, red surface, the patches are signs of thrush. It will need its own oral medication. When the baby swallows this common mouth infection, the fungus traverses the intestine and comes out the other end as a fungal diaper rash. This type of diaper rash often follows the use of antibiotics.

3. Actual blisters, with crusting and oozing, in the diaper area may represent a bacterial infection. Your

doctor may prescribe an oral antibiotic in addition to topical antibiotic ointments.

4. Some disposable diapers contain a gel that absorbs urine. When this gel leaks onto the surface of the diaper, it forms clear beadlike granules that appear to have come from the baby's urine. Of course, they have nothing to do with the baby's urine or general health. The beads are not harmful and can be ignored.

Diarrhea

IT IS FREQUENCY, not consistency, that determines diarrhea and constipation in normal newborns. If a baby has only one or two stools a day, even though they are watery in consistency, this is not diarrhea. However, six or more stools per day is diarrhea, even if they are formed. It is interesting to note that breast-fed babies commonly have looser stools than those who are formula-fed. In addition, some babies will fluctuate between diarrhea and constipation, demonstrating the normal phenomenon of "transitional" stools.

There are many causes of diarrhea. Some of them are:

• Eating too many foods high in fiber, like prunes.

• Bacterial, viral, or parasitic infections, also called gastroenteritis. Sometimes cultures or other tests on the stool are needed to make the diagnoses. Food poisoning is one of these disorders.

• Stress, especially in older children.

• Anatomical problems, such as intussusception (telescoping of one piece of intestine into another). Refer to the section on "Intussusception" in the entry on "Stomachaches" on page 307.

• "Paradoxical diarrhea," when loose stool leaks around the partial obstruction caused by a large, hard piece of stool lodged in the colon. Refer to the entry on "Constipation" on page 80.

• Diarrhea can be a symptom of other illnesses, such as the flu, ear infections, and urinary tract infections.

• Cystic fibrosis, celiac disease, colitis, and various malabsorption illnesses, in which the intestines do not function normally. Refer to the pertinent entries for details.

• Teething is sometimes associated with loose and frequent stools. Refer to the entry on "Teething" on page 321.

• Some antibiotics.

• Lactose intolerance, to milk and dairy products, which can cause diarrhea, bloating, vomiting, and abdominal pain. Babies with lactose intolerance may need a formula without lactose. Refer to the section on "Lactose Intolerance" in the entry on "Stomachaches" on page 307.

Signs of dehydration are decreased urine output (less than three urinations a day or none in eight hours) with concentrated (darker) urine; absence of tears when crying; tenting of the skin after pinching; lethargy; sunken eyes and fontanelle (soft spot); dry mouth and lips.

TIPS:

1. Treatment depends on the cause of the diarrhea. The medications and various diets should be tailor-made for each child, so consult your doctor for diarrhea-related problems.

2. Use good hygiene, such as hand washing, to prevent spread of the disease through the household.

3. For children under one year of age, use commercially prepared electrolyte solutions, like Pedialyte or Ricelyte, for one day. Hold off formula and solid foods. The baby can drink as much clear liquid as he wants. It is usually safe to continue breast feeding, but extra clear liquids should be given between feedings. If he does well, with the guidance of your pediatrician you can

advance him to his regular formula diluted to half its strength. This means that you should prepare his formula as always, but fill only half the bottle with formula and the other half with water. Give this to the baby during the second twenty-four-hour period. By day three, most babies will be ready to go back to solid foods like bananas and rice cereal and to advance to full-strength formula. If the child still has diarrhea, he may need to advance more slowly or to have his formula changed. Your doctor will advise you.

For the older child, I have found, a similar four-day plan is effective.

Day 1: Clear liquids only, such as water, tea, Jell-O, 7-Up, ginger ale, Gatorade, chicken broth, ice pops. The use of fruit juices is controversial, because the sugar in them can cause diarrhea. If they are the only items the child will drink, dilute them with water. No solid foods and no milk should be given on the first day.

Day 2: The BRAT diet. This is not a description of the child, but rather an easy way to remember what to give him on this second day.

    B   stands for bananas.

    R   stands for rice, rice cereal, Rice Krispies, or rice water.

    A   stands for applesauce. The skin of apples contains kaolin and pectin, which are important components of Kaopectate, an over-the-counter medicine for diarrhea.

    T   stands for toast, which includes dry foods like crackers, pretzels, and bagels.

Day 3: If the diarrhea has decreased in frequency, return the child to his regular food but without milk or dairy products. Milk tends to irritate the lining of the recuperating stomach and intestine if it is introduced too early.

Day 4: Reintroduce the milk and dairy products. If, despite this daily regimen, frequent stools persist, notify your pediatrician.

4. It is important to keep up with your child's increased need for fluids. Do not follow the mistaken reasoning that if you don't put anything in his stomach, the diarrhea will stop. The diarrhea, with its loss of water and necessary salts, will continue. Dehydration can occur quickly and is a serious problem. Frequent sips of liquids are important. If he refuses his bottle or cup, give the fluids by dropper into his mouth.

5. In some situations your pediatrician will prescribe medication to alleviate cramps and diarrhea. Don't give any medicine to your child unless you first clear it with your doctor, even if you happen to have it at home. If the doctor suspects that a bacterial infection or a potentially surgical condition may exist, these medicines could be contraindicated. It is better for the intestine to purge itself of a bacterial infection than to be paralyzed by an antidiarrheal medicine, thus keeping the bacteria present for a longer period of time.

Diphtheria

DIPHTHERIA is a serious, contagious, bacterial disease that causes a sore throat, croupy cough, and large swollen glands around the neck. This neck swelling is often so impressive, it has been called a "bull neck." A gray membrane forms over the back of the throat, making it difficult for the baby to breathe. Humans are the only known reservoir for these bacteria. The illness is spread by coughing, sneezing, or close contact. The incubation period is two to five days. Serious complications include pneumonia, paralysis, and heart failure.

About one of every ten people who get diphtheria die of it. Immunizations have almost eradicated this dreaded disease. Eighty percent of cases occur in unimmunized children under fifteen years of age. Regular booster injections of diphtheria toxoid should be given every ten years. See the entry on "Immunizations" for details about this vaccine as well as recommended ages for its administration.

Treatment involves hospitalization for observation, intravenous fluids, antibiotics, and antitoxin.

Ears

Middle Ear Infections – Otitis Media:

THE EAR is divided into three parts: inner, middle, and outer (external). The eustachian tube is a hollow tube connecting the middle ear to the throat. Normally, the mucus and natural secretions drain from the middle ear through the eustachian tube to the throat, where they are then swallowed. If the tube is blocked, the secretions build up in the middle ear and provide bacteria with excellent culture media where an ear infection can develop. Therefore, "fluid in the ear" commonly results in a true ear infection. Similarly, after an ear infection is over, that "fluid in the ear" can linger for a week or two. Blockage of the eustachian tube can be caused by swelling from infection (such as the common cold), allergies, enlarged adenoids, trauma, and rapid changes in air pressure. Although the cold that precedes the ear infection can be contagious, ear infections are not.

Infants and young children are particularly prone to ear infections for several reasons. Their eustachian tubes are shorter than adult tubes, so it is easier for throat infections to travel into the middle ear. Infants also spend more time lying down, a position that encourages the backward flow of milk and other fluids through the eustachian tube into the middle ear. This is why an infant's drinking a bottle while she is horizontal may lead to recurrent middle ear infections. Since a child's immunity is not as developed as an adult's, she is more likely to catch colds, with the potential for resultant ear infections. Finally, very forceful nose blowing can move secretions back up the eustachian tube into the middle ear. Ironically, then, ear infections can result when the eustachian tube is always blocked or always open. Most pediatricians have seen the endearing but heart-wrenching sight of a child walking into the office with a Band-Aid on her ear.

One of the ways to differentiate a middle ear infection from an external ear infection is to pull gently on the pinna, or earlobe, or to push gently on the small cartilage in front of the ear. Neither maneuver will hurt the child with a middle ear infection, but it is painful if an external ear infection is present. Middle ear infections do not result from exposing the child's head to wind or allowing her to get water in the ear. They do not come from forgetting to put a hat on your child. There is, however, a higher incidence of ear infections in children in a household where both parents smoke.

Several things can be done for the child with a middle ear infection.

TIPS:

1. Prescribed eardrops can be applied to decrease the pain. If these are not available, you can use warm mineral oil, olive oil, or even cooking oil. Warm the eardrop bottle by standing it in warm water for three minutes. Do not warm it in a microwave, as the fluid in the center of the bottle can become too hot.

2. A heating pad, wrapped in a towel, can be placed against the affected ear.

3. Acetaminophen or ibuprofen can be administered for relief of pain. If necessary, codeine (liquid or tablet) can be given.

4. Some pediatricians feel that a decongestant also helps to relieve the pressure of a middle ear infection. If

allergies are involved, an antihistamine-decongestant combination may be given.

5. Eliminate the bottle when the child is twelve to fifteen months old.

6. Eliminate the child's exposure to smoking.

7. Many factors enter into the choice of the appropriate antibiotic for middle ear infections. A few of them are the age of the child, cost of the medicine, frequency of administration, taste, side effects, sensitivity of common bacteria to the antibiotic, allergies, and the child's preference for liquid, tablets, or capsules. Just because a certain antibiotic did not work once for a child does not mean that the same antibiotic won't work the next time. The bacteria causing the first infection may have been resistant to the first antibiotic, but the same antibiotic may work for a subsequent infection.

It is important to complete a full ten-day course of antibiotics, even though the child will feel better after one or two days. Otherwise, the bacteria, which may not have been fully eradicated, could grow back, reinfecting the ear. If clinical improvement (lack of pain, decrease in fever) is not obtained after two to three days of treatment, you may need to try another antibiotic. Children with persistence of any symptoms should be checked again after the course of antibiotics. If the eardrum (which is a window to the middle ear) has not healed, another course of antibiotics may be necessary.

It sometimes happens that the child will complain of ear pain at night, when lying down, because the pressure increases when the head is horizontal. In the morning the ear may feel better. Do not ignore this situation, because it may indicate an ear infection.

Occasionally the pressure from the growing infection in the enclosed middle ear may grow and grow until the eardrum bursts. The infected fluid may then leak out of the perforated eardrum and through the canal to the outside. After this clear, milky, or bloody discharge drains, the pain may suddenly disappear. (As a matter of fact, during the years before antibiotics were discovered, ear infections were treated by having the doctor puncture the eardrum to allow the infection to leave.) These small tears in the eardrum usually heal completely.

A child with a middle ear infection can go outside and to school if he is free of fever for one day. Ear infections are not contagious. He does not have to cover his ears. He can go swimming as long as the eardrum is not perforated. He can go on an airplane as long as he is old enough to understand that he must swallow (drink) during ascent and descent to equilibrate the ear pressure.

For children with recurrent (at least four per year) bouts of middle ear infections, a daily prophylactic dose of an antibiotic for a prolonged period of time is sometimes effective in warding off the infections. If these children "break through" the prophylactic antibiotics with more ear infections, your pediatrician may refer you to an ear, nose, and throat specialist. More drugs are not the answer, so to prevent scarring of the eardrum, with possible resultant deafness, the specialist may discuss the option of using myringotomy tubes. These tiny plastic tubes are inserted through the eardrums in a hospital-type setting while the child is under a light general anesthetic. They remain in place until they fall out, six months to two years later. Occasionally they come out too quickly and must be put back. These hollow tubes act as a safety valve by allowing the fluid from any subsequent potential middle ear infection to leak out. Once the tubes fall out, the hole in the eardrum heals completely. If enlarged adenoids are thought to contribute to the blockage of the eustachian tubes, they can be removed at the same time the tubes are inserted.

Every child with recurring ear infections should be given hearing tests. There is usually a temporary decrease in hearing in the infected ear, and audiograms can pick up subtle losses of hearing even before parents notice them. Any persistent documented hearing loss (once the ear infection is resolved) should be brought to the attention of a specialist for consideration of myr- ingotomy tubes. If it is caught early enough, this mild hearing loss is usually reversible. An audiogram should also be part of the work-up for every child with delayed or dysfunctional speech and delayed developmental milestones.

Not all earaches are due to ear infections. Sometimes when a child cuts a new tooth, the brain interprets the pain as coming from the ear. This "referred pain" causes the child to pull at the ear, bang that side of his head, or pull the nearby hair. A low-grade fever can accompany this teething, thus further mimicking a true ear infection. A throat infection may also lead to re- ferred pain as an earache. And a foreign body placed in the ear can present itself as an earache.

External Ear Infections – Otitis Externa or "Swimmer's Ear":

An irritation, infection, scratch, or boil along the length of the ear canal leading inward to the eardrum causes pain when the pinna or earlobe is pulled. Any of these mishaps may follow the inappropriate insertion of a Q-Tip, finger, bobby pin, or other foreign body into the ear canal. The following adage most definitely ap- plies: "The smallest thing to put in your ear is your elbow." (See the next section, which discusses removal of ear wax.)

"Swimmer's ear" gets its name from its frequent oc- currence during the summer months, when children have been in a pool or in the ocean. The exact mecha- nism by which the water irritates the ear canal is not known.

TIPS:

1. Prescribed eardrops (specific for otitis externa) can be applied to lessen the inflammation and pain. Fol- low your pediatrician's directions carefully regarding duration of their use. Never allow the dropper to touch

the ear itself, because it may act as a carrier, spreading the infection elsewhere.

2. Dry heat in the form of a heating pad or hot water bottle (wrapped in a towel) can soothe the affected area.

3. Acetaminophen or ibuprofen can be given for relief of pain. If necessary, codeine can be prescribed.

4. If these tips do not help, your pediatrician may insert cotton or gauze wicks into the ear canal. These will remain in place for two days and enlarge as the eardrops are applied to them in the ear canal. The swollen, saturated wicks enable the medicated eardrops to reach the actual lining of the ear canal. Continue to apply the eardrops for the prescribed amount of time even after the wicks are removed.

5. If swimming triggers the external ear infection, don't let the child go back into the water until the pain is fully gone, even when you pull gently on the pinna of the ear. Once the child is ready to go swimming, your doctor may prescribe certain eardrops to be used prophylactically before and after swimming for the rest of the season to prevent a recurrence of the external ear infections.

6. A common mistake is relying on over-the-counter earplugs to prevent swimmer's ear. These usually let the water in but not out, potentially aggravating the problem. Your doctor can prescribe custom-molded earplugs with a water-tight fit for your child if their use is indicated.

7. Only in rare instances will your pediatrician prescribe oral antibiotics.

Earwax:

Earwax acts as a water-repellent coating of the ear canal to protect it from infection and foreign bodies. The wax usually liquefies and is moved through the canal by the child's chewing movements. It comes out, unnoticed, on its own. The color varies from white to dark brown. Some children have an inherited tendency toward thicker and drier wax, which recurrently plugs the ear canal and can result in a temporary hearing loss. However, once again, the famous adage applies: "The smallest thing to put in your ear is your elbow."

Q-Tips should never be inserted into the ear canal, because they shove the wax farther in. Talk with your pediatrician about using eardrops to dissolve the wax. The time-honored mixture of 1 teaspoon of hydrogen peroxide in 1 teaspoon of water usually helps. Four drops of this mixture (or prescribed eardrops) placed into the ear canal four times a day will soften the wax so that it will come out by itself or with the aid of a gentle washing with lukewarm water. Ear-wax removal kits with directions are available over the counter in drugstores. To prevent the wax from accumulating in children prone to this problem, use the eardrops once or twice every week.

Eating Habits and Picky Eaters

A QUICK glance at a growth chart for normal children will demonstrate how a child's rate of growth for height and weight slows down around one year of age. They continue to grow, but at a much slower rate. There are two basic reasons. First, children become more active at this age—walking, running, falling, climbing—and burn up more calories than they did in their first year of life. Second, their appetites decrease. Most toddlers seem to eat even less than they did when they were younger. They seem to be living on air and water. Yet they grow and develop just beautifully. Do not worry and do not feel frustrated. It's perfectly all right, as long as your child's growth pattern is satisfactory. He will eat as much as he needs to get enough calories for his growth and energy. In the first year of life, an infant will grow an average of 10 inches and will triple his birth weight. It's a good thing that this rate does not continue, or first-graders would be 9 feet tall and weigh 500 pounds. During the second and third years of life, he will grow only about 7 inches and gain 8 to 10 pounds, and may gain only 4 or 5 pounds in each of the next few years.

Choosing to eat or not to eat, as well as choosing what to eat, is how a toddler expresses his individuality and independence. It is normal for a toddler to use mealtime to show that he is master of his surroundings. Some children may go through temporary food fads, demanding only a peanut butter sandwich (with the crust cut off the bread, of course) or a certain juice or only a piece of cheese for each meal. A fad can last a few weeks or even a few months. Go along with it, because his tastes will soon change again. Many studies have shown that if you let your toddler make his own choices, he will thrive, grow, develop, and will not starve. Don't let mealtime become stressful. If the child is not hungry, don't force him to eat. He'll eat more at another meal. About 20 percent of a child's calories are eaten as nutritious snacks. If you evaluate what your child eats over a two-week period, rather than meal to meal or day to day, you will see how well balanced his diet is. If you worry too much about what he eats, you provide him with a powerful weapon to manipulate you. Some pediatricians feel that if a parent acts too controlling, it increases the child's chances of becoming anorectic as a teenager. The golden rule for eating is: *Parents are responsible for the food that is presented and the manner in which it is presented. Children are responsible for how much they eat and even whether they eat.*

Some parents are overly concerned that their infant may get fat if he is allowed to eat as much as he wants. Actually, not feeding the infant enough and keeping him on a low-fat diet when his nutritional needs are greatest are the most common causes of "failure to thrive," evinced by inadequate weight gain and stunted growth. On the other hand, you should resist the urge to wake up a sleeping baby to feed her so that she'll sleep through the rest of the night. You wouldn't like it if I woke you up from a sound sleep and said, "Wake up! You're hungry!" You would respond, in a grumpy voice (after throwing me out of the room), "Leave me alone. I'll wake up myself when I'm hungry." Infants who are pressed to eat will eventually rebel and become angry and irritable.

Each child is different, with a different schedule for maturing. If the mother and her one- or two-year-old are still enjoying breast feeding, it is perfectly all right to continue. When to stop nursing is a decision that only the parents and/or the child should make.

Many children between the ages of one and three start to finger-feed themselves. They like to see, touch, feel, roll, squish, and smell the food before they put it into their mouths. Let your child explore within reason. It is harmless to roll peas and break crackers. Some toddlers use fingers because it is hard to keep a full spoon balanced all the way to their mouths. Allow your baby to dip into her food, rub it into her tray, and scoop it up with her hands. Praise her when and if she finally gets some in her mouth. Short-handled children's forks with round tines are safe.

TIPS:

1. Do not get into the habit of using food to comfort a distressed baby. Sometimes rocking, walking, or offering a pacifier does the trick. Similarly, don't start your toddler down that long path of turning to food for relief of life's traumas. An occasional favorite snack as a reward is safe, but don't make a habit of it.

2. Do not insist that your child finish any particular food or clean her plate. Likewise, do not insist that your toddler sit at the table or in the highchair for long periods of time.

3. Serve smaller servings to toddlers, and use smaller plates for them. Their stomachs are smaller, and they

have a short attention span during meals, so they may need two or three snacks to meet their nutritional requirements. Some appropriate snacks are crackers with peanut butter or cheese, raisins or other dried fruits, yogurt (frozen or plain), slices of cheese, pieces of fruit, and cottage cheese with fruit.

4. Do not worry if your child doesn't have a serving from each food group every day. The food groups are:

• Breads, cereals, and other grains (crackers, pretzels, breadsticks).

• Fruits and vegetables (frozen juice pops, fruit juices—not artificial drinks).

• Meat, fish, eggs, beans, nuts (peanut butter).

• Milk, cheese, yogurt (custard, pudding).

5. Although milk and dairy products are the primary sources of calcium, other good sources are dried beans, sardines, and green leafy vegetables.

6. Have a pleasant atmosphere at mealtime. Minimize distractions like TV and family arguments during the meal.

7. Try to eat the same foods as your toddler. Your example carries more influence than your demands.

8. Do not worry if your toddler's only utensil is her fingers.

9. Remember the golden rule for eating (see above).

10. Do not use snacks or food as a reward. Maybe Dr. Spock was right when he said children would like vegetables if we said, "You can't have your carrots until you eat all your cake." When we bribe children to eat vegetables with the promise of dessert, we imply that vegetables are awful.

11. If the label on the box of cereal lists sugar first, leave it at the store.

12. Take your child to the store and let her choose one or two items from the produce section.

13. Let your preschool child help in preparing the food and setting the table to stimulate her interest in dinner.

14. Present food with a flair. Use a cookie cutter to form animal-shape sandwiches or other funny shapes.

15. Encourage finger foods, but put a piece of plastic or a rubber doormat under the highchair for your own sake. Use sturdy plastic dishes, bowls, and cups. Give the child a two-handled, covered cup with a spout. Utensils with short handles make it easier and less frustrating for toddlers to get food from plate to mouth. Despite all this, your toddler will manage to wear more food than she eats. Enjoy it and take pictures.

16. Offering orange juice as a mealtime beverage or putting a slice of tomato on a sandwich can quadruple the amount of iron the child absorbs during that meal. In addition to being high in vitamin C, orange juice is high in folic acid and potassium.

17. Hard candies, nuts, grapes, hot dogs, lumps of peanut butter, raw carrots, and popcorn are all foods that can cause choking in a young child. A child is between three and five years old before he can master these foods without choking. Teach your child never to talk and eat at the same time.

18. Healthy American children will not become vitamin deficient no matter how inappropriately they eat for a few weeks. Nevertheless, it is safe and harmless to give the recommended dose of daily vitamins.

19. Encourage exercise. Walking or running 1 mile will burn up 100 calories and stimulate a healthy appetite.

Eczema

ECZEMA is an inherited, allergic skin condition (atopic dermatitis) that produces itchy, oozing, reddened scales and crusty patches of skin in a child of any age. In the infant, the cheeks, scalp, chest, back, and outer surfaces of the arms and legs are most often involved. Areas of irritation, such as where elastic rubs against the skin, are also susceptible. Older children can get eczema in the creases of the elbows, wrists, and behind the knees. In the acute stage, the rash is intensely red. It tapers out at the periphery, fading into normal skin. Clear vesicles with open, oozing lesions soon develop from all the scratching, which is why eczema is known as "the itch that rashes."

Frequently there is a personal and/or family history of asthma, hay fever, and food allergies. Food culprits are certain infant formulas, dairy products, eggs, orange juice, wheat, peanut butter, corn, fish, and some medicines, like penicillin or sulfa drugs. Eczema in a wholly breast-fed baby requires that the mother go on a hypoallergenic diet. She should exclude the previously mentioned foods from her diet for three weeks and see whether the baby's eczema clears. If it does, she can reintroduce the foods gradually, one at a time, and watch for recurrences of eczema.

Examples of contact skin irritants are wool, pet fur, soaps and detergents, house dust mites, perfume, jewelry, and grass. Blood tests or scratch tests for specific allergens may reveal the offending allergens. Stress can trigger eczema in the older child. When eczema starts at a very young age (in infancy), it tends to leave after childhood (by ten years of age). If it first starts at eight, nine, or ten years and lasts through puberty, it may linger throughout adulthood.

TIPS:

1. Since a topical steroid cream or ointment is the main treatment for eczema, be sure to pack this cream when you travel anywhere with your child.

2. Keep your child's fingernails short to prevent his breaking the skin when he scratches. You may need to put mittens on his hands if he causes serious skin irritations by scratching.

3. Young children with eczema should be bathed without sensitizing soap. Teenagers should use a moisturizing soap. Never use drying or irritating bubble baths. Ironically, water has a drying effect on the skin, so bathing should be limited to every other day, even less often in cases of severe eczema.

4. After a bath or shower, while the skin is still wet, apply a moisturizing lotion or bath oil. In wintertime, when the skin is usually drier, apply it twice a day.

5. A humidifier in the child's bedroom will help to keep the skin moist.

6. Avoid all clothes or articles with wool. Cotton clothes are preferable. Feather and down pillows can irritate sensitive skin. Refer to the section on allergy prevention in the entry on "Asthma" on page 14.

7. Avoid any sensitizing food.

8. Oral antihistamines may alleviate the itching.

9. Allergy shots against the offending allergens are a last resort.

Erythema Toxicum (Newborn Rash)

ABOUT HALF of all babies develop a rash resembling insect bites on the second or third day of life. These red spots, appearing anywhere on the body, have a small white lump in the center. The palms and soles are usually spared. The rash disappears by the time the infant is seven to ten days old. This "newborn rash" is harmless and the cause is unknown. Although "erythema" means "red" and is appropriate, I don't like the use of the term "toxicum," because it implies something ominous and serious. This rash is neither.

Eyes

Blocked Tear Ducts:

THIS CONDITION, common in newborns, is misunderstood by many parents. A blocked tear duct does not mean that there are no tears, but, rather, that there are too many. Tears are normally made in the upper and outer part of the eye and wash across the eye to keep it moist. The tears then drain through the tear ducts, which are at the junction of the eye and nose, into the nose. That is why, when we cry, we sniffle—our noses are "running" with our tears. When the tear duct is blocked, usually with mucus, the tears are still made, but they have nowhere to drain, so they build up on the eye, which appears wet and runny. These tears are an excellent culture media for bacteria, and "pink eye" (conjunctivitis), with a green or yellow discharge, develops. A concurrent upper respiratory infection sometimes aggravates the problem.

A simple maneuver, performed three times a day, helps to unclog the blocked tear duct. With your clean thumb and second finger, massage the baby's nasolacrimal duct—where the eyes and nose meet. Let your doctor show you this important maneuver. After massaging for two to three seconds, take a cotton ball with lukewarm water and clean away the discharge from near the nose, outward across the eyes. Perform this maneuver three times a day for as many weeks or months as it takes for the tear ducts to open and for one month after the discharge stops. Rarely is it necessary to do this after the baby is a year old. The regimen of daily massaging and cleaning has greatly reduced the need for what used to be one of the most common pediatric surgical procedures: dilatation, probing, and irrigation of the tear ducts by an ophthalmologist.

"Pink Eye"—Conjunctivitis:

Conjunctivitis is an inflammation of the clear tissue covering the white part of the eye, the pupil, and the inside of the eyelid. It can be caused by an infection, allergy, or irritation from dirt, shampoo, smoke, chlorine from a pool, or a foreign body. The white part of the eye becomes red and there is a green or yellow discharge. This condition is very contagious. Wash your hands well and keep the child's towels separate from those of others.

TIPS:

1. If a superficial foreign body (like an eyelash or speck of dirt) is obvious and easily accessible on the white part of the eye, take a clean Band-Aid and touch the foreign body with the sticky surface. If this does not help, patch the eye closed with a piece of gauze (3″ by 3″) and overlying tape. Call your doctor. The eye is patched so that the continuous blinking will not further irritate and hurt it.

2. With most children, it is easier to use eyedrops than eye ointments. Here is an important tip on how to give eyedrops. Before putting them in, clean away any discharge with a moist cotton ball by wiping from near the nose outward across the eye. Have the child lie on his back with his head flat. He can keep his eyes closed at first. Then make a little puddle of eyedrops in the corner where the eye meets the nose. Always be sure to keep the eye dropper away from the eye itself so that the dropper won't transfer the infection to someone else. Once the child opens his eyes on his own, enough drops will enter the eye, even though some may trickle down the cheek. This trick makes giving eyedrops easier than holding the child down with one hand while you pry the eyes open with your second hand and put in the drops with your third hand. In general, eyedrops should be used for at least four days or until forty-eight hours have passed without eye discharge.

Newborns are given antibiotic eye medicine shortly after birth to prevent serious bacterial conjunctivitis. In older children, allergic conjunctivitis requires special eye medicines. Over-the-counter eyedrops, like Visine and Murine, are rarely beneficial for children.

If the eyelid or skin around the eye is swollen and red, call the doctor. Possible causes are trauma, insect bites, topically irritating substances (such as chemicals), allergens, a case of sinusitis, and periorbital cellulitis. The last is a serious bacterial infection that colors the eyelid and surrounding skin red or purple. The infection can spread backward to infect the eyeball and even the brain itself. Although red eyes are common, the more serious complications of periorbital cellulitis are rare.

Whether treating the above problems with compresses, eyedrops or ointments, antihistamines, or antibiotics, keep in mind the benefits of having the toddler or older child wear wrap-around sunglasses. Not only do they protect these sensitive eyes from bright lights, but they also offer some protection when the pollen count is high.

"Cross-Eyed"—Strabismus:

The eyes of newborn babies often move independently of each other. As each month goes by, this should become less noticeable. By the time the baby is three months old, her eyes should be straight. Strabismus is the condition in which one or both eyes wander. Many babies' eyes appear crossed but really are not. This is called "pseudostrabismus"; the bridge of the nose is still so wide that it makes the eyes appear to be close together. One way to distinguish true strabismus from pseudostrabismus is the flashlight test. Shine a flashlight in the center of each pupil. If the eyes are straight, the white dot of reflected light will be seen in the center of the pupils. If one eye turns out, the pinpoint of light will be seen on the inner half of that eye. If the eye turns in, the light will be seen on the outer half of the eye. Either condition of true strabismus should be discussed with your pediatrician.

Styes:

Styes are small abscesses of the eyelash follicles and eyelids. They are red, tender bumps at the base of the lower or upper lashes. The pupil, cornea, sclera (white part of the eye), and the rest of the eyeball are not involved. Treatment includes applying ten minutes of warm soaks four times a day. This may help the stye come to a "point," open, and drain. In addition, antibiotic eyedrops may be prescribed by the pediatrician.

Feet

MUCH HAS been written in textbooks, journals, and lay literature about the correct and pathological positioning of feet because that matter relates to many other parts of the body, such as the brain, spinal cord, hips, knees, toes, and all the bones in between. Given an intact and normal neurological and musculoskeletal system, the following two tips apply:

1. In general, it is preferable for a baby's feet to turn out rather than in.

2. When the child first walks, his feet should still turn outward, resembling Charlie Chaplin's funny walk or the position of a duck's feet. This helps him keep his balance. However, the older a child gets, the more his feet will turn in. If a child's feet start out straight, he often ends up in-toeing or pigeon-toed.

Babies with noticeable in-toeing are commonly put in a Dennis-Brown bar, a brace that turns the feet outward. In severe cases, such as clubfeet, the heel bone and front of the foot will be misaligned. This rare condition is treated with casting and, if necessary, corrective surgery. In less extreme situations, simple daily exercises will help to turn the feet outward.

Since malposition of a baby's feet can signify a problem in another part of the body, it is always best to discuss it with your pediatrician.

On the topic of feet, here's a word about shoes. During the latter half of the first year, when your child begins to stand and cruise, socks or soft slippers or sandals are adequate to protect the feet. Once the child can take four or five steps on his own, he is ready for his first pair of shoes, which will provide warmth and protection. Unless there is a particular orthopedic or podiatric problem, sneakers offer adequate support, and are usually less expensive and more flexible than high-top, hard shoes, which resemble little army boots. Toddlers use their muscles better and have better balance when walking in sneakers. In addition, sneakers allow the foot to "breathe" better than shoes do. This decreases the incidence of "shoe dermatitis," a rash of the feet, resembling athlete's foot but actually caused by sweating. The sweat irritates the toes and soles, causing redness and peeling of the skin. It is best treated by airing out the feet after cleaning them and then applying powder. The sneakers should therefore be flexible, flat, lightweight, and wide in the front for the toes. These first baby shoes can still be bronzed, even if they are sneakers!

Children outgrow shoes rapidly, so the shoe size should be checked every two to three months. The big toe should not rub against the front of the shoe. In addition, check the sides of the feet and shoes for signs of irritation or rubbing. Shoes that are too big can cause blisters, too. Your child's feet should be measured for shoes while she is standing. Socks also need to fit right. If they are too big, they will bunch up and cause irritations.

Flatfeet are common throughout early childhood, because a fat pad lies at the bottom of the arch of the foot. As a matter of fact, all babies are born with flatfeet. They require medical attention if the foot is stiff or painful. Once the fat pad disappears, when the child is around five, a normal arch develops. Babies are often bowlegged and then, when they're between one and three years old, become knock-kneed. Your doctor may be concerned if the condition is severe or occurs only on one side.

Toe-walking is common and of no importance if the child is able to walk normally but just chooses occasionally to walk on his toes. However, if he always toe-walks and can't flatten his feet, this could be a sign of a short Achilles tendon or significant neurological disease.

Fever

THE AVERAGE normal temperature for a child is 98.6° F (37° C). The actual normal temperature ranges from 97° F in the morning to 99.9° F at night. Because an increase in temperature from morning to night also occurs in the sick child, the pattern of high nighttime temperatures complicates the fact that all pediatric problems appear scarier at night.

A low-grade temperature is between 100° F and 100.9° F measured with a rectal thermometer. The rectal temperature, taken for 3 minutes, is the "true" temperature. If an oral thermometer is used, place it under the child's tongue for 3 minutes, then add a half degree F to get the true temperature. If the thermometer is placed under the child's arm (axillary) for 3 minutes, add 1° F to get the true temperature. The forehead "fever strip" is adequate only as a screen, not as a reliable measure of temperature. A special thermometer placed in the child's ear for a few seconds (much like the doctor's otoscope) has recently become available. One should not rely on the old test of hands-on-forehead or lips-on-forehead to determine the height of a fever. Learn how to take your child's temperature, and do so before you call the pediatrician and before you give any medicine to reduce the fever.

These tips may help you control the child's fever and make him more comfortable.

TIPS:

1. Keep him lightly dressed and let him sleep with only a sheet over him. This allows his fever to dissipate and radiate away from his body.

2. Sponge-bathe the child with room-temperature water, either in the bathtub or in the child's bed or crib. Do not sponge-bathe with alcohol or cold water. Cold water closes the capillaries in the skin, preventing the heat from leaving the body. Alcohol does the same thing. In addition, alcohol can be absorbed through the skin, causing intoxication and even coma. Also, alcohol and cold-water sponge baths drop the temperature so rapidly that the child's immature thermoregulatory mechanism can't sustain the lowered temperature, and the temperature shoots back up. A lukewarm bath lowers the temperature at a slower rate, but the lower temperature tends to last longer. The old wives' tale that you should not take a bath when you're sick is not true.

3. Two commonly used antipyretic (fever-reducing) medicines are acetaminophen and ibuprofen. Check with your doctor about their doses and how to use them. Aspirin should be used only on the doctor's recommendation, due to its association with the serious neurological condition called Reye's syndrome. Refer to the entry on "Reye's Syndrome" on page 266. Any of these medicines, when used to lower a fever, should be given only if the temperature reaches 101° F. If it is given when the temperature is lower, it could mask the development of a significant fever.

4. Encourage the child to drink clear liquids, such as water, tea, juices, Jell-O, broth, ice pops, and electrolyte drinks like Pedialyte, Ricelyte, Gatorade, etc. This is important, because the child needs extra liquids to re-

place fluid lost through sweating and to meet the increased metabolic demands a fever places on the body.

5. Do not wake the sleeping child just to take his temperature. When he is sleeping, his metabolism is working at a slower and more relaxed pace—something greatly needed by the feverish child. Waking him may agitate him, increase his metabolic demands, and possibly result in a rise in temperature.

6. Remember, the oral thermometer has the long tubular tip. The rectal thermometer has the round tip.

7. Let's review some tips on taking your child's temperature:

Rectal:
- Shake down the rectal thermometer.
- Coat the bulbous tip with Vaseline.
- Place the child on his stomach. Spread the buttocks to see the anal opening.
- Insert the thermometer one inch into the anal opening for three minutes. Keep the thermometer in place with one hand.
- With your other hand, hold the small of his back to stop him from moving.

Axillary (armpit):
- Use either an oral or rectal thermometer.
- Shake down the thermometer.
- Hold the thermometer tip in the closed armpit for three minutes. Make sure there is no clothing between the skin and thermometer.

Oral:
- Shake down the oral thermometer.
- Gently place the silver tip under his tongue. The child should be five years or older before you use an oral thermometer for him.
- Tell your child to close his lips around the thermometer, but not to talk and not to bite. Keep the thermometer in place for three minutes.

8. Take the child's temperature the same way each time so that you can more accurately compare readings.

9. Wash the thermometer in cold water only. Washing it in hot water could lead to a falsely elevated reading.

Infants under two months of age represent a particularly serious problem when they get a fever. Many of them do not show the typical and important signs of serious illnesses. As a result, it is sometimes necessary to hospitalize these babies to do tests and rule out certain illnesses. In many cases the babies will be started on antibiotics until all the tests show that no serious problems exist. Any rectal temperature greater than 100° F in a baby less than two or three months of age should be reported to your pediatrician immediately. If your baby's temperature is 97° F or lower, notify your pediatrician.

When a toddler or older child has a fever for over twenty-four hours, report the condition to the doctor. Call him if other worrisome symptoms (vomiting, earache, stiff neck, diarrhea, etc.) accompany the fever.

One of the scarier (but not necessarily serious) problems associated with a fever is a febrile seizure, a convulsion. A febrile seizure involves stiffening and twitching of the limbs. It occurs in the first twenty-four hours of an illness to some children between six months and four years of age. Refer to the entry on "Seizures" on page 274.

It is a common misconception that antibiotics treat fever. Antibiotics are potent medicines that specifically fight bacteria. They are not effective against viral illnesses. As a matter of fact, if taken inappropriately, antibiotics can cause serious problems. Any antibiotic can cause vaginitis, diarrhea, stomach upset, allergic reactions, etc. Therefore, never give your child an antibiotic without a doctor's supervision. Children who are independently given an antibiotic by a parent are in a "partially treated" state that frequently makes it hard for the doctor to arrive at a diagnosis. It is best to avoid this "shotgun" or empirical use of antibiotics. Occasionally, the cause of a fever is difficult to determine, even in an untreated child. Try not to insist that the doctor prescribe an antibiotic prematurely. Remember, if it is administered for a viral illness, the antibiotic will kill many beneficial bacteria that belong in our systems, thus causing more problems.

Before leaving the topic of fever, let's review a related topic. If your child needs surgery of any kind, elective or emergency, there are four potential postoperative fevers to be aware of. Some of them can be prevented with good medical, nursing, and parental care.

To make it easy to remember, they are referred to as the 4 W's. In order of usual appearance, they are:

Wind: This refers to the lung infections that may occur after the patient has been lying flat, under anesthesia, and then, after the surgery, for extended periods of time. The child's normal cough reflex is suppressed by the anesthesia, and postoperative pain may inhibit his bringing up accumulated mucus from the lungs. Bacteria can grow in these secretions, causing infections and fever. Moving around, coughing, taking deep breaths, using an incentive spirometer (a bedside portable device the child forcibly blows into), and receiving pulmonary physical therapy (slapping, pounding, and clapping on the back) all encourage the child to bring up these secretions.

Water: This refers to urinary tract infections that may be brought on by the child's lying quietly in bed for several days. If the urine is not completely emptied from the bladder, bacteria can grow in the urine, causing pain on urination and fever.

Wound: There are two types of bacterial infections that can involve the surgical scar.

> **Immediate:** A strep infection usually causes redness, swelling, and a discharge from the scar within the first twelve to twenty-four hours after surgery.

Delayed: Other bacterial infections first become evident two to three days postop.

Walk: This refers to phlebitis, an infection of the blood vessels of the legs. It is a serious complication that also results from the patient's lying in bed for prolonged periods. Thank goodness, it is seen very rarely in the pediatric age range.

Let's clear up some misconceptions about fever:

• The height of a fever does not determine how serious the illness is. Children can have a fever as high as 105° F for a minor viral illness, and a fever of only 101° F for a more serious illness.

• Even though the fever may not initially respond to antipyretic medicines, this does not mean the illness is serious.

• Febrile convulsions (seizures caused by fever) do *not* cause brain damage. They are one of the ways the child's body dissipates heat. The temperature is inevitably lower after febrile convulsions than it was just before.

• Mercury from a broken thermometer is not poisonous. A greater danger may be the sharp glass, though that isn't as much of a threat as one might think.

Fifth Disease

FIFTH DISEASE, also called erythema infectiosum, is the fifth of five diseases of childhood with a similar rash. The others are measles, rubella, scarlet fever, and Filetov-Dukes disease (a mild form of scarlet fever). Fifth disease is a viral infection that affects children between the ages of three and twelve. In its early stages, it has a distinctive rash, which imparts a "slapped face" appearance. That may last up to three days. Although the cheeks are bright red, the skin around the mouth is the normal color. By the second day, a lacy, spotted, sometimes itchy rash develops on the arms, legs, and trunk. It can last for one to two weeks, on and off, worsening after a bath or shower and after sun exposure. The disease turns up in clusters in schools during the late winter and early spring months. The majority of adults have had or have been exposed to fifth disease in their past and are immune. Humans are the only known hosts.

The child with fifth disease is usually not sick, or only mildly ill with a low-grade fever. If there is no fever, she can go to school. The infection is contagious for the few days *before* the rash breaks out, but not while the child has the rash. It is spread by coughing and sneezing. The incubation period is two to three weeks.

If fifth disease occurs during pregnancy, it may cause anemia in fewer than 10 percent of the fetuses. There are no reports of birth defects among newborn infants whose mothers acquired fifth disease during pregnancy. In view of the high prevalence of fifth disease, the low incidence of ill-effects on the fetus, and the fact that avoidance of child care or teaching does not eliminate the risk of exposure, routine exclusion of pregnant women from places where fifth disease is occurring is not recommended. Diagnostic blood tests are available for pregnant women exposed to fifth disease in its contagious pre-rash period. If these women do not have antibodies against fifth disease, the pregnancy will need to be monitored closely.

Children with fifth disease need only supportive treatment. They should practice careful hand washing and should carefully dispose of all used facial tissues with respiratory secretions.

Food

When to Start Your Infant on Solid Food:

JUST A FEW decades ago, it was a status symbol and a sign of accomplishment for parents to brag that their two-month-old infant was already on meats and other solid foods. In those times salt was added to many baby foods to make them taste better. We now know that the earlier babies are started on solid foods, the greater their salt needs and cravings will be later on. Since salt intake leads to hypertension and to kidney and heart problems, it is wiser to begin solids when the baby is four to six months old. After several months, the baby's kidneys have matured to the point where they can deal with the normal salt content of baby foods. Yes, even today, there is naturally occurring salt, called "sodium," in baby cereals and other baby foods, but no additional salt is added.

In many European countries, solid food isn't started until the baby is six months old or even older. In America, many pediatricians have found it best to compromise between Europe's standards and our grandparents' wishes by starting solids when the baby is around four months old. Some babies may be ready at three months, depending on their size and milk intake, while others may be content with just breast milk or formula until they are six months of age. You and your pediatrician can best decide when to start your baby on cereal. Until that time, milk will supply all nutritional needs for your baby.

What Foods to Give Her:

When you introduce food, start with the simplest ones, like cereals, which are easy to digest, and then progress to more complicated foods. This will prepare the intestinal tract each step of the way.

Cereals:

Cereal is the first food offered, since it is easily tolerated, is iron-fortified, and has appropriate vitamins and minerals added. It is a good idea to begin cereal when the baby is no older than six months, since she will require a continuing supply of iron from this point. Begin with rice cereal, which seems to be the best tolerated. After one week of rice cereal, you can introduce other cereals, such as mixed, high-protein, barley or oatmeal. The one caution is that if your baby is constipated, do not feed her rice cereals, which bind. In this case, use one of the other cereals first.

Your Feeding Method:

• Always begin a new food in the morning. If there are any untoward reactions, such as signs of allergies, diarrhea, vomiting, or rash, you or your caregiver will be awake, alert, and present.

• Always feed the cereal with a spoon, not in a bottle. It is important to help your baby learn to chew. Chewing will help to break up any large pieces, which could otherwise plug up the bottle's nipple or, worse yet, slip through the nipple and choke her.

• Increase the amount of cereal by 1 teaspoon per day as follows:

Day 1: 1 teaspoon of rice cereal in the dish in the morning.

Day 2: 2 teaspoons of rice cereal in the dish in the morning.

Day 3: 3 teaspoons of rice cereal in the morning. And so on, up to 9 to 12 teaspoons (or 3 to 4 tablespoons. Three teaspoons equal 1 tablespoon).

• Add breast milk or formula to the cereal in the dish. There isn't an exact amount of milk to add; the best word to describe the cereal-milk mixture is "mushy." You don't want it so thin that it runs off the spoon, nor so thick that the baby has a hard time swallowing and digesting it.

• Offer 1 to 2 ounces of formula or a few minutes of breast first, just to calm your baby. Then sit her down and offer the cereal. When she's done, you can again offer milk to complete the meal.

• After the first week, add a second meal, during the dinner hour. Also, you can try a new type of cereal during breakfast. Again, to make certain that there are no untoward reactions, serve only rice cereal (or another type of cereal if there is constipation) for supper. Once the other cereals have been introduced in the morning and tolerated for four days, they too can be used for other meals throughout the day.

• Increase by 1 teaspoon per day until the baby is taking 3 or 4 tablespoons per meal. By day 9, she will have 3 tablespoons in the morning and 3 tablespoons in the evening. Most babies will show signs of having eaten enough by turning their heads away or spitting up after 3 to 4 tablespoons.

• At the start of the third week, introduce a lunch meal. It can be rice cereal or any of the other cereals that have already been tried and tolerated in the morning.

The above method of starting foods represents a proven, effective, and simple way to help your baby enjoy her first meals.

If at any time, she "says" that she wants only two meals a day, that's fine. If she "says" that she only wants 2 tablespoons of cereal, not 3 or 4, that's fine, too.

Note that you have not yet fed her any fruits or juices. That's for next month.

Fruits:

There are two important rules for introducing new foods that apply for the rest of baby's first year.

FOOD

Rule 1: Any new food should be given to the baby over a four-day period, with no other new food tried at the same time. This way, it will be easier for you to pinpoint the cause of any allergic or untoward reaction. A food that has already been introduced and tolerated can be continued during the four-day test period of a new food. Allergic reactions will occur in the first few minutes or hours after the baby has eaten the troublesome food. These reactions are not subtle; they are hives or severe rashes, wheezing, and swelling of the lips and eyes. A slight diaper rash or mild diarrhea is not an allergic reaction.

Rule 2: During the first two days of this four-day period no new household items should be introduced. This means no new soap, detergent, clothes, furniture polish, floor wax, even a new perfume for Mom or another caregiver. On days 3 and 4, though, you can begin to use these other items.

After a month of cereal, your baby can be started on fruits and juices.

• Fruits such as apples, pears, peaches, apricots, prunes should be offered. Any of these can be tried first.

• Serve pureed, mashed, or blended fresh fruit or commercially prepared jars of baby fruit. Always spoon the food from the jar into her dish. Don't put the spoon from her mouth back into the jar, because the oral bacteria in her saliva may cause earlier spoilage of the contents in the food jar.

• Don't forget the all-important four-day rule detailed above.

• Fruit can be served three times a day, together with the cereal.

• Fruit can be mixed in the same dish with the cereal or each can be fed separately. If you do give them separately, always start with the cereal. Since the fruit is sweeter, the baby may not want to eat the cereal after the fruit.

• On average, babies consume half of a baby jar of fruit per meal, but yours may want more or less. As a matter of fact, your baby may vary her consumption, wanting different amounts at different meals. Allow your baby to help you determine how much she should eat at any given meal.

• After four days of one fruit, you can introduce another while continuing with the tested one.

Juices:

• Whenever you introduce a fruit, you can also introduce that juice. When you start apples, you can give apple juice during the same four-day period; when you start apricots, you can introduce apricot nectar, and so on.

• There are no rules about when to give juice. Your baby can drink juice during or between meals.

• If you use commercially prepared baby juices, she can drink them undiluted, as they come in the bottle. If you use adult juices, dilute them with an equal amount of water.

• Your baby should not be given the strong adult citric acid juices, like orange, pineapple, grapefruit, until she is ten months old. These acidic juices are simply too strong for a baby's stomach.

Vegetables:

After a month of fruits, you can introduce vegetables. Unlike fruits, though, there is a preferred order. Since green vegetables are harder to digest than the yellow variety, you should offer a month of yellow vegetables—carrots, squash, or sweet potatoes, before offering green vegetables.

At this point, you cut back on the cereal by serving it only at breakfast, along with fruit. Lunch and dinner become fruit and yellow vegetables. Most kids will have a half-jar of fruit and half-jar of yellow vegetables for lunch and the other half of each jar for supper. This, however, is just an average. As already stated, some may want more or less per meal, depending only on preference. Don't be alarmed if your baby's skin begins to take on a yellowish tinge. It comes from the vitamin A (carotene) that is absorbed from these vegetables. Note that the whites of her eyes do *not* turn yellow, as they do with true jaundice from an illness.

The following month, start her on green vegetables, such as peas, string beans, broccoli, and spinach, always following the four-day rule. An equal amount of yellow and green vegetables should be used, and there are several ways to do this:

• Offer lunch as yellow vegetables and supper as green.

• *Or* offer yellow and green vegetables at each meal.

• *Or* offer yellow vegetables one day and green vegetables the next day.

Meats:

At approximately eight months of age, your child is ready to start meats, still following the four-day rule.

• Begin with red meats first, like beef and liver, since they are high in iron, which is needed by all babies. Families who want their children to be vegetarian can find iron in beans, egg yolks, peanut butter, raisins, prune juice, sweet potatoes, spinach, and iron-enriched cereals.

• Then introduce white meats—chicken, turkey, and fish.

• Meats should be offered for lunch or dinner, together with a vegetable and fruit.

Dairy Products and Eggs:

This is the last major food group, and should be introduced when the baby is about nine months old. Eggs, yogurt, ice cream, sour cream, cheeses, etc., can all be offered. If they are tolerated well, without vomiting, diarrhea, or rashes, offer cow's milk the following month. Use whole homogenized milk until your child is two years old, since she needs the extra fat for normal neurological development. After she is two years old, switch to a low-fat milk.

TIP:

Save the lids from plastic cups like the ones you get at movie theaters. These are the ones with a cut X for a straw. Whenever you give your child an ice pop or ice cream pop on a stick, turn the lid upside down and insert the stick through the X. You have just created a little platform to catch some of those drips before they land on clothes or the floor.

Food Allergies

A TRUE FOOD allergy is an adverse reaction that involves the body's immune system. The allergenic food component becomes an antigen by provoking an antibody response. The resulting allergic reaction may be immediate (within minutes) or delayed (up to three days later). It is separate and distinct from "food intolerance," in which the abnormal response does not involve the immune system. For example, an antigen-antibody response to cow's milk protein results in true milk allergy. However, the deficiency of an enzyme called lactase results in lactose intolerance, which does not involve the formation of harmful antibodies. Refer to the section on "Lactose Intolerance" in the entry on "Stomachaches" on page 307.

True food allergies are rare, affecting about 5 percent of children and less than 1 percent of adults. Since they most frequently affect young children, it is good to delay the introduction of solid foods, and then offer them from one food group at a time. This enables the gastrointestinal tract to mature at an appropriate rate and may prevent some food allergies from developing. Introducing allergenic foods (cow's milk, eggs, nuts, shellfish) early in the first year of life may increase the incidence of infant eczema. Children with food allergies sometimes have other allergic conditions, such as asthma or hay fever. Since food allergies can be inherited, parents and siblings may have food allergies too, but not always to the same food. When the first food allergy symptoms occur in the first year of life, the child tends to outgrow the problem by three years of age. Allergies to peanuts, fish, and nuts may persist for life.

The most common symptoms are hives, rashes, and swelling of the lips, tongue, and mouth. Other symptoms are runny nose, wheezing, abdominal pain, vomiting, diarrhea, bad breath, headaches, irritability, and anaphylactic shock (sharp drop in blood pressure and breathing difficulty). Babies with milk allergy may also be poor feeders, may have blood in the stool, and may be irritable and cry excessively. Attention deficit disorder and behavioral disorders have not been proven to be caused by food allergies.

Only a few foods cause 95 percent of these problems. They are nuts, peanut butter, milk, soybeans and soy formula, wheat, eggs, and fish (lobster, crab, and shrimp). Although chocolate, strawberries, corn, and tomatoes have traditionally been blamed for allergic reactions, actually they are rarely the cause.

It is difficult to test which foods are causing the allergic symptoms, because skin tests are inconclusive. A negative skin test does not conclusively eliminate a certain food as the culprit. Diagnosis, then, is based on the history, along with clinical testing through an elimination diet. Drop the suspected food from the diet for two weeks. If the symptoms disappear, give the child a small amount of the suspected food. (Do this only if the child did not have a severe or anaphylactic reaction to the food.) The same symptoms should appear within a few hours.

Since allergy shots (desensitization) are not effective, the major treatment for food allergies is avoidance of the offending food. This avoidance does not, however, have to be total. Tolerance levels of offending foods vary among children. For example, some children with milk allergies may tolerate the small amount of milk found in dairy products like butter and cheese and in bread. Some children can tolerate milk after it has been heated, as in soups, puddings, and cakes. If too much of these are eaten, though, or if straight milk is drunk, the symptoms will appear.

If a given food has been eliminated from the child's diet and he is symptom-free for six months or more, you can gradually reintroduce the food to see if symptoms recur. If they do not, gradually increase the amounts to normal levels.

Milk, wheat, and soy are the most difficult food allergens to avoid because they are major components of the typical American diet. Infants with milk allergy can take a soybean or casein formula substitute. Consumers should realize that some products labeled "wheat-free" may contain gluten, which can be a wheat protein. Children allergic to wheat must be wary of malt, a common flavoring and coloring agent. Most dry breakfast cereals contain malt or malt extract. These children must also avoid wheat germ, bran, farina, and many flours (white bread, all-purpose, cake, self-rising, whole wheat, graham, and enriched flours). The soybean, a legume, used to be hypoallergenic, but it currently causes allergy problems because of its frequent use in formulas, flour, oil, and nuts. A child allergic to soy may be allergic to other legumes, such as kidney beans, string beans, pinto beans, black-eyed and green peas, chickpeas, lentils, carob, licorice, and those ever troublesome peanuts. Soy is also found in some paints, candles, varnishes, adhesives, and blankets. An allergist and a registered dietitian can educate parents about food allergies, acceptable food selections, and food groups to be avoided.

TIPS:

1. If you are breast feeding, eliminate the food your child is allergic to from your own diet. Protein from the

cow's milk drunk by a lactating mother can enter the breast milk and affect the baby. Ironically, breast-feeding mothers are told to drink extra milk, but if the baby has milk allergy, the mother should go on a milk-free and dairy-product-free diet. Many of the babies outgrow the problem by six to twelve months.

2. If a child is allergic to one food, be cautious about other foods in that same food group. For example, children allergic to peanuts may react to soybeans, peas, or other beans.

3. For children with milk allergy, use juices, apricot nectar, or cream substitutes with dry cereal. As a snack, serve ice pops or fruit ices instead of ice cream.

4. Since milk is the major source of calcium, children with milk allergy should have other foods high in calcium. Some are beans, orange juice, broccoli, sardines, and dried beans.

5. For children with wheat allergy, use cornstarch instead of wheat flour to thicken gravies and sauces. Other substitutes are rice and oat flour and pasta products made with corn. Natural food stores are excellent sources of these foods.

6. When keeping a food diary or starting an elimination diet, include drugs, toothpaste, mouthwash, and chewing gum.

7. For children who are sensitive to food additives, try home gardening, canning, and freezing of homegrown fruits and vegetables to ensure that the food contains only known products.

8. If the reaction to a certain food was severe (causing anaphylaxis), the child should wear a Medic Alert bracelet stating the allergen. There should be an Epipen (an epinephrine-loaded syringe) at home and one in school.

Frostbite

THE POPULARITY of outdoor winter sports has heightened the incidence of frostbite. Frostbite typically occurs in the face, ears, and extremities after prolonged exposure to cold. Microscopic ice crystals form in the various tissues and clog the blood vessels. As a result, oxygen and nutrients cannot make their way to the surrounding tissues and skin. The skin at first becomes red and then turns pale or blue. When the damaged skin thaws, blisters may form. If early care is not obtained, gangrene can develop.

TIPS:

1. Rapidly warm the affected pale skin by putting the injured part in very warm water. Do not massage the damaged area. Do not rub with snow or ice. The warming can be painful.

2. Acetaminophen, ibuprofen, or sometimes codeine is needed for pain relief.

3. In severe cases, hospitalization is necessary so that intravenous fluids and medications can be given and aggressive care devoted to the skin. Only in rare instances of infection is amputation or excision of tissue necessary.

4. Patients with frostbite should be given tetanus prophylaxis if they have not had an immunization within the previous five years.

5. Be sure to cover your child's ears and as much of his face as possible in subfreezing weather. Mittens offer more warmth than gloves. Avoid clothing with tight elastic cuffs that could impinge on the circulation. Boots and two pairs of socks are advisable. Layers of clothing preserve warmth. Since most of the body's

warmth escapes through the head, the child should always wear a hat with earflaps.

Growing Pains

GROWING PAINS are dull, vague aches, usually in the legs. They occur in 15 percent of children and are of no medical significance. They begin when the child is between two and eight and stop when the adolescent stops growing. There is no relationship between the rate of growth and the intensity of growing pains. The pain is in the leg muscles (the midportion of the upper legs and the calves) rather than in the joints. There is no joint redness, swelling, or heat, and there is no associated fever. The pain is intermittent, developing late in the day or at night, and worse on more active days. This leads some doctors to feel that growing pains are due to overexertion. Another theory is that muscles and bones grow at slightly different rates, resulting in the aching soreness. There is no limp and the child's gait is normal. All laboratory tests and x-rays are normal.

TIPS:

1. Rest
2. Massage or heat (hot water bottle or towel)
3. Acetaminophen or ibuprofen
4. Reassurance

Hair Loss (Alopecia)

MOST NEWBORNS lose all or some of their scalp hair and body hair (the lanugo) when they are between one and six months. Since this usually results from rubbing (against sheets while sleeping, or against people while being held and played with), distinct "bald spots" may appear. Once babies spend more time upright, such as sitting when they are between six and nine months old, these bald areas fill in and the hair grows back within twelve months. Some newborns have small patches of alopecia as part of hairless birthmarks of the scalp. The prognosis for regrowth varies in each case.

Older children may lose hair through trichotillomania, the habit of twisting or pulling the hair, especially when they are tired, going to sleep, or watching television. By breaking the hair shafts, they create discrete patches of baldness. The scalp is most commonly involved, but eyebrows, eyelashes, and pubic hair may be affected. The problem is similar to nail biting and other tics. Instead of being completely bare, the patches will have short hairs, broken off at various lengths. Traction on the hair, from tight ponytails, braids, cornrows, pigtails, and curling with a hot iron, also can produce bald areas. If hats, helmets, or headphones rub against a particular area, hair loss may result.

A more common cause of alopecia is a fungal infection called ringworm, manifested by itchy round patches on the scalp. Refer to the entry on "Ringworm" on page 267. Impetigo and eczema can produce similar patches of baldness. Refer to those respective entries. In rare cases the hair loss can be the symptom of an underlying illness, such as a thyroid disorder, lupus, or anorexia, or it can be a side effect of drugs such as hor-

153

mone pills, heparin, and too much vitamin A. In these cases, the hair loss typically occurs six to ten weeks after exposure. Anticancer medications and radiation therapy cause hair loss one to three weeks later. With correction of severe anemia and malnutrition, the hairs slowly grow back.

TIPS:

1. Don't panic. Although the average person loses 50 to 100 hairs each day, this is a small fraction of the 100,000 hairs the average person has. Some loss is normal.

2. Your doctor and/or dermatologist will diagnose and treat the underlying cause. Oral and topical medications are sometimes prescribed.

3. If your child is self-conscious, let her wear a hat until the hair grows back.

4. Hair should be washed with a mild shampoo every day or so, but don't comb or brush harshly. Use a soft hairbrush.

5. Avoid tight rubber bands, head bands, barrettes and "scrunchies," which apply traction on the hair.

6. Don't scold or punish the child for hair-twisting behavior. It will only be replaced by a different nervous tic. Try to distract her with another activity, one that requires both hands.

Head

Soft spot (fontanelle):

A BABY'S head is made up of several individual bones loosely joined together. There is a diamond-shaped soft spot at the point where several of these bones join in the front part of the top of the head. It may be as small as the tip of your pinky or as wide as one to two inches. This fontanelle closes when the baby is between nine and fifteen months old as the bones fuse. A smaller triangular soft spot can be felt at the back of the head. This fontanelle closes within the first six months of life. In some babies, either fontanelle is so small that it is barely discernible. If the baby's head is growing normally, it doesn't matter. Underneath the soft spot is a thick, sturdy membrane and a fluid-filled space, both of which protect the brain. You can sometimes see or feel the fontanelle pulsating along with your baby's heartbeat. It is also normal for it to protrude while the baby is crying. If the bulging persists when the child is quiet and in an upright position, it could signal excess pressure in the baby's brain. On the other hand, if it stays sunken, it could be a sign of dehydration. Ask your pediatrician if you are concerned about either extreme.

Do not be afraid to touch the fontanelle or to shampoo and brush the overlying hair. Too often, cradle cap forms in this area because parents are afraid to scrub the scalp. Treat the soft spot like any other part of the scalp.

Cephalhematoma:

On the way through the birth canal during labor and delivery, the baby's head gets banged around quite a bit. As a result, a soft, swollen bump may form on one or both sides. This cephalhematoma is a boggy mass of fluid and blood under the skin but outside the skull. It is not associated with brain damage and can be touched safely. It may take weeks or months to fully disappear as the blood gets absorbed by the body. If it occurs on both sides of the head, the pediatrician may get an x-ray to rule out a fracture. Even if there is a fracture, usually nothing needs to be done if the head grows normally and the fracture is not displaced downward.

Hydrocephalus:

Hydrocephalus, which means "water on the brain," is caused by an excessive accumulation of fluid inside the brain. The fluid squashes the brain tissue against the skull, causing the skull bones to separate. It can develop due to a congenital or an acquired narrowing (from infection, tumor, or bleeding) of the passageways that the spinal fluid normally traverses in and around the brain. As a result, the fluid backs up, causing the problem. The soft spot will be wide open and bulging. Scalp veins will be enlarged. The forehead will appear broad, and the eyes will deviate downward. One of the earliest signs is the rapid growth of the head beyond expected values, so a baby's head circumference should be measured regularly.

In the older child, the skull bones are already joined, so the internal swelling will cause the following symptoms: irritability, lethargy, poor appetite, vomiting, headache, change in personality, and gradual worsening of school performance. Most cases of hydrocephalus require neurosurgical intervention. Most hydrocephalic children are pleasant and mild-mannered but are at risk for developmental and learning disabilities.

Microcephaly:

Microcephaly is defined as an abnormal smallness of the head, which reflects an abnormal smallness of the brain. The many causes of microcephaly fall into two groups: primary (genetic), and secondary (nongenetic, acquired, and infectious). The primary types are usually identified at birth and have an associated family history of microcephaly. The agents that cause secondary microcephaly can affect the baby either in utero or after birth, especially during the first two years of life. This is another reason that it is important to measure a baby's head circumference regularly. An infectious injury to the brain after two years of age is less likely to produce significant microcephaly. Blood and urine tests, chromosome studies, and x-rays may be needed to determine the cause. Genetic and family counseling are advisable, because many cases of microcephaly are associated with mental retardation.

Headaches

HEADACHE is one of the most common neurological complaints of children. This chapter will focus on frequent or recurrent headaches. Viral illnesses, meningitis, sore throats, ear infections, and fevers in general can cause headaches that disappear when the infections leave. Some children get headaches from sitting in a hot, stuffy room and will benefit from going out in the fresh air. In addition, many children get headaches if they haven't had enough sleep the night before.

There are many other reasons that children get frequent headaches. Here are a few, with some of their characteristics.

Migraine:

Migraine headaches occur in 10 percent of all children, and the number increases in adolescence. They constitute more than half of frequent or recurrent headaches. Eighty percent of these children have a strong family history of migraine. Some children can tell when their migraine is starting because they get an aura—a visual clue (e.g., halos around lights), or a certain smell sensation, or even vertigo (spinning sensation) just before the headache starts. Cluster headaches are considered similar to migraines, but they occur in groups. They are usually one-sided, like migraines, and are associated with a teary eye or runny nose on the side of the headache. Migraines may be as infrequent as once every few months or as common as three to five times a week. There is usually no known predisposing factor or cause. Many teenage girls get migraine headaches before their menstrual periods. For some children and teenagers, the headaches are so severe that they undergo fainting spells, numbness of their fingers, abdominal pain, slurred speech, temporary loss of vision, and memory loss. Pediatricians and neurologists usually make the diagnosis based on the history and physical exam, but they will occasionally need to order a CAT scan or an MRI scan to rule out a brain lesion.

Any treatment of the headache should be started as close as possible to its onset. Some medicines that help migraine headaches are acetaminophen, ibuprofen, Fiorinal, and ergotamine. Other medicines that can be given daily to prevent the headaches are propranolol, phenobarbital, Dilantin, Elavil, and Periactin. Some children benefit from biofeedback and relaxation therapy. Since migraine headaches are not allergic reactions, special diets or allergy shots usually do not help. However, some foods can trigger the headaches in children who are sensitive to them. Chocolate, cheese and other dairy products, foods with MSG (monosodium glutamate), and drinks with caffeine should be avoided by children who react badly to them. Some children feel better after resting in a dark room.

Tension:

It is often difficult to distinguish between migraine and tension headaches. Here, too, a physical exam is usually normal. Stress is more likely to play a role in tension headaches than in migraines. Whereas migraines tend to involve the front and one side of the head, tension headaches tend to affect the back of the head and neck. Tension headaches also tend to be continuous, getting better and worse throughout the day, but not disappearing. It is not always easy to determine what the child is worrying about. Problems with school, friends, parental fights or divorce, something seen on television, even the anticipation of a fun event can trigger tension headaches. (Many actors have them just before they go on stage.) Acetaminophen, ibuprofen, codeine, or biofeedback and relaxation therapy may ease the headache, and it is helpful to have the child lie down in a dark, quiet room.

Sinusitis:

Characteristics of sinus headaches are runny nose, frontal location of the pain, which worsens when the child bends his head down, a cough, and a postnasal drip. Treatment includes pain medicines, decongestants, and antibiotics. Rarely is surgical drainage necessary. Refer to the entry on "Sinusitis" on page 287.

Eyes:

Eye strain can cause headaches that usually occur in the afternoon or night. They are frontal in location. An ophthalmologist will check vision, eye muscle balance, and eye pressure for glaucoma.

Teeth:

I have seen the patient whose dental cavity causes a headache, so be sure dental visits are up-to-date.

Epilepsy:

Headaches can precede or follow epileptic seizures. They are treated with the anticonvulsants used for seizures.

Trauma:

Refer to the entry on "Head Trauma" on page 161, as headaches can be part of the postconcussion syndrome. The headache can last for weeks, even months. If the headache follows acute trauma, it may represent a serious intracranial bleeding problem, and medical attention should be sought.

Tight headbands:

Tight headbands can restrict the scalp and cause headaches.

Temporomandibular joint:

TMJ syndrome involves pain radiating from the temples into the face and sometimes in the ear, too. Occasionally the child can feel a click—or you can hear it—

in front of the ear as the child chews. A vicious cycle develops: the TMJ pain causes grinding of the teeth, which in turn causes a worsening of the TMJ headache. A consultation with a TMJ specialist may be needed.

Low blood sugar:

Some children, just like some adults, experience headaches two or three hours after a meal or whenever they are hungry. An appropriate snack (fruit, crackers, peanut butter, etc.) will do the trick.

Carbon Monoxide:

If your child always gets a headache when riding in the car, it is not necessarily due to motion sickness. Carbon monoxide may be leaking into the car, so have it checked. It can seep into the house if a car in an attached garage is allowed to run for a long time. Carbon monoxide, an odorless, colorless gas, can also enter homes from faulty fuel-burning appliances, such as furnaces, room heaters, and grills. All such appliances should be inspected annually by qualified technicians for cracks or blocked vents. A carbon monoxide detector can be bought at hardware stores and installed near the bedrooms. It will trigger an alarm before carbon monoxide reaches a dangerous level.

Tumors:

Fortunately, brain tumors are a very rare cause of headaches, occurring in only 1 out of 40,000 children. Characteristics of brain tumor headaches are pain in the morning that may wake the child from sleep; concentration in the back of the head; a worsening caused by straining or sneezing; projectile vomiting, and seizures. They sometimes bring about personality changes as well as problems with walking, vision, and speech. As was not true with the previously described headaches, your pediatrician may be able to detect signs of a sizable brain tumor on physical exam. Treatment is individualized and beyond the scope of this chapter, but it usually consists of surgery, radiation therapy, and che-motherapy.

Imitation:

Just as young children love to imitate their parents' and older siblings' good habits, they also like to mimic their bad habits. I have sometimes determined that a child needs glasses by seeing a younger sibling, maybe a toddler, squint his eyes in imitation. Similarly, children may complain of headaches when imitating parents or older siblings who frequently do the same. Although we must never ignore a child's complaints, we should remember that kids love to imitate.

Head Trauma

SOONER OR LATER, almost every child will sustain a head injury through falling, banging, being in an accident, or, in some unfortunate cases, through abuse. Most children recuperate fully, even after what sounds like a loud knock on the head. Since accidents (cars, bicycles, roller skates, etc.) are the major cause of head trauma, the hallmark of prevention is the use of safety items, such as car seats and restraints, helmets, and other protective devices. With the growing acceptance of stylishly designed helmets, it is no longer considered "nerdy" to wear them. Their use should be uniformly insisted on. Indeed, some states have mandated their use.

A frequent question after a child sustains a head trauma is "How can I tell if it's anything serious?" Since the brain is encased by a hard and relatively inflexible skull, we rely on external signs that may suggest serious consequences (such as internal bleeding) involving the brain. I will ask parents of an otherwise healthy child who has sustained a head injury to check for the following 4 signs:

1. Loss of consciousness: Did the child black-out or faint immediately after the injury?

2. Recurrent vomiting: Sometimes kids vomit once after an injury because of "nerves" or fright or just the commotion of the incident. Does the vomiting persist? I advise parents to give a child only clear liquids for 6 to 12 hours after significant head trauma to minimize the risk of aspiration of food in case of vomiting.

3. Are the pupils equal?: The pupils (the black center of the eyes) should be equal in size. Note if one is larger than the other. Some children normally have one pupil slightly larger than the other, so it is important to know your child's normal baseline pupillary comparison before evaluating for head trauma. Pupils normally become smaller when you shine a flashlight (or any light) on them. All pupils should constrict in light and dilate in the dark.

4. Check arms and legs: Note whether the child cannot move any extremity.

If even one of these four signs is present, call your doctor immediately. He will want to evaluate the child for more serious problems; even if there is no evidence of internal bleeding, the child may have sustained a concussion, the condition that results from a jolt to the brain. The resulting nausea, dizziness, and headache can last anywhere from a few hours to a few days. This is the postconcussion syndrome. It is self-limiting and rarely serious. If all four signs are normal, you can let your child sleep if he wants to. However, after a real hard fall or knock to the head, it is a good idea to wake him every three to four hours overnight to check on the same four signs. Minor head bumps do not require such frequent checking.

Two other findings to look for are:

1. "Battle" sign: Black and blue marks behind the ears.

2. "Raccoon" sign: Black and blue marks and swell-ings of the upper eyelids.

Either of these may indicate a skull fracture.

There are other reasons to seek medical attention. If the child has a seizure (convulsion), has amnesia (loss of memory), cries continuously, is very pale, has blood or a watery fluid coming from the nose or ears, or com-plains of blurry vision, call your doctor. Those signs may indicate a subdural hematoma, a rare condition in which bleeding in the skull occurs slowly. It may result in chronic headaches, recurrent vomiting, or changes in personality over a period of several months after the injury.

The scalp is full of blood vessels, which is both good and bad. It's bad because if there is a cut, the scalp tends to bleed a lot—which is scary to see. It's good because the scalp heals well and quickly, even if stitches are needed to close a laceration. The outward flow of blood also helps to draw bacteria away from the wound. Employ the usual first-aid measures to clean any abrasion.

Blunt trauma to the scalp often results in a golf ball–size blood clot, or hematoma, under the skin. Applying ice or another cold compress with gentle pressure will minimize the swelling. A hematoma on the forehead or skull tends to be pronounced because there is no soft tissue (like surrounding muscle) to hide the swelling. As the blood from a forehead or nasal hematoma settles through gravity, the child may get "shiners," or black and blue marks around each eye. In time, they too will disappear.

Heart Murmurs

FEW THINGS shock parents more than the pediatrician's statement that their child has a heart murmur. Don't panic and don't worry. As many as a third of all normal children have heart murmurs that do not reflect any pathology of the heart. They are merely the normal sounds of blood flowing through the heart and aorta. It is important for parents to know about the existence of these "innocent" or "functional" murmurs so that they won't be surprised when a new doctor, examining the child for an illness (perhaps during a vacation), casually mentions that he hears the murmur. Such benign murmurs get louder when the child has a fever, is excited, or has exercised. Half of these murmurs disappear in adolescence or earlier, so only a sixth of all adults still have them.

If the murmur has more serious characteristics, or if the child has symptoms involving the cardiovascular system (blue color, easy fatigue, shortness of breath, poor growth), further testing will be needed. A consultation with a cardiologist may be appropriate.

Heat Rash

HEAT RASH, also called prickly heat, occurs when excess sweat plugs up the ducts of the sweat glands. The glands build up with pressure until they burst, releasing sweat under the surface of the skin. The area around each tiny sweat gland then reddens and swells. Many of these together form the classic heat rash, clusters of tiny red bumps. The rash is not contagious.

Hot, humid weather and overdressing the child are

precipitating factors. The parts of the body most frequently involved are the neck, face, shoulders, elbows, groin, the area behind the knees, and anywhere there are creases in the skin.

TIPS:

1. This is not the time to use ointments, creams, or lotions. Wash the area with soap and cold water. You can then leave the skin alone or apply a little powder (cornstarch, baby powder) to keep the skin dry.

2. Avoid overdressing the child. Don't use shirts or tops that are tight around the neck, a common site for prickly heat.

3. Do not keep the baby's room temperature warmer than your own bedroom's temperature. If you need air conditioning, so does the baby. A fan (with a protective shield) will prevent the room air from becoming stuffy.

4. Use clothes with natural fibers, like cotton, that breathe easily.

Hemophilia and Other Bleeding Disorders

THE BODY calls on an amazingly sophisticated and complex mechanism to stop unwanted and unexpected bleeding. There is a continuous balance controlling the normal flow of blood and the necessity of clot formation. Among the factors involved in forming a clot are the contraction of the blood vessel walls, the presence of functioning platelets (small sticky fragments in the blood that contain chemicals important in stopping bleeding), and the availability of different coagulation (clotting) factors, labeled I to XIII. Diseases that lower the platelet count cause bleeding under the skin and easy bruising (see below in this entry). Vitamin C deficiency (scurvy) also causes easy bruising.

Hemophilia:

If one of the clotting factors is congenitally reduced, or if it becomes defective through malnutrition or infection, normal clotting does not occur. The child will suffer from easy bruising and life-threatening bleeding tendencies. Although there can be deficiencies of many of these coagulation factors, *hemophilia* refers to the three most common congenital deficiencies. Hemophilia A, or classic Hemophilia, refers to the deficiency of Factor VIII, also called the "antihemophilic" factor. Hemophilia B refers to the deficiency of Factor IX, also called the Christmas factor. Hemophilia C refers to the deficiency of Factor XI, also known as plasma thromboplastin antecedent.

Hemophilia A represents 80 percent of all cases of hemophilia. This congenital deficiency of Factor VIII is rare, occurring in 1 in 5000 male births. Of these cases, 80 percent show a positive family history of hemophilia A. The remaining cases represent a new mutation of the gene on the X chromosome, which results in hemophilia. Since males have only one X chromosome, they will have hemophilia A if that chromosome contains the faulty gene. Since females have two X chromosomes, if one X chromosome is involved (through heredity or mutation), the healthy X chromosome produces enough Factor VIII to form clots. These women "carriers" may not have the full complement of Factor VIII, but bleeding does not occur if over 30 percent of the "normal" amount of Factor VIII is present. A carrier usually has 30 to 75 percent of normal activity. Therefore, women who are carriers for the hemophilia gene do not have bleeding problems but may transmit the defective gene to their children. (Theoretically, a hemophilic father and a carrier mother could have a daughter who inherits the two faulty X chromosomes from both parents, resulting in hemophilia A. This is so rare that hemophilia A is considered a disease of males.) Each male baby from a carrier mother has a 50 percent chance of having the disease. Fetuses at risk can now be diagnosed through amniocentesis as early as ten to twelve weeks into the pregnancy. All such families should receive genetic counseling.

Once bleeding begins, it will continue until first-aid measures are applied or the missing factor is given. The severity of the blood loss depends on where the bleeding starts and on how much Factor VIII is available in the body. Severe bleeding occurs if there is no Factor VIII or less than 1 percent of normal Factor VIII activity. Moderate cases of bleeding occur in a child who has 1 to 5 percent of activity. Mild bleeding occurs in a child with 5 to 25 percent of normal activity. Cuts of the tongue or lip, which are rich in blood vessels, could bleed for hours or even days. Recurrent bleeding into joints—knees, elbows, and ankles—causes pain, swelling, decreased movement, and, eventually, crippling deformities. Bleeding into the head and abdomen constitutes a life-threatening emergency. A child in the mild category may bleed only after significant trauma, such as tooth extractions, surgery, and major injuries.

Factor VIII does not cross the placenta, so if the baby does not make his own factor, bleeding could be noticed in the newborn period. All babies are given a shot of vitamin K (ironically, to help clotting) shortly after birth. Hemophilic babies may bleed more than usual after this shot. Surprisingly, only 50 percent of hemophilic babies will bleed profusely following circumcision. Apparently enough "tissue juice," platelets, and other clotting factors are available to promote clotting after the other circumcisions. The remaining children with hemophilia will demonstrate their bleeding tendencies when they first cut and injure themselves while crawling, walking, and falling. The diagnosis is made through blood tests that show whether there is a deficiency of the clotting factor.

The aim of treatment is to replace the missing clotting factor—in this case, Factor VIII—at a level that promotes clotting. Concentrates of Factor VIII are given intravenously to transfuse these children following a bleed. Unfortunately, Factor VIII is destroyed by stomach juices and so cannot be taken by mouth. Because the transfused clotting factor lasts only twelve to twenty-four hours, repeated transfusions may be needed for severe bleeds. Parents and adolescents can be trained to give intravenous infusions at home. Transfusions are also necessary just before elective dental and surgical procedures. Routine first-aid measures (applying cold, pressure, and elevation of a bleeding arm or leg) should always be used.

Since the factor concentrates are derived from whole blood, there is a risk of the patient's contracting hepatitis B, hepatitis C, or AIDS. Newer and safer methods of preparation are now being used to lower these risks. In the near future, a synthetic Factor VIII will be available. Since it is not derived from human blood, it will not transmit harmful viruses that might be present in human blood.

Recently, DDAVP (Desmopressin), as nasal spray or intravenous medication, has been found to increase Factor VIII in patients with mild and moderate hemophilia A up to 25 to 50 percent above their baseline. Desmopressin is recommended only for minor bleeding episodes; patients with severe deficiencies do not respond to it.

Hemophilia B (Christmas disease, Factor IX deficiency) makes up 12 to 15 percent of all cases of hemophilia. The remaining few cases are hemophilia C (Factor XI deficiency). The clinical manifestations are the same as for hemophilia A. Diagnosis is made by the blood test revealing which clotting factor is decreased. Since some newborns normally have a mild reduction of Factor IX for 1 to 2 months, hemophilia B cannot be diagnosed until a repeat blood test shows reduction of Factor IX persisting at three to four months of age. Treatment for hemophilia B and C consists of routine first-aid measures plus the intravenous administration of the missing clotting factor.

TIPS:

1. The crib and playpen should be well padded.

2. Aspirin, which promotes bleeding, must be avoided.

3. Hemophilic children, like all children, should be immunized against hepatitis B. Immunizations are usually tolerated well by hemophilic children when immediate cold pressure is applied to the vaccine site for an extended period of time.

4. Each hemophilic child should wear a Medic Alert bracelet clearly stating which type of hemophilia he has.

5. The child should sleep on a low bed over carpeted floors. No floor at home should be slippery, and all floors should be uncluttered.

6. Avoid hazardous toys and those with jagged edges. Furniture should be "rounded off."

7. All children with bleeding disorders should refrain from competitive contact sports. They should wear helmets during any physical activity.

8. A famous pediatric rule is "Black and blue marks on the lower legs of a child are signs of a healthy child." This means that the child is getting the normal amount of exercise and activity, with the inevitable minor bruising. It also means that the child is not being ignored or neglected. However, if black and blue marks are frequently seen elsewhere or are on the legs in excess, bleeding disorders need to be considered. Finally, and most unfortunately, even hemophilic children can be abused. The diagnosis of child abuse in a hemophilic child could be overshadowed and overlooked by the medical drama of the bleeding event. Suspicion of child abuse must always be kept in mind.

Appropriate management can permit many hemophilic children to grow and develop normally, and to lead happy and productive adult lives.

Idiopathic Thrombocytopenic Purpura (ITP):

"Ecchymoses" and "purpura" are the medical terms for black and blue marks. As noted above, bruising is a normal and common phenomenon of childhood. However, a deficiency in platelets (see above), called thrombocytopenia, can result in easy bruising and frequent nosebleeds. Petichiae, small red spots under the skin that result from microscopic bleeding, develop in clusters over the body when the platelet count is low. Petichiae can be distinguished from other red rashes in that they are flat and do not blanch when pressed. Pressing a clear glass against the rash enables you to see whether or not the spots blanch. A few petichiae sometimes occur on the face of a healthy child with a normal platelet count after the increased pressure of vomiting or strenuous coughing, which breaks small blood vessels. (Such petichiae appear on the faces of a healthy mother and her newborn due to the straining of childbirth.) However, when the platelet count is low, showers of petichiae appear spontaneously over large parts of the body. There could be life-threatening internal bleeds following even minor trauma to the head, chest, or abdomen.

When the cause of a certain medical condition is not known, it is called idiopathic. Idiopathic thrombocytopenic purpura (ITP), then, is a disease in which the body makes antibodies that kill its own platelets for unknown reasons. This condition often follows a viral syndrome, like the common cold, the flu, or a sore throat. ITP is less serious than hemophilia in that the vast majority of affected children recuperate completely in a few months. The diagnosis is usually made through a blood test that shows the lowered number of platelets. Sometimes a piece of bone marrow must be removed from the hip or shin bone so that it can be examined to confirm the diagnosis of ITP. Since platelets are first formed in the bone marrow, tumors that fill the marrow (such as leukemia) could squash and damage the platelets, resulting in a low platelet count. In this case, the bone marrow examination will show the abnormal cancer cells.

Treatment for ITP sometimes consists of mere observation and an emphasis on safety precautions. Some children require steroids, which raise platelet counts. Gamma globulin (a concentrate of antibodies), given intravenously, also raises the platelet count. As a final resort, in rare and extreme cases, the child's spleen (which acts as a filter to remove these platelets) is surgically removed. Although this is major surgery, it results in a permanent rise of the platelet count.

Henoch-Schönlein Purpura:

When the walls of many blood vessels become inflamed, a constellation of symptoms may develop. Hives may appear on the legs, arms, and buttocks, and change, after two to three days, to purpura (see above). Many children complain of colicky abdominal pain and of joint pains, especially in the knees and ankles. Blood can be seen in the stools and in the urine, reflecting the involvement of the blood vessels of the intestines and of the kidneys. Blood tests will show a normal platelet count and normal clotting factors. This disease, called Henoch-Schönlein purpura, may follow a viral or bacterial infection or indicate a drug allergy. It resolves spontaneously in a few weeks. There is no specific treatment, but acetaminophen and/or ibuprofen can be given for joint pain. Steroids are reserved for the rare cases with severe abdominal or neurological involvement. If there is no kidney damage, the long-term prognosis is excellent.

Hepatitis

HEPATITIS is an infection of the liver, an organ in the upper right part of the abdomen, which becomes enlarged and tender to the touch. Many different viruses can cause hepatitis. The two most recognized viruses that infect children's livers are hepatitis A and hepatitis B. However, as if these alone aren't enough of a problem, researchers have discovered at least three more viruses that cause hepatitis, called, therefore, hepatitis C, D, and E. Since the liver is sick, it cannot excrete the yellow chemical, bilirubin, from the body. When this chemical builds up in large amounts in the skin, it causes jaundice. If the infection is mild and the liver is not very sick, jaundice does not occur. Some viruses cause a more severe illness than others. Other infectious causes of hepatitis include the Epstein-Barr virus (which causes infectious mononucleosis), toxoplasmosis, syphilis, cytomegalovirus, rubella, herpes, and chickenpox.

Hepatitis usually begins with nonspecific symptoms, such as fever, headache, general achiness, decreased appetite, and diarrhea. The urine often appears dark, because it contains large amounts of bilirubin byproducts, and the stools appear lighter (clay colored), because the malfunctioning liver cannot transport the bilirubin to the intestine. Soon, hives, joint pains, nausea, vomiting, and abdominal pain develop. Jaundice, first noticed in the whites of the eyes, follows shortly. In young children, the transition to the jaundice phase is usually accompanied by improvement or disappearance of the other symptoms. However, there is great variation in intensity of symptoms from patient to patient. In children, the jaundice usually lasts one to two weeks, after which recovery is prompt. Children less than three years old develop hepatitis with little or no jaundice.

Following is a summary of the similarities and differences of the various hepatitises.

Hepatitis A:

Also called infectious hepatitis, hepatitis A is an ancient disease described by Hippocrates. The illness can last from a few weeks to several months. Regardless, the hepatitis usually completely resolves and does not cause chronic liver disease. The incubation period is two to six weeks. Transmission is through the fecal-oral route, and through contaminated water and food. The virus is shed in the stools until shortly after the jaundice develops. Therefore, hepatitis A is considered contagious until one week after the jaundice develops. Children with hepatitis A may return to school once the jaundice is gone. Hepatitis A is only rarely transmitted through the use of blood, blood products, and contaminated needles and syringes. This is because the hepatitis A virus stays in the blood a very short time, and there is no carrier state.

Hepatitis B:

Also called serum hepatitis, hepatitis B has a more recent history. The incubation period is two to six months but the symptoms are the same as with hepatitis A. It causes chronic liver infection (evidence of liver disease for more than six months) in 3 to 13 percent of adults. However, this risk approaches 90 percent in infants born to mothers who have hepatitis B. It is the most common and important cause of neonatal hepatitis. (To date, there has been no documentation of perinatal transmission of hepatitises A, D, or E.) About 5 percent of newborns who acquire hepatitis B from their mothers do so while in utero. These infections cannot be prevented. However, 95 percent of the sick infants manifest the infection weeks or months later. Possible routes of perinatal transmission are leakage of the virus across the placenta during labor; ingestion of amniotic fluid or maternal blood; breast feeding—especially if the mother has cracked nipples.

Almost 50 percent of children who get hepatitis B before the age of five years will develop chronic liver disease. Hepatitis B is also a leading cause of cirrhosis and liver cancer. The infection and its complications can be prevented. Refer to the entry on "Immunizations" for the hepatitis B vaccine schedule. Although the American Academy of Pediatrics recommends immunization for infants and adolescents, many pediatricians believe that children of all ages should be immunized. There are several reasons.

• Selective immunization of high-risk groups over the past ten years has not decreased the transmission of hepatitis B virus.

• Hepatitis B during childhood has a high rate of becoming chronic, increasing the risk for cirrhosis and liver cancer. Therefore, those children beyond infancy should not wait until adolescence to be protected.

• The vaccine is safe and gives long-term immunity.

• The vaccine can be given during regular office visits together with other immunizations.

• The vaccine produces a better antibody response in children than in adults.

• There is a greater chance of getting children back for repeat doses than there is of getting adolescents to return for booster shots.

• Children under eleven years of age get smaller and therefore less expensive doses.

Transmission of hepatitis B occurs through contaminated needles as well as the following routes: oral-oral (the friction associated with kissing occasionally is enough), sexual, and intimate physical contact of any type. The virus is found in saliva, semen, and many other body fluids, but not in stool. (It is not spread by the fecal-oral route.) Child-to-child transmission can occur within households. Tattooing and acupuncture have also been responsible for transmitting hepatitis B. It is endemic in institutions for the mentally retarded because of the close, cramped quarters in which they live.

Chronic hepatitis B virus carriers usually have no history of hepatitis and are not sick. Their condition is discovered "by accident" when they donate blood or have blood tests for other reasons. They can still transmit the virus to others.

Since hepatitis B is common in Asia, Africa, and South America, infants adopted from these areas may have obtained the virus from their mothers and therefore should be tested.

Hepatitis C:

Previously called "non-A, non-B hepatitis," hepatitis C was recognized as a separate entity during the 1970s. Jaundice usually does not develop with hepatitis C, and other symptoms are milder than in hepatitis A and B. The incubation period is one to four months. It frequently progresses to chronic liver disease. In the United States, hepatitis C is the cause of 30 percent of all acute hepatitis cases and the majority of posttransfusion hepatitises. Transmission occurs through contaminated blood products. People at risk are transfusion recipients, including thalassemics (those with an inherited form of anemia particular to people of Mediterranean descent), hemophiliacs, and hemodialysis patients, intravenous drug users, and health care workers. The ability to detect hepatitis C in donated blood has lessened the incidence of transfusion-related hepatitis. Recently published reports suggest that perinatal transmission can occur.

Hepatitis D:

The hepatitis D virus exists only in the presence of a hepatitis B infection. In other words, hepatitis B must be occurring at the same time; the hepatitis B virus transports the hepatitis D virus around the body. The symptoms are more severe than those of acute or chronic hepatitis B. Hepatitis D is lethal in 2 to 28 percent of cases, as compared with less than 1 percent for hepatitis B. It can progress to chronic liver disease. Transmission is the same as for hepatitis B, except that there is no known perinatal transfer. The incubation period is one to two months unless hepatitis B starts simultaneously, in which case the incubation period is the same as for hepatitis B (two to six months). High-risk groups are intravenous drug users, hemophiliacs, and institutionalized mentally retarded patients.

Hepatitis E:

The cause of hepatitis E is similar to that of hepatitis A, but it is rare in children. Like hepatitis A, it is self-limiting and does not cause chronic liver disease. Unlike hepatitis A, it can be devastating in pregnant women. Whereas hepatitis A is lethal in under 1 percent of pregnant women, hepatitis E has a mortality rate of 10 to 20 percent in pregnant women. It is spread along the fecal-oral route through contaminated water and food. With the exception of a few imported cases, hepatitis E has not shown up in the United States. The incubation period is six weeks. Ultimate prevention depends on good hygiene and the development of a vaccine against hepatitis E.

Only rarely does any of the five viruses cause severe fulminant hepatitis. This condition, which occurs one to four weeks after onset of the initial hepatitis, is characterized by irritability, confusion, restlessness, bleeding problems, and even coma.

Treatment for all forms of hepatitis is essentially supportive. As with other viral illnesses, antibiotics are of no value. A well-balanced diet is helpful. Keep the child isolated until one week after the onset of jaundice. Hospitalization may be needed for severe fulminant hepatitis. (See above.) Prevention remains the most important therapy. Stress good hygiene to minimize the risk of fecal-oral spread. Clean the toilet bowl well, especially after your child uses it. Parents and caretakers may contaminate their hands by changing the diapers of a baby with hepatitis A, and this can make day care centers sources of hepatitis A infection. Because hepatitis A and B viruses can survive on inanimate objects for a month or more, environmental hygiene is also important. (However, since the fecal-oral route is not a mode of transmission for the hepatitis B virus, children who are hepatitis B carriers may attend day care. Aggressive behavior, such as biting or scratching, should be assessed on an individual basis.) Wash hands well after every bowel movement. Use separate towels, glasses, dishes, and toys.

Hepatitis A can be prevented or suppressed with a shot of immune (gamma) globulin given before you travel to areas of the world where hepatitis A is endemic or after a known exposure. Therefore, individuals intimately exposed to patients with hepatitis A (such as household contacts or close friends) should receive immune globulin. If two weeks have passed since the last exposure, immune globulin is not indicated. People who have only casual contact, like most classmates, do not require it. All cases of hepatitis should be reported to health authorities. Researchers are currently trying to develop a vaccine against hepatitis A. The hepatitis B vaccine also supplies effective prevention for hepatitis D.

People with certain exposure to hepatitis B should receive hepatitis B immune globulin together with the first of the three doses of the hepatitis B vaccine. This immune globulin is given to all newborns of mothers who are hepatitis B positive, along with their first dose of hepatitis B vaccine. Immune globulin may also be useful after accidental exposure to blood from someone who has hepatitis C, but it has not been found beneficial when given after exposure to hepatitis E virus.

Finally, it is likely that our alphabet game will not end with A, B, C, D, and E, as other viruses that cause hepatitis are identified.

Hiccups

IF YOU'RE like most parents, hiccups will probably bother you more than they affect your child. They are a normal, physiological phenomenon, of no medical concern for your baby.

The diaphragm is a thin dome of muscle separating the lungs from the abdominal cavity. As a matter of fact, the stomach lies directly underneath the left side of the diaphragm. When the stomach fills and enlarges with food or air, as it may after crying, it rubs against the diaphragm, triggering spasms called hiccups.

There are many "cures" and old wives' tales for these frequent occurrences, but one physiologically correct way to stop your child from hiccuping is to give her a pacifier. Your baby's sucking action sends a signal to her stomach that food is on its way down. In response, her stomach will hasten its attempts to empty itself, making room for more food. But since the pacifier "fooled" her stomach, and no food enters, the stomach shrinks down and no longer rubs against the diaphragm. The source of irritation moves away, and the hiccups stop.

Always remember, though, that even if you do absolutely nothing, the hiccups will stop by themselves as the child's stomach shrinks on its own.

High Blood Pressure

HIGH BLOOD pressure (hypertension) is rare in children. When present, it causes headaches, irritability, nosebleeds, and vomiting. Over a period of time, it takes its toll on the heart, brain, and kidneys, and it increases the chance of heart attack or stroke. Several factors contributing to high blood pressure are family history, smoking, and high-fat and high-salt diets.

Blood pressure is routinely measured during annual physical exams. It is a painless test. If a child or teenager is nervous before the physical exam, or before he receives blood tests and shots, this could temporarily elevate his blood pressure, so it should be checked again before the child leaves the office and repeated a few days later. If the hypertension is a reflection of the child's obesity, weight loss will help it return to normal levels. Since the kidney is the main organ responsible for controlling blood pressure, many kidney diseases result in hypertension. Some examples are glomerulonephritis, infections, tumors, and congenital abnormalities of the kidneys. Hyperthyroidism (elevated thyroid hormone) also elevates blood pressure.

It is important that the correct size of blood pressure cuff be used on a child and teenager. The cuff should fully encircle two thirds of the upper arm, from shoulder to elbow.

If the blood pressure is high, your doctor will order a urinalysis, urine culture, blood tests, and sonogram or x-rays of the kidneys. Treatment involves one of the following or a combination of them: weight loss, a low-salt diet, stress management, medication, appropriate exercise, and, rarely, surgery. A pediatric nephrologist (kidney specialist) may be consulted.

179

If your five-year-old masters the ability to pronounce the name of the machine that takes her blood pressure, give her a hug and a kiss from me. It is a **sphygmoma-nometer!**

Highchairs

WHEN a child can sit unsupported while eating solid foods, he'll need a highchair. There are many styles and types of highchairs, but there is one feature that you must be sure to look for.

Purchase a highchair with a spring-action removable tray. This feature enables you to remove the tray from the highchair in one step, *using only one hand*. You can hold the baby in the other hand, so the baby is placed in the highchair *without being left unsupervised even for a moment*. This simple feature prevents an active baby from falling from the highchair while the parent uses both hands to retrieve and replace the tray. As the child gets older, the tray can be removed and the highchair placed near the table so that the child feels like part of the family.

Other important features to look for:

• Safety straps, including a crotch strap, that are easy to use.

• Legs with a wide stance to decrease the chance of the chair's tipping over.

• Ease in being folded and stored safely.

• A tray with adjustable positions to accommodate the child's growth.

Hips

Congenital Dislocation of the Hip:

A DISLOCATABLE hip is an abnormal condition in which the top of a baby's leg bone can easily be manipulated out of its hip socket. As part of a newborn's physical exam, your pediatrician will perform certain maneuvers to determine whether one or both of the baby's hips can be easily slipped out of place. The earlier this condition, not a painful one, is diagnosed and tested, the better the prognosis. If undetected, a limp and perhaps arthritis could develop. Ultrasound and/or x-rays of the hip are sometimes needed to confirm the diagnosis and to follow the condition. Ten to 20 percent of these babies have a family history of congenital hip dislocation. It is most common in firstborn white females delivered in a breech position.

Since there is also a higher incidence in multiple births (twins, triplets), the cause is felt to be mechanical: malposition (such as breech) in the uterus and overcrowding. The left side alone is involved 60 percent of the time; the right side alone, 20 percent; both hips, 20 percent. The risk of recurrence with normal parents and an affected sibling is 6 percent; with one affected parent, 12 percent; with one affected parent plus one affected sibling, 36 percent. A sonogram or x-ray can confirm the diagnosis and act as a baseline for comparing and following the hip in the future.

Treatment initially consists of the use of two diapers at one time to keep the legs turned outward in a froglike position. This forces the top of the femur into its normal alignment in the hip joint. An orthopedist will then prescribe a Pavlick harness, which is effective in keeping the baby's legs in the desired frog-like position. It will be used for four to six weeks and, in most cases, can then be gradually discontinued. The harness has

Velcro closures on the shoulder and leg straps, and it does not hurt the baby. If this treatment fails, or if the diagnosis is delayed until after the baby is six months old, traction followed by surgery may be necessary.

Toxic Synovitis of the Hip:

Toxic synovitis is a common, self-limiting inflammation of one hip that causes the child to limp for one or two weeks. It may be due to a recent viral infection, like a common cold, that has settled into the hip joint. It is four times more common in males, and it usually occurs when the child is between three and six years old, but I have also seen ten-year-olds with toxic synovitis.

Sometimes this hip problem presents itself as tenderness in the knee, a type of referred pain. Part of the nerve going to the knee passes over the inflamed hip joint, which irritates the nerve and sends the mistaken signal that the pain originates in the knee. The child has no other complaints, and, aside from the pain he feels on moving his leg, the physical exam is normal. There is either no fever or only a low-grade one (100 to 101° F). X-rays and blood tests are normal, although sometimes an x-ray will show an increased space between the bones of the affected hip joint. If the diagnosis is uncertain, an orthopedist may insert a needle into the hip joint to remove some fluid, which will be tested to rule out more serious problems, like septic (bacterial) arthritis.

TIPS:

1. Rest the leg until the pain is gone.

2. Ibuprofen or acetaminophen may provide pain relief. Antibiotics and steroids are not helpful for toxic synovitis.

By the way, I hate the use of the term "toxic" synovitis for this relatively harmless condition. Try not to let this ominous adjective scare you. The condition is not likely to recur, and it leaves no residual problems.

Hives

HIVES, also called urticaria, are raised, red, itchy welts on the skin in circular, wavy, or multishaped patterns called erythema multiforme. They can be as small as shirt buttons or as large across as ten inches. Hives may move from one part of the body to another, but they are not contagious to other people. They may disappear in minutes or last for days. They may appear as an allergic reaction to such things as medicine (penicillin, aspirin, laxatives, decongestants, vitamins, sulfa drugs, codeine), foods, pollen, bee stings and insect bites, and even emotional tension. The most likely times for the onset of drug-induced hives are within twenty-four hours after starting the medicine or any other ingested allergen and between seven and twenty-one days later. Hives often are part of concurrent or recent viral or parasitic illnesses, including hepatitis, infectious mononucleosis, and arthritis. Other illnesses associated with hives are lupus and hyperthyroidism. Some of the foods that cause hives are nuts, peanut butter, fish, shellfish, shrimp, eggs, milk, and cheese. This is why foods should be introduced gradually—one new food every four days—to every infant. Sometimes the culprit is an added food coloring or spice. The actual cause of hives is determined in only 30 percent of the children who get them. If travel has been part of the child's recent history, it may be beneficial to obtain a stool sample and have it examined for parasites. If the itching does not interfere with the child's ability to sit in class and concentrate, he may go to school.

Cold urticaria, hives that develop as a response to cold weather or to a cold-water swim, develop on warming, as when a child returns home from a winter outing. An easy way to diagnose cold urticaria is to press an ice cube against the skin for a few seconds; a hive will appear as the skin warms up afterward. Children who get cold urticaria should wear thick gloves and a face stocking or ski mask; and the family should consider moving to warmer weather.

A common misconception is that an allergic reaction always follows the first exposure to a food or drug. But hives can appear when the child has had the allergen once, twice, or many times before. For unknown reasons, he can suddenly become allergic to a familiar item.

A frequent scenario is that a first bout of hives will come and go without our ever being sure what caused it. If a second or third bout develops, a pattern can then be discerned and the culprit determined. If necessary, an allergist can try to determine the cause through skin and laboratory tests.

The allergic reaction can also cause joint swelling and pain, wheezing, and swelling of the lips, eyes, and eyelids. These require medical attention.

TIPS:

1. Oral antihistamines relieve the itching, redness, and swelling.

2. In severe cases, oral or injectable steroids will be needed.

3. Cold compresses and cool baths relieve itching and decrease swelling. Treatment with Aveeno oatmeal bath is also soothing.

4. If the hives are severe or if wheezing develops, your child should wear a Medic Alert bracelet, stating the medicine or food he must avoid. In this rare case, there should also be an Epi-pen (injectable epinephrine) available at home and in school for emergencies.

Hospitalizations:
Do's and Don'ts

PEDIATRICS has increasingly become an "out-patient" specialty. Many surgical procedures can now be done on a "same-day" basis so that the child does not have to stay overnight in the hospital. Unfortunately, some children have problems that do require observation and treatment in a hospital setting. For them and their parents, I offer this list of "do's and don'ts" to make the hospital stay as comfortable as possible.

DO:

1. Speak truthfully but simply to the child. Children who understand what is happening to them and who have the emotional support of their family and hospital staff do better than those children without this support.

2. Each hospital has its own rules and regulations about parents sleeping over. Whenever possible, especially with a child less than six years of age, a parent should stay overnight.

3. Since a child enjoys being surrounded by familiar persons and routines, try to bring favorite dolls, books, toothbrush, hairbrush, pajamas, and toys from home. She may also like to have a favorite picture or poster at her bedside. If the child is in the process of being toilet trained (and if the hospital allows), bring her own potty from home so that she doesn't undergo yet another "trauma," having to use the hospital's toilet. She may even prefer using her own toilet seat cover rather than the hospital's bedpan.

4. Group tours of nursery and pediatric wards in local hospitals for young schoolchildren help acclimate the children to possible hospitalizations. The visits can

eliminate the unknown factor in a child's "mind's eye" and lessen the mystery of these imposing and over-whelming buildings. Similarly, a visit to the hospital before an expected stay to meet the people who will be offering care and to ask questions about what will happen helps to dissipate some of the child's and parents' anxiety.

5. Real medical equipment that may be encountered during a hospital stay should be provided for hands-on experiences in a school-type setting. Play sessions with dolls should be encouraged.

6. During the hospitalization, each parent should ask the nurses how he or she can help in the child's care. Bathing, feeding, and changing a child can often be done by the parent. The long hospital day is a time for a parent to be patient, understanding (of the child and the hospital routine), and creative. Schoolteachers are usually cooperative about supplying schoolwork that can be done in the hospital.

7. If recurrent blood tests are needed during the hospitalization, reassure your child that the body keeps replenishing its own blood supply. There is no fixed amount of blood taken for tests that could leave her depleted. This is a common but often unspoken concern of children.

DON'TS:

1. Children may internalize conversations they hear on TV shows about seriously ill or dying hospitalized people. Be careful, then, about such conversations, especially around the time of the child's hospitalization.

2. Hospital routines and last-minute changes of scheduled surgery, x-rays, tests, etc., often strain the relationship between parents and the hospital staff. If you keep this in mind, you can minimize another source of anxiety. Don't lose your cool! Your child will pick up your feelings.

3. Don't give the child anything to eat, especially

from outside the hospital, unless you first clear it with the child's nurse.

4. Do not discard the child's urine and stool unless so requested by the nurses.

5. Every child's routine is disrupted by a hospitalization. Immediately after discharge, a child may revert to thumb sucking, bed-wetting, clinging, and sleeping problems. It may take a day or two (or three) for her normal sleeping and eating habits to return. Don't be too demanding at first. She'll soon resume her old, comfortable routine and behavior. Some children actually benefit by proving to themselves, their family, and friends that they made it through a hospitalization, illness, or surgical procedure with flying colors.

Humidifiers

DO YOU EVER find that your throat is dry when you wake up and you can't wait for that first glass of orange juice or cup of coffee? Well, we adults normally breathe approximately twenty times per minute. A baby breathes twice as fast. Imagine how much drier her throat gets! In addition, it is a fact that the average American home in winter is drier than the Sahara Desert, and since babies don't wake up to orange juice or coffee, we must supply the humidity with a humidifier or vaporizer.

Actually, any source of humidity will do, even an open pot of water sitting on a radiator, but then you must be careful about other children burning their hands or spilling the hot water. If you already own a humidifier, it's probably fine. If you are planning on buying one, a cool-mist vaporizer is preferable over the warm-mist variety. It makes the room feel less like a steam bath, and it also supplies a cooler environment, which is preferable if the child should have a fever.

Always follow the directions for cleaning the device.

Uncleaned, stagnant water can serve as a breeding ground for fungi and bacteria. If you clean the machine properly and as frequently as recommended by the manufacturer, this should not be a problem.

Humidifiers can be used year-round. In cold weather, our windows are closed and the heat is on, resulting in dry conditions. In warm weather, air conditioning makes us comfortable by lowering the temperature *and* getting rid of the humidity in the air. We have just seen, though, that babies need some humidity. A reasonable compromise would be to keep the air conditioning on and have a humidifier in the room as well. The baby's room temperature should be the same as the parents' room temperature. If you require air conditioning or heat, so does your baby.

Some people assume incorrectly that a humidifier will prevent or cure various illnesses. A humidifier is soothing and may help with some respiratory problems, but its main role is to make the baby comfortable. Medicine added to the humidifier or vaporizer makes the room smell therapeutic but is not necessary for your baby's comfort.

Imaginary Friends

WHEN PLAYMATES are not available, the two- to three-year-old may invent friends to play with. They are generally harmless, and the pretense gives the child practice in speech, play, and friendship. These pretend friends tend to appear at the same times as other forms of make-believe. Around 50 percent of all preschoolers have invisible playmates, who may have names and full-blown personalities. They usually hang around until your child is six or seven years old.

Imaginary friends enable a child to exert some control over his life. They can be bossed around without backtalk, and they can act as scapegoats for a child dealing with loneliness, boredom, and anxiety. Imaginary friends allow a child to be upset yet still obey his parent's rules.

There is no evidence that having imaginary friends indicates a personality disorder. The only time it represents a problem is when the child with these pretend friends has trouble with normal, age-appropriate socialization or academic performance. If having imaginary friends does not cause problems outside the child's home, they're harmless and will go away.

Eventually, even the most faithful playmate fades away, usually when a child's thoughts of make-believe become private, around the age of six.

TIPS:

1. Support your child's imagination without overdoing it. If you take the playmate too seriously, the child may feel that he has lost control of his own creation.

2. Don't let the imaginary friend take the blame for any wrongdoing. If your child does something wrong, include both culprits (child and imaginary playmate) in the punishment or appropriate management of the problem. If your boy spills cereal on the floor and blames his imaginary friend, explain to him that there are consequences to his actions and that he should set a good example for his friend. He and his friend should be involved in the clean-up.

Immunizations:
Part 1 (Schedule)

THE FOLLOWING is the schedule for immunizations our practice currently recommends. Since the recommended ages for administering these vaccines can change, and since new vaccines may be added to the schedule, be sure to check with your pediatrician about all immunization updates. There can always be minor variations from one baby to another. It is a good idea for you to keep a copy of the dates of your baby's immunizations at home for future reference. I have included routine tests that are commonly performed. Refer to the entry on each disease for the child's possible reactions to the immunization.

AGE	IMMUNIZATION/TEST
2 Weeks	Hepatitis B, #1 (given to newborns in some hospitals before discharge rather than at 2-week office visit); urinalysis (yearly)
6 Weeks	Hepatitis B, #2
10 Weeks	Polio, #1; DPT, #1; Hib, #1
4½ Months	Polio, #2; DPT, #2; Hib, #2
6½ Months	DPT, #3; Hib, #3
7½ Months	Hepatitis B, #3
8½ Months	Hematocrit (yearly fingerprick blood test); Lead test (every other year until the child is six). The frequency of recommended lead testing varies in different locations. Check with your pediatrician.
9½ Months	Tuberculosis test every year
15 Months	MMR, #1; Hib, #4
18 Months	DPT, #4; Polio, #3
Over 4½ Years	DPT, #5; Polio, #4
Over 5 Years	MMR, #2 (Some pediatricians administer the second MMR around twelve years.)
Every 10 years	DT booster
DPT =	Diphtheria, Pertussis, Tetanus
DT =	Diphtheria, Tetanus

Hib = *Haemophilus Influenzae* type B

MMR = Measles, Mumps, Rubella

Immunizations:
Part 2 (Information)

THE SUCCESS of immunizations in controlling many common childhood infectious diseases in the United States is one of the most important medical developments in the twentieth century. The following figures demonstrate this dramatic improvement.

Diphtheria:	206,939	cases in 1921,
but only	2	cases in 1991
Measles:	894,134	cases in 1941,
but only	9488	cases in 1991
Mumps:	152,209	cases in 1968,
but only	4031	cases in 1991
Rubella:	57,686	cases in 1969,
but only	1372	cases in 1991
Pertussis (whooping cough)	265,269	cases in 1934,
but only	2575	cases in 1991
Polio:	21,269	cases in 1952,
but	0	cases in 1991 (although there were 8 vaccine-associated cases in 1991)
Tetanus:	1560	cases in 1923,
but only	49	cases in 1991

The eradication of smallpox from the entire world is further proof of the benefits of immunization programs. Vaccines work by strengthening the child's immune system. A baby is born with antibodies against some diseases, but many of these antibodies last only a few months. Vaccines boost the immune system's ability to make new antibodies. Although no vaccine is completely free of all potential adverse effects, several decades of their use have demonstrated their excellent safety profiles. When many people are vaccinated, everyone benefits, because the chance for spread of the disease is reduced. In the small number of children who develop illnesses in spite of being vaccinated, the symptoms are much milder and less dangerous.

Let's clear up several misconceptions about immunizations.

1. In most cases, multiple vaccines can be given without impairing the ability of any of them to work effectively and without increasing the risk of adverse reactions.

2. There are only a few reasons to hold off giving immunizations: concurrent moderate or severe illness; a previous allergic reaction to that specific immunization or to one of its components; a live virus vaccine (e.g., oral polio vaccine) to pregnant women or to children living with a patient who has AIDS or with an immunocompromised patient. These children should receive the inactivated polio vaccine shot, called the "killed" vaccine. The risk of live virus vaccines causing harm to the fetus is theoretical and has never been proved. Certainly, all vaccines can be given to healthy children of healthy pregnant women. Since young children may have as many as six to eight colds each year, neither the colds nor mild ear infections should interfere with the immunizations. So if your child has a cold on the day of his appointment, he should still get his shots. Both the American Academy of Pediatrics and the Centers for Disease Control recommend that children with minor illnesses should be vaccinated, regardless of the degree of fever, especially if it is uncertain that they will return.

3. Concurrent antibiotic treatment is not a reason to withhold immunizations.

4. Premature babies should be immunized at the usual chronological age.

5. Breast feeding is not a reason to withhold immunizations from a healthy mother or her baby.

6. According to the Advisory Committee on Immunization Practices, immunizations can safely be given to children with a family history of convulsions or crib death.

7. The Traveler's Hotline can supply up-to-date information on required immunizations for those traveling to any country. The telephone number is 1-404-332-4559.

Here is a list of important points about individual vaccines:

DPT Vaccine:

The combination of diphtheria, pertussis, and tetanus vaccines into one shot works as effectively as three separate shots. Most children have little or no problem from the DPT shot. Some may have mild fever or soreness, redness, and swelling at the site of the injection, and some may be cranky for a day or two. Rarely will a high fever and irritability develop. Even less often, a child may have a convulsion, although this is due to the fever and not directly due to the DPT vaccine. The chance of a nonimmunized child getting whooping cough is 1 in 3000. However, the chance of getting a convulsion with temporary neurological problems is only 1 in 2 million! The American Academy of Pediatrics, the Advisory Committee on Immunization Practices, and the Centers for Disease Control have all concluded that the DPT vaccine does not cause chronic neurological damage. A new type of DPT vaccine, called acellular, has been licensed for use in the eighteen-month (dose 4) and four- to five-year (dose 5) age groups. Studies are currently under way to evaluate its effectiveness in the younger age groups. It has fewer local and systemic reactions. For children with seizure disorders or those with a family history of seizures, acellular DPT is strongly recommended. If your child had a slight reaction after one DPT vaccination, give acetaminophen just before the next DPT shot and every four hours after as needed to control fever or irritability. If your child does develop a high fever (over 104°F) or a convulsion after the DPT vaccine, he should subsequently receive only the DT vaccine, leaving out the P.

The **DT vaccine** (combined diphtheria and tetanus vaccine) should be given to adults every ten years. It is not known to cause any problems for pregnant women or their unborn babies. Nonimmune pregnant women should receive the vaccine, because babies born under unclean conditions (and not all deliveries take place exactly as or where planned) to women who are unprotected against tetanus are at risk of getting tetanus as a newborn.

Polio Vaccine:

This vaccine comes in two forms: oral (live) vaccine and injection (killed) vaccine. They are equally effective, although the live virus can be shed for one month in the stools after the child has had the oral vaccine. The last reported case of nonvaccine-induced polio in the United States was in 1979. The shot is saved for people with cancer, children who are immunosuppressed (e.g., with AIDS), or children whose household contacts are immunosuppressed. The risk of paralysis in healthy children following the oral vaccine is 1 per 7.8 million doses. Similar statistics apply to household contacts of the child who receives the oral vaccine. The advantage of the oral polio vaccine (aside from the obvious ease of administration, and avoiding another shot to the child) is that it stimulates the gastrointestinal tract to make antibodies against polio. This prevents future shed of the virus in stools following subsequent polio exposures. Breast feeding does not interfere with the oral polio vaccine's success, so no interruption of breast or bottle feedings is necessary. IPV, the inactivated polio shot, should not be given to a person who is allergic to neomycin or streptomycin. Neither vaccine is known to cause any problems to unborn babies. IPV can cause a little soreness at the site of injection. Your doctor may recommend an additional dose before you take a trip to any country where polio is common. Since thousands of people still get polio every year in other parts of the world, it remains a threat for travelers and a risk for all Americans through importation into the United States. We must not let down our guard; we have to continue aggressive immunization against this disease.

MMR Vaccine:

The measles, mumps, and rubella (German measles) vaccines are usually combined into one shot. Most children will not have side effects, although some may have temporary soreness at the site of injection. The first MMR is not given until the baby is fifteen months old, because he acquires the mother's antibodies against these diseases while still in utero, across the placenta. These antibodies leave the baby by fifteen months. Some children develop a rash, fever, or stiff joints one to two weeks after the shot. The child with these symptoms is not contagious, so no one can catch measles, mumps, or rubella from his reactions to the vaccine. The symptoms usually disappear after one or two days. These side effects occur more often after the first MMR vaccine than after the second, which is given to preschoolers or to adolescents. It is not recommended that pregnant women be given the MMR vaccine (a live vaccine), even though it has not been proved to cause problems for pregnant women or their unborn babies. The mothers should receive this shot after their babies are born. It is safe, however, to give the MMR shot to a child whose mother is pregnant. Any woman who has received an MMR shot should not get pregnant for three months. In 1990, there were twenty-five cases of "congenital rubella syndrome" in Southern California. Refer to the entry on "Rubella" on page 269 for details of congenital rubella syndrome. Over half the mothers of these babies missed opportunities to have rubella testing and vaccination after a previous abortion or after the delivery of a previous child.

The MMR vaccine is made in chick embryo cell cultures. People with severe allergic reactions to eggs (hives, swelling of mouth and throat, difficulty in breathing) should not receive this vaccine. If the reaction to eggs is mild, or if the person is allergic to chickens or feathers, it is safe for him to receive the MMR vaccine.

Hib Vaccine:

This vaccine protects against the *Haemophilus influenzae B* bacteria, one of the leading causes of meningitis, epiglottitis, arthritis, and pneumonia in children. The bacteria attack 1 out of every 200 children in the United States before they are five years old. It is contagious and spreads through day care centers and nursery schools. The vaccine has a very low rate of minor side effects, such as a mild fever or slight swelling at the site of injection. Recently it has become available in a shot that combines it with the DPT vaccine.

Hepatitis B Vaccine:

In the United States, there are three hundred thousand new cases of hepatitis B each year. The estimated one million persons with hepatitis B virus in this country are potentially infectious to others and can pass it along through sexual contact, intravenous drug use, household contact, occupational exposure, and perinatal transmission. Eight percent of the infections occur in infants and children. Up to 25 percent of all Americans have had a hepatitis B virus infection by the time they are thirty. Immunization of infants and children is expected to provide long-term immunity, but this vaccine does not protect against hepatitis A, hepatitis C, or other viruses known to infect the liver. Vaccines against hepatitis A are currently being developed. The hepatitis B vaccine, given in three shots, is generally well tolerated, without any serious adverse reactions.

Flu Vaccine:

The flu vaccine, which protects against the many strains of influenza virus, is given to children with chronic diseases like asthma, diabetes, kidney or heart disease, sickle cell disease, thalassemia, cystic fibrosis, as well as to immunocompromised children. In these children, the flu could exacerbate the underlying problem, resulting in serious consequences. But the majority of children need not have the vaccine. Its side effects (fever, soreness at the site of injection, muscle aches, irritability) make it inappropriate simply to modify a disease that is generally milder in children than in adults. Immunization of adults who are in close contact with high-risk children is an important way to protect these children. This includes hospital personnel and household contacts (parents, siblings, and caregivers). People for whom skin testing confirms allergies to chickens or eggs should not receive the flu vaccine.

Pneumococcal Vaccine:

This vaccine protects against pneumonia and meningitis caused by the pneumococcal bacterium. It is recommended for children with sickle cell disease, AIDS, and kidney disease, and for those who do not have a spleen, either because of disease or surgery. It is given to these children when they are over two years of age and is repeated every 6 years.

Typhoid Vaccine:

For travelers to areas where typhoid is endemic, a new oral live vaccine is available. It protects as effectively as the typhoid shot, with only minimal side effects, such as abdominal discomfort, nausea, and vomiting.

Smallpox Vaccine:

This vaccine is no longer routinely used, because its side effects are greater than the chance of getting the disease, which has not occurred anywhere in years.

Chickenpox Vaccine:

A vaccine against chickenpox is expected to be licensed for use by the general pediatric population within the next 2 years.

Impetigo

IMPETIGO is an infection of the skin caused by the staph or strep bacterium. These bacteria often live on our skin, but if they invade a cut, rash, bite, chickenpox or herpes lesion, or other break in the skin, they can cause an infection. This is a common scenario after a cold, when the child wipes his nose with his fingers and infects the surrounding skin. Impetigo occurs most frequently in the warm summer months. It is contagious to other people and can easily spread to susceptible areas on the child's body. Small red pimples rapidly become blisters, less than 1 inch in diameter, with clear or yellowish fluid. They often open and drain, forming sticky, heaped-up, honey-colored crusts, and new sores and swollen glands develop nearby. Itching and burning are usually mild. Poststreptococcal kidney problems and scars on the skin can develop. However, acute rheumatic fever, another complication of strep infections, has not been reported as a result of impetigo.

Treatment includes washing with an antibacterial soap (Dial or Safeguard) three times a day, followed by the application of an antibacterial ointment (such as Neosporin or Bactroban). Oral antibiotics may be prescribed by your pediatrician. It is important to teach good hygiene to your child. Keep the fingernails short to reduce the risk of his spreading the infection to other parts of his body. Have him use a washcloth and towel not used by the rest of the family. Change bed linens daily. The child can return to day care or school only when the lesions are dry and scabbed over. Open, draining lesions are still contagious. The incubation period is two to five days.

Influenza

INFLUENZA, also called the flu, is a winter infection caused by any of several different viruses. Children develop fever, chills, headaches, sore throats, runny noses, coughs, muscle aches and pains all over the body, and, in some cases, vomiting and diarrhea. Although these acute symptoms last two to five days, the lethargy and weakness may last for two weeks. During the worldwide influenza epidemic of 1918, approximately twenty million people died. Nevertheless, influenza can be considered a disabler rather than a killer, because it is seldom the direct cause of death. As with any viral illness, the body's resistance is reduced, and secondary bacterial infections like bronchitis, pneumonia, ear infection, and sinusitis can develop. Influenza can exacerbate the underlying problem in children with asthma, chronic bronchitis, diabetes, cystic fibrosis, heart or kidney disease, and sickle cell anemia.

Influenza is spread by direct contact, coughing, and sneezing. Children are contagious from twenty-four hours before the onset of symptoms until the major symptoms are passed and until they have been free of fever for at least twenty-four hours. The incubation period is one to three days.

TIPS:

1. The same precautions should be taken to prevent the flu as the common cold. Antibiotics do not cure influenza, but they are used if secondary bacterial infections develop.

2. Refer to the entry on "Fever" on page 134. Note that neither ibuprofen nor acetaminophen is associated

with Reye's syndrome. Either one can be used for fever reduction and pain relief. Do not use aspirin.

3. Encourage your child to drink extra fluids.

4. Encourage your child to rest in bed, especially if he has a fever.

5. Refer to the entry on "Cough Medicines" on page 86.

6. Discard used tissues with as little direct handling as possible.

7. Teach good hygiene, such as covering the nose and mouth when coughing and sneezing. Wash hands well. Use separate eating and drinking utensils.

Only temporary immunity follows the flu, and since there are several viruses that cause it, having had one kind does not protect you from catching another. Similarly, vaccines give protection for some months, but only against certain influenza viruses. Therefore, the live weakened vaccine is changed from year to year, depending on what influenza strains are expected to cause that winter's epidemic. The vaccine is given in one or two doses (usually separated by one month) beginning in September or October. One third of those who are vaccinated complain of soreness at the vaccine site for up to two days. Fever and muscle aches due to the vaccine occur infrequently. At present, the vaccine is recommended for children with chronic illnesses like asthma, cystic fibrosis, chronic bronchitis, heart or kidney disease, diabetes, sickle cell anemia, and cancer. The influenza vaccine is considered safe for pregnant women, and it can be given to children with concurrent minor illnesses. It may be administered simultaneously with other routine vaccines, although each injection should be given at a different site on the body.

Jaundice in the Newborn

THE RED blood cells in our bodies live to the ripe old age of 120 days. Then they die and break apart, emptying their contents into the bloodstream. One of their components is a yellow pigment called bilirubin, which makes its way to the liver, where it is "changed" by the enzyme glucuronyl transferase. After this change, the bilirubin can be excreted from the body. Babies, while still in utero, do not yet have glucuronyl transferase, so the unchanged bilirubin goes into the mother's blood via the umbilical cord, and the mother's enzyme changes the baby's bilirubin so that she can excrete it. Once the baby is born and the umbilical cord is cut, the baby has no way to get rid of all the excess bilirubin from red blood cells that have just died. Some babies need four or five days to produce the enzyme. Until that time, the unchanged bilirubin accumulates throughout the body, including the skin, so many babies develop a slight yellow tinge, first visible in the eyes and face. If the bilirubin continues to rise, the yellow color will spread down the chest, abdomen, groin, and legs.

The baby's bilirubin is measured by a test of blood usually drawn from the baby's heel. About a fifth of all babies are yellow enough to need this blood test. A rough correlation between height of bilirubin and where it is seen on the body is as follows:

Bilirubin in 4–8 (mg/100 ml) range: Seen on head, neck, and eyes.

Bilirubin in 5–12 (mg/100 ml) range: Seen at chest level.

Bilirubin in 8–16 (mg/100 ml) range: Seen down to groin and thighs.

JAUNDICE IN THE NEWBORN

Bilirubin in 11–18 (mg/100 ml) range: Seen down to lower legs.

Bilirubin greater than 15 mg/100 ml: Seen throughout the body, including palms and soles.

The yellow color disappears in reverse fashion, so the face is the last to clear.

Years ago, before this process was understood and treatment was available, the brain was one of the internal organs also "stained" yellow. A serious condition, called kernicterus, resulted and was a leading cause of mental retardation. Today, this condition is practically unheard of.

One of the ways doctors used to get rid of elevated bilirubin from a baby's blood was through an exchange transfusion. Two tubes were inserted into the baby's blood vessels—one to draw out the blood with the elevated bilirubin, and the other to replace it with fresh blood containing normal amounts of bilirubin. Due to modern medical advances, and some very sharp nuns, this procedure is rarely done anymore.

About forty years ago, several nuns who were caring for newborns made the observation that those babies who stayed in the middle of the nursery got jaundice a lot more often than those who were near the windows. This important finding led to the discovery that a certain wavelength of light helps to rid the baby's exposed skin of the excess bilirubin. This "phototherapy" is used in nurseries today in the form of bulbs that shine in the baby's isolette. Although the exact mechanism of how the light works is not known, phototherapy has alleviated the need for more drastic ways of decreasing the bilirubin. The higher the baby's bilirubin level, the longer (usually two to four days) it takes for the bilirubin to drop under phototherapy. There are exceptions to this, so it is difficult to predict how long the jaundiced baby will require phototherapy. Some doctors suggest that parents call medical supply companies that rent the phototherapy equipment for home use. Nurses or paramedical technicians will visit the home daily to draw and measure the baby's bilirubin and will report the results to the pediatrician.

It is important not to confuse this jaundice with the yellowish tinge the skin assumes as the baby of four to eight months eats yellow vegetables, such as carrots, squash, sweet potatoes, and corn. This harmless condition is caused by the carotene (a vitamin A precursor) in these foods. The key differentiating point is that the eyes do *not* turn yellow in the child eating these vegetables. No treatment is necessary, as the color will disappear by itself when other foods are introduced.

There are, however, other important causes of newborn jaundice that elevate the bilirubin. If red blood cells break down more rapidly than normal, as they do in certain anemias (like sickle cell anemia), or if there is a mismatch between the mother's blood and the baby's, then the baby's liver will be overloaded with bilirubin. In neonatal hepatitis, the liver itself is sick and can't deal with the bilirubin in the normal fashion. In some rare cases, the mother's breast milk can interfere with the child's excreting the bilirubin. As a result, these breast-fed babies require a few more days to clear the substance. But most breast-fed babies do not require any special treatment. Your doctor will be on the lookout for other rare causes of jaundice.

If your baby is allowed to go home with a slightly elevated bilirubin, you can follow these few tips to lower it.

TIPS:

1. Give the baby extra fluids in the form of water, formula, or breast milk. They will help to "wash out" the excess bilirubin.

2. Expose the baby to indirect sunlight by undressing him and keeping him near a sunny window.

3. In rare situations, your pediatrician may recommend that you stop breast feeding for a day or so.

4. If your newborn's yellow color spreads down to his abdomen, groin, or legs, call your pediatrician. The

baby should be viewed unclothed in natural sunlight by a window. The point at which your pediatrician will be concerned depends on many factors: height of the bilirubin; size and gestational age of the baby; health of the baby; how well and what the baby is eating; family history of similar or related problems; the rate at which the bilirubin is rising.

Kawasaki Disease

KAWASAKI disease, also called mucocutaneous lymph node syndrome, was described in Japan by Dr. Kawasaki. This rare, noncontagious disease occurs in children under five years old, and its cause is unknown. One of its hallmarks is a high fever that lasts for one to two weeks. The palms of the hands and soles of the feet redden, and during the second and third weeks of illness, the fingers and toes peel. There is a diffuse rash over the body, and the white parts of the eyes become red. The lips redden and crack, and the child complains of a sore throat. Swollen lymph glands develop in the neck. The most serious complication of Kawasaki disease is damage to the coronary arteries, the arteries that supply blood to the heart muscle. One percent of untreated children suffer fatal heart attacks. Since this cardiac damage may occur weeks after the onset of the disease, the children need to be followed for extended periods, with clinical, laboratory, x-ray, or echocardiogram testing for signs of this complication.

Intravenous gamma globulin, given in a hospital setting, and oral aspirin are effective in shortening the duration of the disease and in preventing damage to the coronary arteries. Antibiotics and steroids do not help.

Kawasaki disease sounds like but should not be confused with Coxsackie viruses, which cause blisters in the mouth. Coincidentally, Coxsackie viruses cause hand, foot, and mouth disease, which also brings about rashes on the hands and feet.

Learning Disabilities, Hyperactivity, and Attention Deficit Disorder

ABOUT 15 percent of all school-age children have learning disabilities. Of those, 25 percent have attention deficit disorder, with or without hyperactivity. Learning disabilities and attention deficits are two distinct problems, though they frequently occur together. As a result of their frustrations and failures, children with these problems develop a low self-image and have difficulties with friends, classmates, and family.

A learning disability is the type of difficulty associated with a particular skill. Some examples are dyslexia (reading problems), dysgraphia (writing problems), and dyscalculia (problems with math). Classwork and homework are not the only areas in which learning disabilities manifest themselves. Sports (baseball, basketball, hopscotch), art, and music are also involved.

Attention deficit disorder applies to the difficulty children have in concentrating and paying attention. Sometimes they are uncontrollably fidgety, that is, hyperactive, and this problem can affect their relationships with family and friends. Some children "outgrow" these problems, and some adults continue to have the difficulties throughout life. Many of these adults have good attention spans but remain restless and need to keep busy. Clever teenagers and adults can channel their endless energy to their advantage. The ideal goal is to build up their self-esteem by maximizing their strengths and not focusing on their weaknesses.

Learning Disabilities:

Information enters the brain to be processed through all five senses, but seeing (visual) and hearing (auditory) are the two most important for learning.

Visual Perception Disabilities: Examples of this are writing reversed letters or words, like ɘ for *e, d* for *b, was* for *saw.* The child will have difficulty catching or hitting a ball, doing puzzles, using a hammer and nail, or jumping rope. Some three- to four-year-olds with this reversing problem are able to correct themselves by the time they are five or six. Visual motor disabilities interfere with the child's ability to coordinate his eyes and hands to copy an object he sees.

Auditory Perception Disabilities: The child will confuse words like *blue* and *blow,* or *ball* and *bell.* "How are you?" may be heard as "How old are you?" He may not be able to identify fine distinctions in sound, like those between *p* and *b.* He may also have difficulty focusing on one person's voice (e.g., his teacher) if there is background noise. Calling his name and making eye contact with him help this child to focus.

Abstraction Disability: The child understands only the literal meaning of a word or phrase. He cannot grasp the abstract meaning of "It's raining cats and dogs," or "Don't be such a chicken." He will take jokes too literally and won't understand puns and sayings.

Sequencing Disability: This child will confuse the sequence of thoughts, events in a story, lists, or numbers. He may see *23* but write *32.* He may spell *belt* as *betl.* He will frequently rearrange digits in a telephone number.

Organization Disability: Although many children are slightly disorganized, this child takes the cake! His locker and desk in school are always a mess. His room is even more disheveled than the average child's. His notebook is crammed with folded and torn papers —all in the wrong places. He never remembers homework assignments or test dates, and always forgets to bring home the books he needs for that night's work. It is a good idea for the parents of this child to buy or rent an extra set of textbooks on each topic at the beginning of the school year. That set should always remain at home. Although this does not teach responsibility, it will at least save the child the inevitable reprimand when he forgets to bring home the necessary book on a given day. Another suggestion is that the parents and teacher pass between them a notebook, *not* to be used by the child. Through this daily communication, the parents can know what assignments are due and when, and the teacher can get a feel for how much time the child spent doing homework and how difficult he found it. It is also helpful for the parent to give the child a note, every day, clearly stating what books or papers he should remember to bring home.

Memory Disability: The child with short-term memory disability will know a spelling list the night she studies it but forget it the following morning. She may understand a math concept in school but forget how to do the problems that night. Yet she'll remember in detail things from two or three years ago.

Attention Deficit Disorder (ADD):

ADD is not a learning disability. It is a related disorder frequently found in children with learning disabilities, and ADD must be treated separately. It is five times more common in males than in females, but many experts feel that since girls are less disruptive, they tend to go undiagnosed. ADD runs in families. If one child is diagnosed with ADD, there is a 30 percent chance that one of his siblings will have it and a 30 percent chance that one of his parents will have it. There are no blood tests or x-rays to confirm the diagnosis of ADD. Psychoeducational tests are the best way to define a type of learning disability as well as to diagnose ADD. Of the three types of behavior that characterize children with attention deficit disorder—hyperactivity, distractibility, and/or impulsivity—only one is needed to diagnose ADD. For example, a child can be distractible and/or impulsive, but not hyperactive.

Hyperactivity: The child appears to be in constant motion—tapping his feet, snapping his fingers, swinging his legs, wiggling his body. He may look clumsy, with poor control of his fine motor movements.

Distractibility: This child has problems filtering out the many forms of information (noises, sights, tastes, smells, etc.) that enter his brain simultaneously, and he is therefore easily distracted and unable to focus on the important matters at hand; that is, he has a short attention span. A normal attention span is three to five minutes per year of a child's age. A five-year-old should be able to pay attention for twenty to twenty-five minutes. Ritalin, a medication commonly used for this type of problem, actually stimulates the "filter" in the brain to allow only the important and relevant information to get through. Dexedrine and Cylert are similar medicines. It is important to note that these medications do not lead to drug addiction. In fact, since a significant percentage of untreated children tend to slip into a bad crowd, these medicines may prevent drug abuse.

Impulsivity: This child acts before he thinks and does not consider the consequences of his actions. He has a short fuse and gets angry easily. It is hard for him to learn from past experiences.

Another way to understand the difference between ADD and a learning disability is that ADD makes students *unavailable* for learning because they are too hyperactive, distractible, or impulsive. A learning disability makes them *unable* to learn, due to a problem with one or more of their processing skills.

It is important to be aware of some warning signs of attention deficit disorder and learning disabilities. These include the child's feeling inadequate or dumb; being easily frustrated; getting into fights easily; being depressed; complaining of frequent headaches or stomachaches. Some children avoid stressful learning situations by becoming the class clown. Others avoid embarrassment or failure by appearing bossy or in need of being in control. Treating these symptoms, though, does not cure the problem. You can't put out a fire by blowing away the smoke. If a child's ADD is not recognized and addressed early, he will have to overcome ten years of parents and teachers yelling at him. Pinpointing the problem is done by a team of professionals, consisting of psychologists, special education experts, neurologists, and the child's pediatrician. They may determine whether there is need for a speech pathologist, occupational therapist, or other professionals.

The best form of learning is the one-on-one exchange between the child and a parent, teacher, tutor, or special ed expert. The positive feedback the child gets for asking a good question aids his emotional and mental development. Within the school setting, some children do better in a regular classroom, but are "pulled out" during the day for special education help. Others do better in a special resource room from which they are "mainstreamed" into a regular classroom for part of the day. Still others need to be in a full-time, self-contained, special ed program.

One of my eight-year-old patients has accepted the responsibility of coping with his ADD in a very responsible manner. He told his third-grade teacher that he has ADD and that it would be helpful if he could sit near her. "And if you don't mind," he said to her, "when you are saying something important, could you please get my attention by tapping me on the shoulder?"

Sometimes your child's doctor will prescribe medication. The appropriate type, dosage, and frequency of medication will depend on the observations by the child's parents and teachers as well as feedback from the child himself. The medications are usually aimed at decreasing the hyperactivity, distractibility, and/or impulsivity of an attention deficit disorder. They help with the learning disability only by making the child more available for learning; they do not correct the specific learning disability. There is no evidence that dietary management, megavitamins, sugar restriction, or supplementary trace minerals are effective, and allergies do not play an important role in these problems. Parents are usually surprised to learn that the sugar in fruit is the same as the sugar in cereal, honey, brown sugar, even the same as white sugar itself. They all end up as glucose, and usually do not cause hyperactivity.

TIPS:

1. Don't feel guilty or blame yourself. Children are born with different traits, and most can channel their energies usefully and become productive adults.

2. It is helpful to keep to schedules and routines, especially for the disorganized child with a short attention span. Keep the times for wake-up, meals, chores, naps, and bedtime as regular as possible.

3. Give these children a few chances to burn off some of their excess energy throughout the day.

4. Since some of these children find it hard to focus on more than one thing at a time, don't give them a series of complex commands. If there is something you want them to do, arrange your requests in sequence and say them in simple and uncomplicated terms. Similarly, encourage your child to play with one toy at a time, because too many toys may be distracting.

5. Even these children need limits set for socially unacceptable behavior, like biting, kicking, and hitting. Negative behavior should consistently be confronted with firm discipline. Positive behavior should always be rewarded. Pick your battles realistically. Although you should not allow your child to kick others, don't expect him to keep his hands and feet still.

6. Parents tend to have more patience than older siblings. Spend some private time reading and telling stories to the younger child with these problems.

7. Not only is time-out an effective disciplinary measure for many children, but parents of difficult children also need some time-out to clear their own heads. Try to schedule time to do things for yourself. An occasional baby sitter and an evening out are greatly needed by exhausted parents.

8. The IQ, intelligence quotient, is an inaccurate instrument for prediction. Group testing is much less accurate than individual testing. A child who does poorly on a group IQ test should take an individually administered intelligence test. It more easily takes into account whether a child's poor performance is due to his having a cold, being tired, or truly having a learning disability. The IQ is not an indelible number that will be carried throughout life. The best use of IQ tests is in developing an appropriate educational program for your child. Most children with attention deficit disorder have a normal IQ. However, those with learning disabilities may lag behind on certain areas of the IQ tests.

9. Listening and sequencing skills can be strengthened by progressing through the following age-appropriate activities: looking at picture books; reading stories; coloring pictures; encouraging play with building blocks, puzzles, dominoes, card games, and board games; matching picture games; playing checkers and tic-tac-toe.

With appropriate help for these problems, these children can overcome their hyperactivity, distractibility, and impulsivity. They can improve their learning disabilities and lead healthy, happy, and productive lives.

Lice

LICE ARE tiny insects that go from person to person under close contact or through infested combs, brushes, hats, and clothing. They move very rapidly and can infest the head, body, and pubic area; the last is frequently involved in adolescents. We will discuss the more common problem of head lice. Lice are not a sign of uncleanliness or poor health habits. They can lodge on anybody. The adult louse lays up to ten egg sacs (nits) daily in human hair, and these are found at the root of the hair, especially on the back of the neck, or on surrounding clothes, as white or gray particles resembling dandruff. However, they stick to the hair much more firmly than does dandruff. After one or two weeks, the eggs hatch, and more lice appear. It is easier to see the white nits than the tiny gray lice. Their bites itch greatly, resulting in scratching, with its potential for infection of the skin. Tender, swollen lymph glands in the back and sides of the neck may develop.

Your pediatrician will prescribe a medicated shampoo or cream. After the treatment, remove dead eggs with a fine-toothed comb or tweezers. A vinegar rinse 15 minutes before using the comb will loosen the nits from the hair. Repeat the medicated shampoo treatment in 1 week to get any remaining eggs. Clothes, sheets, and pillowcases should be put through a double rinse. Washing clothes removes lice, and ironing clothes destroys nits. Boil brushes, curlers, and combs, and clean hats and bicycle helmets. If a particular hat, coat, or other item cannot be washed, set it aside in a plastic bag for two to three weeks. The nits cannot survive that long. If the parasite infects the eyelashes, apply Vaseline twice a day for a week. If the lice persist in the eyelashes, a doctor may have to remove the lice with great care. A lice insecticide spray kills lice and eggs on furniture, carpeting, mattresses, and other household items that can't be washed or dry-cleaned. Examine the head of everyone at home. All family members and close contacts should be treated at the same time. Contact for even less than a second is sufficient to transfer the lice. Notify the child's teacher. Reinfestation from classmates and playmates is common. Lice generally cannot survive away from the host for more than forty-eight hours; eggs generally do not survive away from hair for more than seven days.

Children can return to school or day care the morning after their first treatment, because the risk of transmission is promptly reduced by treatment. "No nit" policies requiring that children be free of nits prior to returning to school are not effective in controlling head lice.

Limping and Joint Problems

A CHILD LIMPS, or walks with an abnormal gait, when pain or weakness prevents him from putting his weight down on the affected leg. A limp is always an abnormal finding, not something the child fakes. The following list discusses the more common, and some uncommon, causes of limping and joint problems.

Trauma:

Cuts: Refer to the entries on "Bites and Stings" on page 27 and "Stitches" on page 306.

Splinters: If the end of a splinter is sticking out of the skin, you can remove it with a pair of tweezers. Other superficial splinters work themselves out in one or two days if heat is applied for a half-hour three or four times a day. If a splinter doesn't work itself out, place a piece of ice over the area to numb the skin. Then distract the child and use a clean, sharp sewing needle to gently break the surface of the skin, thus exposing the splinter. Be sure the needle has been sterilized by a cleaning with alcohol. When the splinter's tip is exposed, pull it out with tweezers. Refer to "Bites and Stings" on page 27 for first-aid measures. If you are unable to remove the splinter, your doctor will take it out under a local anesthetic.

Blisters: Refer to the entry on "Burns" on page 43.

Sprains and strains: Ligaments are bands of thick, fibrous tissue that connect one bone to another bone. Tendons are similar tough tissues that connect muscles to bones. A sprain occurs when the ligaments and/or tendons that support a joint tear because of too much pressure on and twisting of the joint. A strain is essentially a mild sprain, in that the ligament is merely stretched or only a few of its fibers are torn. The injury causes the ligaments and tendons to swell, so the entire joint becomes swollen and painful. An x-ray will be normal because the bones are not involved in the injury, and ligaments and tendons do not show up on x-rays. Tendonitis—inflammation—of the Achilles tendon, in the back of the foot, is a common cause of limping in the athletic child. Since worn-down shoe heels can stretch this tendon, a few days of rest (and a new pair of shoes) will usually help the child. A cold compress, elevation of the affected part, and an Ace bandage on the joint are appropriate first-aid measures. Ibuprofen will help to relieve the pain.

Fractures: Refer to the entry on "Bones" on page 32.

Shin splints: Muscle pain along the front of the lower leg can follow strenuous physical activities, such as marathons, some track-and-field exercises, and even long walks. Rest, cold compresses, and ibuprofen usually do the trick.

Injections: Children who receive a shot (for immunization or medication) in the leg may limp from the pain for one or two days. By the time the child is old enough to walk, immunizations can be given in the deltoid muscle of the upper arm, thus avoiding a cause of limping.

Infection:

Cellulitis: A bacterial infection of an area of skin and its underlying supportive and connective tissues can cause redness, swelling, and pain. When this occurs anywhere on the leg, the child will limp. Cellulitis requires oral and/or intravenous antibiotics.

Osteomyelitis: Osteomyelitis is a bacterial infection of the bone itself due to a penetrating injury of the overlying skin, or to a blood-borne infection from a cut elsewhere in the body, which then settles in the bone. The area is tender and swollen, and the child may develop a fever. The diagnosis is made by x-rays and bone scans. Sometimes surgery is needed to clean out the infection and take cultures. Treatment consists of intravenous antibiotics for four to six weeks, either in a hospital setting or at home through one of the recently established home-treatment programs. Nurses or paramedical personnel come to the child's home to start and care for intravenous catheters, and to administer the needed medications, under a doctor's written supervision.

Arthritis:

Arthritis is the hot, red, swollen, and painful condition of a joint. Arthralgia is the term used to describe a tender joint that is without heat, redness, or swelling. Arthritis can be acute, meaning that its onset is sudden and it occurs only once or twice. If it is chronic, there may be decreased movement and even deformity of the joint. Limping develops when arthritis affects the back, hips, knees, ankles, or toes. Arthritis can be due to trauma (see above), viral or bacterial infections, rheumatic fever, juvenile rheumatoid arthritis, and drug reactions.

Viral infections: Arthritis occurs as part of many common viral illnesses, such as the flu, rubella, and measles. As these illnesses abate, the joint pains and swellings also subside. Toxic synovitis is a common type of arthritis (usually of the hip) that follows some viral illnesses. Refer to the entry on "Hips" on page 181 for a discussion of toxic synovitis.

Bacterial infections: When the infection in a joint is caused by bacteria, it is referred to as a septic arthritis. The arthritis associated with Lyme disease is an example of this. Refer to the entry on "Lyme Disease" on page 219. If this type of arthritis is not treated rapidly, the infection may destroy the joint and spread to the bone. The doctor makes the diagnosis by inserting a sterile needle into the joint, with the patient under anesthesia, and removing and culturing the pus. He will then prescribe intravenous and/or oral antibiotics.

Rheumatic fever: Arthritis is part of the syndrome referred to as rheumatic fever. Refer to the section on "Rheumatic Fever" in the entry on "Sore Throat (Pharyngitis) and Tonsillitis" on page 299.

Juvenile rheumatoid arthritis (JRA): The cause of JRA (also called Still disease) is unknown. It is a chronic disease with flare-ups and remissions. Sometimes only one joint is involved, sometimes many. About 250,000 American children have JRA. Although the disease goes into remission for many children during puberty, some patients continue to have active arthritis as adults. These children may develop fever, rashes, swollen glands, enlargement of the liver and spleen, inflammation of the eyes, and heart problems. Often they experience aches in the neck and upper back, with decreased range of movement. The arthritis pains tend to be worse in the morning or after long periods of inactivity, such as watching TV or studying. Blood tests help in the diagnosis. Treatment involves medications (anti-inflammatory, gold compounds, steroids), and physical and occupational therapy. Swimming is one of the best exercises for these children, because the involved joints can exercise without having to bear the weight of the child's body. Splints may be needed to prevent contractures (permanent bendings) of the joints. Surgery is reserved for severe joint involvement and for correcting disabling deformities. Most children with JRA lead active and productive lives, attend school, socialize, and participate in noncontact sports.

Drug reactions: Arthritis is sometimes an unexpected side effect of, and an allergic reaction to, certain medications. Stopping the suspected drug usually reverses the reaction.

Other Problems:

Growing Pains: Although growing pains usually do not cause a limp, they are included in this list because they can be confused with the more serious disorders listed here. Refer to the entry on "Growing Pains" on page 152.

Ingrown toenails: Refer to the entry on "Nails" on page 232.

Shoe problems: Limping can be caused by shoes that are too tight or narrow. A pebble or a nail sticking into the shoe can cause a limp. Calluses may indicate tight or irritating shoes. Two important tips are to bring the shoes your child normally wears for the doctor to check, and to see whether your child limps both with and without these shoes.

Plantar warts: Refer to the entry on "Warts" on page 372. Other podiatric problems, such as "heel spurs," may require a consultation with a specialist.

Osgood-Schlatter disease: Refer to the entry on "Osgood-Schlatter Disease" on page 246.

Other Rare Problems:

Tumors: Bone tumors, as well as leukemia, cause persistent, severe pain. They are diagnosed by x-rays.

Legg-Perthes disease: This rare condition occurs when a disruption of the blood supply to the femur (thigh bone), for unknown reasons, results in damage to the bone. Hip pain and limping develop, with decreased movement of the hip joint. X-rays are helpful in making the diagnosis. Weight-bearing is a problem for these children, who must use crutches, sometimes for several years. Rarely will surgery be required.

Toe-walking: It is important to distinguish between those children who *choose* to walk on their toes and those children who *have to,* because they can't bend their feet upward. If the Achilles tendon, in the back of the foot, is too tight (as part of a clubfoot or a more serious neurological problem), the child is not able to stretch his foot flat on the ground. When many children first learn to walk, they choose to toe-walk, though they can easily stand with their feet flat on the ground. Soon they will start walking normally. If the Achilles tendon remains tight, physical therapy, special orthopedic appliances, and surgery may be needed.

Congenital dislocation of the hip: Refer to the entry on "Hips" on page 181.

Slipped capital femoral epiphysis: The epiphysis is the growth plate at the end of each bone. In some obese adolescents, chronic stress from weight-bearing may cause the epiphysis at the head of the femur (thigh bone) to slip. Limping, limitation of movement of the hip, and hip or knee pain develop. The slipped epiphysis is visible on x-rays. Orthopedic surgery to stabilize the hip is usually needed.

Henoch-Schönlein Purpura: Refer to the section on "Henoch-Schönlein Purpura" in the entry on

"Hemophilia and Other Bleeding Disorders" on page 165.

Systemic lupus erythematosis (lupus) and dermatomyositis: For unknown reasons, children with lupus and dermatomyositis develop antibodies against their own organs. The kidneys, central nervous system, muscles, and skin are frequently involved. When the joints are affected, arthritis develops. Blood tests aid in the diagnosis. These are multifaceted disorders requiring multidisciplined therapeutic approaches.

Sickle cell anemia: Arthritis may occur during flare-ups of this condition. Refer to the entry on "Anemias" on page 6.

Lyme Disease

LYME DISEASE is a widespread illness caused by the bite of a deer tick that is infected with a spiral microscopic bacterium called *Borrelia burgdorferi*. The tick is tiny—approximately the size of the period at the end of this sentence. After it feeds and fills with blood, it grows to the size of a small pea. Lyme disease peaks during the summer and early fall. Although it has been reported in at least forty-three states, it is primarily evident in the Northeast, the Midwest, and in California. Cases tend to cluster in wooded areas and adjacent grasslands. It is spread in the wild by deer, mice, and raccoons, but domesticated dogs, cats, and horses carry the tick closer to home. Most specialists agree that the tick must be attached to the child for more than twenty-four hours for the disease to be transmitted.

The incubation period is from three days to one month, during which time the typical "target" skin rash may develop. A little dot at the site of the bite gradually enlarges to form a ringlike lesion, with a clear or pink center. The rash is not itchy or painful, but it can range from five inches to twenty inches in diameter and can last for three to six weeks. Since children are often bitten on the scalp, the hair may hide the rash. The child may complain of headaches, joint pains, and of being tired, and he may develop a fever, swollen glands, a sore throat, and "pink eye." Sometimes there are more severe cardiac or neurological complications, such as an abnormal heart rhythm, meningitis, and paralysis of some nerves. The most common manifestation is Bell's palsy, a drooping of one side of the face. About half of these kids will develop one or more swollen joints several months after the bite. These bouts of arthritis can come and go for months. In between, the children will feel fine.

The diagnosis is made by combining the history, physical exam, clinical course, and appropriate blood tests. Antibiotics are used to treat Lyme disease. In severe cases, these medicines may need to be given intravenously. Patients with active disease should not donate blood.

When camping or walking in wooded areas, wear a hat, long pants, and a long-sleeved shirt. Tuck the pants into the socks to close the ankle area. Place tape over the tops of the socks to prevent ticks from falling in. If the pants and socks are light in color, it will be easier to find a tick. Remove the tick immediately by getting a grip on its head with sharp, pointed tweezers. Remove the head and body with gentle upward pressure (not with sudden jerks), trying not to squeeze the tick. If you don't have tweezers, tie a loop of thread around the tick's jaw and gently pull upward. Remove all parts of the tick's body and head. Don't use a cigarette to remove the tick, because that may promote the spread of bacteria from the tick into the bite. Since ticks breathe only a few times per hour, it is not helpful to smother them in Vaseline, fingernail polish, or alcohol. That will not hurt them or cause them to loosen their grip. After you've removed the tick, wash the area thoroughly with soap and water, and apply an antibiotic cream.

When hiking or camping out, check for ticks every

four hours, and after the hike (or every day of the trip) examine all of the skin and hair for ticks. Since the bite is painless, the tick may go unnoticed by the child. Once you get the tick, save it in a clean jar in case your doctor wants you to bring it to be identified. On a label write your child's name, the date, and "tick for identification." If the child got the tick in an area where Lyme disease is endemic, and if the tick is identified as one that can carry the Lyme bacteria, your doctor may choose to start an antibiotic prophylactically, although this remains controversial.

Always use insect repellents as directed, and spray tick repellent on clothing, including shoes and socks. Permanone is a tick repellent that should be sprayed only on clothing. DEET can be used on clothing and on skin. However, concentrations of DEET vary in different repellents from 5 to 100 percent. Since DEET can be absorbed through the skin and cause neurological problems like seizures, use it only with the following precautions:

• Do not use DEET on raw or sunburned skin, because it is more readily absorbed in these areas.

• Use only repellents with less than 10 percent DEET directly on skin. Even then, try to avoid contact with the eyes or mouth.

• Do not use DEET on the skin of children under two years old.

• Do not use DEET more often than twice a day.

Check your pets regularly for ticks, and wash domesticated pets with an antitick soap during the summer months.

For more information on Lyme disease, call: 1-800-886-LYME.

Masturbation

MASTURBATION is the self-stimulation of the genitals for pleasure by rubbing them with a hand or another object. Rocking body movements, grunting, flushing, and sweating may accompany this stimulation, followed by pallor and a relaxed, quiet period. A child may masturbate several times a day, once a week, or less often. It is frequently done when the child is tired, bored, watching television, or under stress.

Masturbation is not intellectually, emotionally, or physically harmful. It does not cause blindness and will not make the penis fall off! It also does not mean that the child will become promiscuous or sexually deviant. Masturbation is merely a natural extension of the child's curiosity about body parts, self, and sexuality. It is a normal precursor of adult sexual satisfaction. It is an almost universal activity around puberty in response to the normal rise in hormones and sexual drive. However, since it is not socially acceptable to masturbate in public, a parent should teach the child to limit the behavior to the privacy of his bedroom or bathroom.

TIPS:

1. Limit masturbation to private rooms, but do not try to curtail it completely.

2. Parents should never say that this behavior is "dirty" or "bad." Never should the child be punished, physically abused, or restrained (e.g., hands tied, hands kept in makeshift straitjackets) for masturbating. Such inappropriate overreaction by a parent can only lead to emotional harm and contribute to a child's unnecessary guilt feelings. If the five- or six-year-old child masturbates in public, distract him with a toy or other activity. If the intensity and frequency of masturbation interfere

with age-appropriate socialization, speak to your pediatrician. It could reflect a more serious problem, such as depression or sexual abuse.

3. Children do not suddenly, one day around puberty, wake up and become interested in sex. Even five- and six-year-olds have an innocent, healthy curiosity about sex. Refer to the entry on "Sensitive Topics" on page 277, for guidelines on discussing these issues with your child.

4. Extra physical contact, like hugging and cuddling, sometimes lessens the child's need to masturbate frequently.

5. Be truthful, relaxed, and casual when answering your child's questions about sex. Peter Mayle's book *Where Did I Come From?* can be used as a textual and pictorial steppingstone to discussions of sexual matters. Use proper terminology for sex organs and behavior, and convey positive, not shameful, feelings about these body parts.

6. Avoid tight and irritating underwear and clothes.

7. Rarely, pinworms cause itching, which is relieved by masturbatory actions. Ask the pediatrician if it is appropriate to test for pinworms.

Measles

MEASLES, also called rubeola (but not to be confused with rubella, or German measles), is a contagious viral illness that causes fever, a "barking" cough, pink eye, photophobia (pain when the eyes are exposed to light), joint pains, and a rash. The rash starts on the face and shoulders and spreads to the whole body; it lasts for one to two weeks. The incubation period is two weeks. Early in the disease, Koplik's spots (white spots inside the lining of the mouth) can be found. Measles is spread by coughing and sneezing. Children are contagious from three days before the rash appears until five days after it appears. Do not send your child back to school until two or three days after the rash has faded. Rare complications include ear infections, pneumonia, and encephalitis. The child will have lifelong immunity after getting the disease. A teacher of mine once told me that he could diagnose measles over the phone, because no other illness provokes such a harsh, intense cough.

TIPS:

1. Treat the fever as described in the entry on "Fever" on page 134.

2. Cold compresses to the eyes are soothing. Keep the room dimly lit. The photophobia can be so intense that the child may not want to read or even watch television (believe it or not!). Your doctor may prescribe eyedrops or cool compresses. Sunglasses may be helpful.

3. Encourage the child to drink extra fluids.

4. Antibiotics are used only for complications like ear infections or pneumonia.

5. Babies, immunosuppressed children, and nonimmune pregnant women may be given a shot of immune globulin (a specific type of gamma globulin) to prevent or modify the disease. This supplies protection for up to three months.

6. Use a cool-mist vaporizer in the room.

7. A decongestant can help the child sleep by suppressing the cough.

8. For details of the measles vaccine, refer to the entry on "Immunizations" on page 189.

Measurements and Doses

IN ORDER to make things easier and to be absolutely certain that you give your child the exact doses prescribed by your pediatrician, check this chart.

1 cc	=	1 ml
120 drops of water	=	1 teaspoon
1 teaspoon	=	5 ml
*2 teaspoons	=	1 dessert spoon = 10 ml
1 tablespoon	=	15 ml = 3 teaspoons
1 ounce	=	30 ml = 2 tablespoons = 6 teaspoons
1 kilogram (kg)	=	2.2 pounds (lbs)
1 inch	=	2.5 centimeters (cms)

*Since we all have different sizes of teaspoons in our homes, get a 5 cc syringe and be sure that your medicine teaspoon measures 5 cc. Some dessert teaspoons are larger. Refer to the safety tips on "Giving and Taking Medications" on page 381.

Meningitis

FEW WORDS in a doctor's vocabulary evoke the terror in a parent that *meningitis* does. This is perfectly understandable, since any problem involving the brain is scary to talk about. However, if identified and treated early, and if preventive measures are taken, most cases of meningitis can have a good outcome.

The brain and spinal cord are covered by a thin layer of tissue called the meninges. Fluid under the meninges, called cerebrospinal fluid, bathes the brain and spinal cord. Meningitis is the term for infection of the meninges. The cerebrospinal fluid reflects this meningeal infection. To test the fluid, a sterile needle is inserted through the lower back and pushed through the meninges into the space containing this cerebrospinal fluid. In older children, a local anesthetic is given first (like a dental anesthetic) to decrease pain from the needle stick. In babies, the risk of side effects from the local anesthetic precludes its use. The fluid is drawn into a syringe or tube and is tested for signs of infection. This procedure is called a spinal tap or lumbar puncture. If the fluid, which is normally as clear as water, is cloudy or filled with pus, or if the lab reports indicate infection, the child has meningitis. Early results (within the first two hours) can suggest a diagnosis of viral or bacterial meningitis, or of no meningitis at all if the spinal tap is normal. However, the definitive test is the culture, which takes about three days, the time needed for the bacteria, if present, to grow. In the hands of a competent and skillful doctor, a spinal tap is relatively safe and free of complications. In these situations, the risk of not doing a spinal tap and not diagnosing meningitis is greater than the minimal risk associated with the procedure.

Just like a sore throat, bronchitis, and pneumonia, meningitis can be caused by viruses or bacteria. Viral meningitis is usually not serious. Bacterial meningitis is more serious, even potentially fatal, but it can be treated successfully if diagnosed early enough.

In a baby under two months of age, the only symptoms of meningitis may be fever, irritability, and a full or bulging soft spot (fontanelle). The neck muscles are not yet strong enough to demonstrate the classic "stiff neck" of meningitis. This is why most babies under six to eight weeks of age with a fever will require a spinal tap to rule out this serious disease. Remember, if it is caught early enough, it is treatable. In an older infant and child, the hallmark of meningitis is a stiff neck. The stiffness and pain of the back of the neck are felt when the child moves her head forward and tries to touch chin to chest. Other symptoms include headache, lethargy, fever, inability to tolerate bright light, vomiting, and, in severe cases, convulsions and coma. Long-term problems to be looked for are hearing loss and learning disorders.

As is true of other viral illnesses, antibiotics do not help viral meningitis. Frequently, however, antibiotics will be started until the bacterial cultures are negative for the three days following the spinal tap. At this point, the doctors may feel certain that the initial cause was viral, and will stop antibiotics. If the child was taking oral antibiotics before the spinal tap, even for just one day, the spinal tap may not grow out bacteria, and the disease could be misinterpreted as being due to a virus. This is called "partially treated" meningitis, and the child may need to be treated as if bacteria did grow from the culture. In this case, or if bacteria actually do grow from the culture of the spinal fluid, the child will need intravenous antibiotics for seven to fourteen days. That is one reason that no child should be given antibiotics except under the direction of a doctor.

The incubation period for viral meningitis is three to six days, but children with viral meningitis are contagious only while they are acutely ill. The disease is not very contagious, and those who have had contact with these children do not need to take medicine and do not have to be isolated.

For bacterial meningitis, the extent of contagion, the incubation period, and the treatment both for the child and for the immediate contacts all depend on which bacteria are causing the problem. One common troublemaker is the virulent bacterium called *Haemophilus influenzae* type B (Hib). An effective vaccine is routinely given to all children against this bacterium. If an unvaccinated child does get Hib meningitis, his household contacts and day care classmates under the age of four years should receive an oral antibiotic as a precaution. However, other contacts, and classmates over four, are not at risk and do not need prophylactic antibiotics.

Children with certain chronic medical problems, such as sickle cell anemia, absence or removal of a spleen, etc., are prone to infections, including meningitis, caused by a bacterium called *Streptococcus pneumoniae* (the pneumococcus bacterium). This is not the same strep bacterium that causes the strep throat. The pneumococcal vaccine against this bacterium is recommended only for these high-risk children.

Mononucleosis

INFECTIOUS mononucleosis, also called the kissing disease, is a viral infection caused by the Epstein-Barr virus. It acquired its nickname because its spread requires intimate contact, such as kissing. It is interesting that although adolescents living in close contact in schools, colleges, the military, etc., are prone to mono, only rarely does it occur in two family members at the same time. The incubation period is from one to two months, but since the onset of symptoms is vague, it is difficult to pinpoint. Symptoms last for two to four weeks, but occasional cases linger for three to six months.

Symptoms can be so mild that they are confused with a common viral syndrome. They can, however, be severe enough to necessitate hospitalization for intravenous fluids and for treatment of complications. Frequent symptoms and findings are fever, sore throat and inflamed tonsils with white patches, skin rashes, weakness and fatigue, aching of the arms, legs, and back, swollen glands in the groin, under the arm, and in the neck (including the back of the neck), swollen eyelids, and an enlarged spleen. The enlarged tonsils and adenoids may block the airway, causing difficulty in breathing. Occasionally, more severe neurological complications, like Bell's palsy of the face or encephalitis, can develop. The Alice-in-Wonderland syndrome sometimes appears; the patient experiences perceptual distortions of space and size.

The diagnosis of infectious mononucleosis is made by combining history, physical exam, and blood tests. The heterophile blood test for mono is positive in 80 percent of cases and will commonly be negative if drawn too early in the course of the illness, that is, in the first week of symptoms. A different blood test, which measures antibodies against the Epstein-Barr virus, is more accurate but more expensive.

Treatment consists mainly of ways to make the patient comfortable. It is important for him to rest, but he does not have to be confined to bed. He should drink many fluids to prevent dehydration. Throat pain can be alleviated with gargling (a half-and-half mixture of mouthwash and water), using Chloraseptic spray and lozenges or other hard candies, and taking acetaminophen or ibuprofen. Sometimes codeine will be needed. Soft foods are easier for the patient to swallow. Since the illness is viral, antibiotics are of no help. For more serious cases, corticosteroids, like prednisone, are necessary. Steroids can be taken safely, as prescribed, for short periods, one week or less. Since straining to have a bowel movement might injure an enlarged spleen, laxatives may be necessary.

Patients may resume calm outdoor activities and may return to school if there is no fever for twenty-four hours and if they feel well enough to concentrate. However, if the spleen is enlarged, it is important that they not resume gym or contact sports for at least two weeks after the spleen has shrunk to its normal size *as determined by a doctor's physical exam*. Otherwise, the child risks rupturing the spleen, a life-threatening complication.

Since some antibodies against mono remain elevated for life, blood tests cannot be relied on to determine whether one is better or well enough to resume all activities. Mononucleosis can be so debilitating that it may take up to six months before your child feels like his old self again. The status of chronic mononucleosis, or chronic fatigue syndrome, is still controversial, as most cases do not seem to be related to the Epstein-Barr virus.

Motion Sickness

THE INNER ear contains organs that help control our balance. Motion sickness occurs when certain movements make the brain confuse information it receives from the inner ear with information from the eyes. Various rocking movements can trigger this: roller coasters, swings, rides in buses, cars, planes, or boats. Some children just feel nauseated; some actually vomit; some occasionally faint. Motion sickness is hereditary.

TIPS:

1. Have your child close his eyes and lie down. This will lessen the stimulation to the brain. Alternatively, let the child sit in the front seat of the car, bus, or boat and focus on the distant horizon, avoiding the stimulation from the nearby rapidly moving scenery. Some children benefit by wearing sunglasses. Discourage activities like reading and playing games in the car. Don't allow any smoking in the car, and keep a window slightly open for good ventilation. Likewise, on a bus or plane turn on the overhead fan. Carry strong brown paper bags with you to contain vomit.

2. Some over-the-counter medications, like Dramamine Junior, and some antihistamines, like Benadryl, help to control symptoms. They should be given about a half-hour before starting the trip.

3. Don't talk about motion sickness in front of the child. The mere suggestion of it can sometimes worsen the symptoms.

4. It is best for the child to eat a little just before setting out. An empty stomach can cause hunger pains, which contribute to nausea. His having eaten some-

thing beforehand may also prevent his overeating in the car. However, don't have the child travel on a full stomach.

5. Sitting over or close to the wings of an airplane cuts down on the rocking motion. Similarly, try to sit in the center of a boat.

Mumps

MUMPS is a viral, contagious illness that causes fever, headache, joint pains, and swollen, painful salivary glands—the parotid glands—on the side of the face, just at and above the jaw. The swelling may occur on one side of the face or may involve both sides. The throat may feel dry because the salivary glands have temporarily stopped producing saliva. Pickles, lemons, and other sour foods can cause pain in the swollen areas. Occasionally, within two weeks after a boy has developed mumps, the testes may swell, causing pain. It is extremely rare for these patients to become sterile. The ovaries, too, can become inflamed, causing abdominal pain. The incubation period is three weeks, and lifelong immunity is obtained after one contracts the disease.

Mumps is spread by coughing, sneezing, and direct contact. The child becomes contagious one day before the facial swelling starts and remains contagious until three days after the swelling has subsided. He does not have to be isolated from household members but should remain at home. Don't send him back to school until five days after the facial swelling has gone down. Rare but serious complications include meningitis, encephalitis, pancreatitis, and deafness. These complications occur more frequently in adults than in children.

TIPS:

1. Treat the fever as described in the entry on "Fever" on page 134.

2. Encourage the child to drink extra fluids. Let him use a straw if this is easier for him. Give him ice chips or ice pops to suck. Milkshakes and yogurt are easy to swallow. Avoid fruit juices, tart beverages, and spicy foods.

3. Encourage him to rinse his mouth if it's dry.

4. Apply local warmth (like a hot water bottle in a towel) to the affected side(s). Some children prefer cool compresses. Use whichever is more soothing.

5. Antibiotics are not used for this or other viral illnesses.

6. Keep a cool-mist vaporizer in his room.

7. Treatment for the involved testes or ovaries includes bed rest and acetaminophen.

8. For details about the mumps vaccine, refer to the entry on "Immunizations" on page 189.

Nails

Cutting Baby's Nails:

JUST AS some parents have a hard time taking their baby's temperature, others break into a panic at the thought of clipping their infant's nails. Yet some newborns' fingernails and toenails grow so quickly that they need to be trimmed once or twice a week. Babies can scratch themselves (sometimes dangerously close to their eyes) with long or jagged fingernails. Here are some tips to help you get through this "monumental" task.

TIPS:

1. Make it a fun project by having both parents participate. One can hold the baby's fingers steady while the other parent snips and files. Smile at the baby, laugh at each other, enjoy spending time with your baby! The baby will pick up these positive "vibes."

2. A good time to trim nails is after the baby's bath. The baby is relaxed, and the bath will have softened the nails. Some parents prefer doing it while the baby is sleeping.

3. Use a pair of infant scissors with blunted ends, as well as a soft, small emery board. Cut the nails straight across, but round the corners with the scissors or emery board.

4. Although hair and nails generally grow faster in the summer than in the winter, some babies' toenails take a long time before they need clipping. This is normal.

Ingrown Toenails and Paronychia:

Some newborns and older children develop ingrown toenails, especially on the big toes. The edge of the nail grows into and irritates the surrounding skin, causing localized tenderness and redness, occasionally with pus accumulating in the corner. In the older child, shoes that are too tight will push the nail into the skin.

TIPS:

1. Apply warm soaks to the area three or four times a day (each lasting ten to fifteen minutes) with a washcloth to soften the nail and draw out the infection.

2. Elevate the foot to relieve some pressure and pain.

3. Apply an antibiotic ointment (e.g., Neosporin) to the nail and skin. Cover it with a Band-Aid.

4. If the infection persists for three days despite this treatment, or worsens even sooner, see your pediatrician, who may prescribe an oral antibiotic. If the problem recurs, it may be necessary to have the ingrown part of the nail surgically removed, a procedure usually done in a doctor's office.

5. While the toenail is healing, have your child wear a sandal, loose slipper, or open-toed shoe. (A hole can be cut out of an old shoe.)

The term *paronychia* applies to any infection of skin surrounding a fingernail or toenail. It may be caused by the child's picking or biting the nail and the nearby skin. Bacteria enter, especially if the finger is wet, and a painful, red swelling develops. Occasionally, pus drains from the infected area. Treatment is the same as for ingrown toenails.

Nail Biting:

Thumbsuckers are not more likely to become nail biters than nonthumbsuckers. Refer to the entry on "Thumbsucking" on page 339. Although nail biting can result in the formation of a paronychia (see above), it should not be considered a sign of more serious psychopathology. It is a habit that may persist throughout life. Treatment is the same as for thumbsucking. Positive reinforcement, such as rewards for not biting nails, is more effective than reprimands and punishments.

Nervous Tics

ALL CHILDREN, at some time, demonstrate repetitive movements that can be described as habits or spasms. They are more pronounced in children who are shy and very self-conscious. If they occur to such a degree that they affect the child's relations with friends (e.g., being teased) or if they interfere with his academic performance and self-esteem, then they require medical and psychological intervention. Following is a list of just a few of these tics.

Bruxism: Teeth grinding, also called bruxism, is one of those nervous habits that drive everyone crazy, but it doesn't at all bother the child who's doing it. It can be brought about by dental malocclusion or by the child's feeling frustrated, unable to verbalize his anger, resentment, or everyday stress. Bruxism can make dental problems worse by wearing away the teeth's superficial enamel. It can cause headaches by contributing to jaw muscle fatigue and temporomandibular joint pain. Calming the child and distracting him helps to alleviate the problem. A dentist or orthodontist may supply a plastic appliance for temporary relief. Praise and rewards to the child for lengthening the periods that he does not grind are more successful than reprimands. Psychological referral may be appropriate if there are underlying emotional problems. Bruxism can also be the child's response to the anal itching of pinworms. (Refer to the entry on "Pinworms" on page 257.)

Head banging: Rhythmic head banging or rocking may take place when the child is alone or asleep. These self-stimulating movements sometimes reflect a lack of loving attention and tactile stimulation for these children. Similar activities include hair twisting and pulling as well as excessive masturbation. They signal the need for professional help only if they interfere with normal age-appropriate activities. Refer to the section on "Head Banging" in the entry on "Sleeping and Bedtime Problems" on page 289.

Stuttering: Refer to the entry on "Stuttering" on page 316.

Repetitive Muscle Tics: Hitting or biting parts of one's own body, blinking the eyes, making grimaces, smacking the lips, clearing the throat, shrugging—are all examples of nervous tics that may start out as intended movements but can become recurrent mannerisms that help the child deal with tension and stress. These tics do not occur while the child is asleep. Parents should try not to focus on the tics and not to reprimand their child, because the tics are involuntary, not deliberate. As a matter of fact, it is a good idea to reassure the child that he will soon be able to gain control over the tics and make them go away. Positive reinforcement, like rewards and compliments for increasing periods without tics, is more successful. Avoid stimulant medications, such as some decongestants, which can increase the tendency.

Gilles de la Tourette Syndrome: This rare condition demonstrates the extremes of tics. The children and adolescents with the syndrome exhibit compulsive barking and shouting of obscene words. Haloperidol is a medicine that has been effective for some of these patients.

Newborn's Appearance

THE PICTURES of "newborn" babies in magazines and baby books are usually of babies who are six months old. They are, inevitably, gorgeous. In the real world, newborn babies have a lot of "normal peculiarities." Don't be disappointed when you first see your new baby. Underneath the blood, vernix (see below), and amniotic fluid is your own gorgeous baby. Within one to two weeks, most of the "normal peculiarities" will disappear.

Skin:

At birth, babies are covered with a white, thick, "cheesy" material called vernix. This protective covering is washed off after birth, though some of it always manages to stick behind the newborn's ear. Simply wash it away. Although the skin is initially pink and the baby has a ruddy complexion, if the baby becomes cold, the skin can be pale, mottled, or bluish. The hands, feet, and tip of the penis are most likely to exhibit this bluish color, on and off, for a few weeks. Due to the pressure in the birth canal, some babies are born with black and blue marks all over their faces. These purple discolorations will fade over one to two weeks. After a few days, the skin may develop a yellowish tint.

Refer to the entry on "Jaundice in the Newborn" on page 201. Black babies are lighter-skinned at birth than they will be later. Fingertips and earlobes indicate the true color.

A newborn's skin is thicker than it will be at any other time in his life, because of the superficial layers of skin that accumulated during the nine months in utero. In the first weeks of life, the skin may seem dry and scaly. What's happening is that every time the baby rubs against something, the skin sheds some of the outermost layers. Although this gives the appearance of dryness, don't use ointments, creams, or oils, because they will only plug up the small sweat glands, causing pimples and a heat rash. Bathe the baby daily in pleasantly warm water with a gentle shampoo and soap. (Don't be afraid to shampoo the soft spot on the head.) As the superficial layers of skin are shed, the soft, delicate, thin, "newborn" skin will appear.

A baby's face should be washed daily with a mild soap, just like the rest of the body. After all, the face is more exposed to dirt than the parts of the body that are covered all day. Powder is helpful over the trunk and extremities, especially in creases and in areas of friction. It is appropriate to apply a barrier cream (such as Desitin or A and D Ointment) to the diaper area to protect the skin from urine, stool, and sweat. Wipe the cream away completely (especially from the hip and thigh creases) and reapply with each diaper change.

Some babies are born with fine hair on their backs and shoulders. This lanugo will normally rub off during the first month of life.

Refer to the entry on "Birthmarks" on page 25, and to the Index for individual rashes.

Nails:

Refer to the entry on "Nails" on page 232, for care of fingernails and toenails and for treatment of ingrown toenails.

Head:

A baby's head has a larger diameter than any other part of its body. As a result, the head is the most likely part of the body to reflect the trauma of passing through the narrow birth canal. Commonly, the head molds into a long, narrow "conehead." This shaping is most marked in firstborn infants. It also occurs if the head was stuck in the birth canal, necessitating a Caesarean section. The molding goes away in a few days, leaving a nice round head.

A large bump on the back or side of the newborn's head, called a cephalhematoma, reflects the banging and friction between the baby's scalp and the mother's birth canal. The resulting bruises can be one-sided or bilateral. They are usually harmless, and the overlying scalp can be touched, cleaned, and washed just like the rest of the head. These accumulations of fluid and blood are not associated with brain damage and will disappear in two to three months.

If forceps are used to pull the baby out, they may leave red or purplish pressure marks anywhere on the head or face. These will disappear in a few days.

It is normal to feel, and sometimes see, ridges across the top, sides, and back of a baby's head. They may represent normal "bumps" of the skull, or they may be the areas where one skull bone meets another. Sometimes these areas, called sutures, overlap. They will usually even out in a few weeks.

It is an old wives' tale that a baby will lose his hair if he doesn't wear a hat every time he goes outside. Actually, it is normal for most newborns to become temporarily bald. Refer to the entry on "Hair Loss" on page 153.

Eyes:

Newborns are able to see, but they have difficulty in focusing. By the time they are one month of age, they can focus for a distance equal to their arm's length. Each month, that distance increases. By six months they can see clearly a distance of twelve feet. One-year-olds see almost as well as adults.

The eyelids may be puffy due to the pressure on them while the baby traveled through the birth canal. This swelling will disappear within three days.

Caucasian babies are usually born with bluish-gray eyes. Black babies usually have brownish-gray eyes. The permanent color of the iris cannot be determined until the baby is six months old. The sclerae (whites) of a baby's eyes may turn yellow. Refer to the entry on "Jaundice in the Newborn" on page 201. Sometimes the pressure in the birth canal causes small blood vessels to burst in the whites of the eyes. These red streaks and blotches will disappear in two to three weeks.

If one or both eyes are always watery, the baby may have one or both tear ducts blocked with mucus. Refer to the section on "Blocked Tear Ducts" in the entry on "Eyes" on page 129.

Strabismus (crossed or "lazy" eyes) is discussed in the section on "Strabismus" in the entry on "Eyes" on page 129.

If one eye appears larger than the other and there is a hazy or fuzzy film over the iris, the colored part of the eye, the baby may have congenital glaucoma, an internal increase of pressure in the eye. Another cause of cloudiness of the eye is a cataract. Both conditions require medical and ophthalmological attention.

Birthmarks on the eyelids are discussed in the entry on "Birthmarks" on page 25.

Nose:

Initially, babies are "obligate nose-breathers." This means that, because of their anatomy, they have to breathe through their noses, not their mouths. Unfortunately, even the slightest bit of nasal mucus or a small foreign body, like lint, can block the nasal passageway and make the breathing sound stuffy or snorty. The nasal congestion is similar to what the baby experiences with a cold. Frequent suctioning of the nostrils with a nasal aspirator or catheter can further irritate the nose, causing more congestion. In all these cases, infants easily resort to mouth breathing. Similarly, a sneeze does not necessarily represent a cold or an allergy in a baby. It is the baby's reflex mechanism for clearing away foreign bodies, just as we clear our throats. If the baby is able to close his mouth around a nipple and suck well, then he is breathing fine through his nose, no matter how stuffed he sounds. A humidifier or vaporizer in the bedroom is all he needs.

Many newborns have tiny white bumps on their noses, cheeks, foreheads, and chins. These plugged skin pores, called milia, will disappear within two months through normal washing. No lotions, creams, or ointments are needed.

Ears:

Often a newborn's ears are soft and folded over. They will assume their normal shape after a few weeks. Since ears and kidneys are formed at the same embryonic stage, any congenital anomaly of the ear may lead the doctor to order tests to rule out a problem with the kidneys. Some babies are born with a skin tag or dimple just in front of one ear or both. They are of cosmetic significance only as long as they do not become infected.

Mouth:

The friction of sucking sometimes produces a callus or blister on the upper lip. It will disappear when the baby drinks from a cup. No treatment is necessary.

Refer to the entry on "Tongue-Tie" on page 347.

Little white cysts, called Epstein's pearls, are frequently seen on the hard palate, the roof of the baby's mouth. These blocked mucous glands will disappear within two months.

"Natal" teeth may be present at birth. Ten percent of these are extra teeth, and 90 percent are normal primary (baby) teeth that have erupted too soon. The extra teeth should be removed before they loosen and pose the danger of choking. The primary teeth will have to be removed, too, if they get loose.

Breasts:

Many male and female babies have swollen breasts for the first few months of life. This is due to the mother's hormones, which cross the placenta and stimulate the baby's breasts. Sometimes these enlarged tissues actually secrete milk (called witch's milk) through the nipples. Do not be alarmed and do not squeeze the milk out, because that could cause an infection. Once the umbilical cord is cut, so that mother's hormones no longer enter the baby, these tissues will shrink and stop secreting milk.

Chest:

The lower tip of the sternum, the breastbone, is a small piece of bone called the xiphoid process. Since, in the newborn, it is only loosely connected to the rest of the sternum, it seems to protrude and move on its own in the area where the chest meets the abdomen. It will eventually flatten out, although it may still be felt easily in many older children and adults.

Abdomen:

A baby's abdomen is larger than his chest, so all babies have pot bellies, as do most children until they are two to four years of age. At that age the muscles on either side of the abdomen join together to flatten the abdomen. Even thin two-year olds have pot bellies. This is also why umbilical hernias are so common. The contents of the midline umbilicus, the bellybutton, protrude until the overlying muscles join and push back this hernia. The hernia (not to be confused with an inguinal or groin hernia) may last for a few years but is harmless. Taping coins on an umbilical hernia or applying a belly band is of no therapeutic value. Surgery is reserved for the rare cases in which these hernias persist, causing cosmetic and psychological problems.

Umbilical Cord:

The clamp on the newborn's umbilical cord is removed before the baby goes home from the hospital. Otherwise, your pediatrician can remove it in the office. The cord itself will wither, dry, and fall off within the first two to three weeks. Sometimes a little piece of the base of the umbilical cord will remain. Your doctor can cauterize this granuloma with a silver nitrate stick to sterilize it and help it fall off sooner. Keeping the umbilical cord dry prevents it from getting infected and makes it fall off sooner. This is why, when you are sponge-bathing the baby, you should try to keep the cord dry. Once it falls off, you can submerge the baby's body in the bath. Many parents like to roll down the top of the diaper so that the urine and stool do not contaminate the umbilical cord. Rubbing alcohol should be applied with a cotton swab to the base of the cord (where it attaches to the abdomen) twice a day to keep it dry and clean. Stop applying the alcohol once the cord falls off. It is not unusual for the umbilicus to bleed slightly, on and off, for a few weeks after the cord falls off. If the skin around the bellybutton reddens, swells, or develops a foul odor, consult your pediatrician.

Vagina:

Refer to the entry on "Vagina" on page 366. The vagina, clitoris, and hymen frequently appear swollen in the newborn because the mother's stimulating hormones have crossed the placenta. These swellings will decrease in two to four weeks. A whitish or blood-tinged discharge (called false menstruation, or pseudomenses) sometimes occurs in the first or second week as the lining of the baby's uterus sheds in response to the withdrawal of the mother's hormones. This should not recur. The hymen commonly has pronounced skin tags, which also decrease in size as the effects of the mother's estrogen subsides over two to four weeks.

Penis:

Refer to the entry on "Penis" on page 248. Erections are normal in a newborn. They usually occur when the bladder is full, so if your baby has an erection . . . watch out and reach for the diaper!

Scrotum:

Just as the newborn female's genitalia sometimes appear swollen, so too do the genitalia of newborn boys. A swollen, enlarged scrotum is usually a temporary response to maternal hormones or to the trauma of bumping around in the birth canal.

Some baby boys have a hydrocele. This is a painless collection of clear fluid squeezed into the scrotum during birth. It may take up to a year for the fluid to be fully absorbed by the body. If it changes size or has a bluish discoloration, the scrotum may also contain a hernia, which will require medical attention.

Refer to the entry on "Testes" on page 333.

Back:

It is both common and normal for a small dimple or pit to appear at the base of the spine, sometimes hidden by the upper part of the fold of the buttocks. This sacral dimple will require medical attention if it issues a discharge or if there is hair or a lump near it. Although it should not be probed or poked, it can be washed and cleaned as part of the regular bath.

Hips:

Refer to the section on "Congenital Dislocation of Hip" in the entry on "Hips" on page 181.

Legs:

It is normal for babies to be "bow-legged," that is, to have their lower legs curved inward. This is because of the cross-legged position the baby assumes in utero. The bowing is most obvious when the baby is one year old, but the legs will straighten out in most children by two years. If the feet complete the bow by turning inward, they are "pigeon-toed" and may need exercises, special shoes, braces or splints, and, in severe cases, casts to straighten the legs. It is normal for feet to turn outward. If the feet are flexible and easily movable in all directions, they are normal. Refer to the entry on "Feet" on page 132.

Nosebleeds

A NOSEBLEED (also called epistaxis) can frighten a child, but it is rarely serious. In addition, it usually looks as if more blood is lost than is the case; a little blood can spread over a wide area. When the blood vessels inside the nose become fragile (from a dry environment, common cold, allergies, trauma, etc.), they easily bleed. Check under your child's fingernails for signs of dried blood, evidence that he has been picking his nose. The nose may bleed again within the next few days with very little trauma, so don't be surprised if there is blood on the pillowcase the morning after a nosebleed.

The importance of a nosebleed is whether it signifies a bleeding tendency. Is the child prone to other bleeding problems? Is there blood in his stool? Do his gums bleed easily when he brushes his teeth? When he gets a cut on his skin, does it continue bleeding beyond the expected length of time? If the answer to these questions is no, then the nosebleed is probably not of clinical importance.

Old wives' tales abound on how to treat a nosebleed. Sound medical advice, however, dictates the following:

TIPS:

1. The child should be sitting erect, with his head straight—not tilted down, which could increase the

blood flow to the nose, and not tilted back, which could cause him to swallow the blood. Swallowed blood upsets the child's stomach and may make him vomit.

2. Using a cold compress, pinch the sides of the nose together, below the hard, bony part. Don't put ice directly on the nose or face, because it could irritate the skin. Wrap the ice in a wet washcloth or other covering. Do not put the cold compress under the nose, behind the head, or on the forehead.

3. Hold the pressure on the nose for *ten minutes without peeking.* If one relieves the pressure every minute or two to check on the bleeding, a clot will not be able to form.

4. Keep a cool-mist vaporizer in the child's bedroom. The humidity will soothe the inner lining of the nose.

5. That night, gently place some petroleum jelly (Vaseline) just inside the nostril to help prevent drying.

6. Your doctor may suggest the use of Neosynephrine nosedrops after the nosebleed or later that night to help shrink the involved blood vessels. Nosedrops should never be used for more than four days, because at that point they begin to irritate the inner lining of the nose and cause a nasal discharge. Overmedication with nosedrops is called rhinitis medicamentosum.

7. Keep your child's fingernails short to lower the chance of irritation during the finger's inevitable trip into the nose.

8. Aspirin should be avoided, as it increases the body's tendency to bleed. This could make nosebleeds last longer.

If the nosebleeds keep recurring, your doctor may decide to cauterize the lining of the nose with a silver nitrate stick. If this does not help, he may want to do some blood tests and refer you to an ENT (ear, nose, and throat) specialist. In addition, your pediatrician will check your child's blood pressure for hypertension.

The day after a nosebleed, it is prudent to check that a large clot (hematoma) has not stayed in the nose. It can make it uncomfortable for the child to breathe and can become a culture medium for bacteria. A serious infection can result. Simply shine a flashlight into the involved nostril. If a large, dark, boggy mass—the clot—blocks your view into the nostril, notify your doctor.

Finally, don't be surprised if the child's stools are very dark for the next day or two. The discoloration is due to the blood that was swallowed from the nosebleed.

Osgood-Schlatter Disease

YOUNG adolescents who are physically active are prone to an overuse syndrome of the tibial tubercle—the small elevation one to two inches directly below the knee. Drs. Osgood and Schlatter described this condition. Both tubercles are often tender to the touch and swell with pain when the child runs, jumps, uses the stairs, or kneels. The problem is caused by the strong quadriceps thigh muscles pulling at their insertion on the tibial tubercle. Involvement in sports, together with a growth spurt, may separate pieces of cartilage from bone. The knee joint itself is not involved.

Since the problem will usually disappear when the adolescent stops growing, temporizing measures are appropriate. Any sports or activities that induce pain or require kneeling should be restricted. Stretching exercises before strenuous activities are helpful. If the teenager refuses to curtail activities, he may need a knee-immobilizing splint or cast to "force" him to rest. Cold compresses, oral analgesics, and anti-inflammatory medications are also helpful. Although the long-term prognosis is excellent, a small bump may remain at the tibial tubercle.

Pacifiers

PACIFIERS are perfectly all right for a baby to use. Sometimes babies just want to suck, and don't want or need milk or food. The sucking reflex remains for several months after birth, during which time a pacifier can be useful to calm the baby. It is not a good idea to put sugar or other sweet items on the tip of the pacifier.

On the other hand, once your baby reaches six months, when the sucking reflex is already gone, or once his first teeth erupt, you should be aggressive about throwing the pacifier away, because pacifiers can cause problems with the teeth. The pressure of the pacifier against teeth can, after prolonged use, result in bottle mouth syndrome. Even the permanent teeth may be malformed, misshapen, and weakened. Refer to the entry on "Bottle Mouth Syndrome" on page 34. Aside from contributing to tooth problems, prolonged pacifier use is felt by some experts to cause a tongue-thrust habit. If your child needs a security or "love" object, offer a doll, stuffed animal, or a blanket. The child's stopping the pacifier at an early age will avoid his psychological pain at having it taken away later, when he is more attached to it.

TIPS:

1. Since you will stop allowing a pacifier at the proper time, it doesn't matter if you offer a Nuk, Premie, or any other type *as long as it has the large (at least one-and-a-half-inch diameter) protective ring barrier behind the nipple* to prevent your baby from swallowing and aspirating the pacifier. Many home-made pacifiers don't have this protective ring. Their use should be discouraged.

2. Do not tie a pacifier around your child's neck or hand, as there have been reports of strangulation by the string.

3. Avoid pacifiers with a liquid center, because some have been found to be contaminated with bacteria.

Penis

Care:

AT BIRTH, the newborn's entire penis (shaft plus glans or tip) is covered by the foreskin. The foreskin will separate from the glans, but this may take up to five or ten years. The foreskin may retract by itself as the baby has erections, which are normal from birth on. All boys discover their penises as they become aware of their bodies and may retract the foreskin themselves. It is common and normal for the foreskin not to retract easily early in life. The foreskin is retractable in 25 percent of babies six months old, 50 percent of those a year old, 80 percent by two years, and 90 percent by five years. Do not forcibly retract or manipulate the foreskin. That can cause pain and bleeding and may sometimes worsen the problem by forming new adhesions (tight connecting bands) between the foreskin and glans. Only a gentle retraction of the loose foreskin once a week, during a bath, is needed.

The whitish pearls, called smegma, which accumulate around the inside of the foreskin are normal skin cells and oils that are shed from the glans and the inner lining of the foreskin. The foreskin and penis should be bathed and sponged daily, which will gently wash away the smegma. No special care, such as use of Q-Tips, is required. Soap and water will suffice. Once the foreskin can fully retract, cleaning beneath it should be part of the daily bath.

New parents sometimes worry when the tip of the penis seems to "disappear" or "go in" and hide from sight. Actually, the penis is perfectly fine and is not shrinking in size at all. It is merely being engulfed by the surrounding fat pad of the lower abdomen and then being covered by its foreskin. Gently pushing down on the surrounding fat pad will make the penis reappear and reassure you that it is fine.

Frequently the protected tip of the penis and outer surface of the foreskin become irritated by contact with urine and stool in the diaper or detergent in the underpants. This may occur on hot, humid days or during bouts of diarrhea. Gentle, frequent soap washes and applications of an antiseptic ointment, like Neosporin, three to four times a day will help the healing. Change diapers frequently. Use a thin coating of barrier cream such as Desitin, Balmex, or A and D Ointment to protect the penis and perineum from contact with urine, stool, and sweat, even when there is no irritation.

Circumcision:

Circumcision is the surgical removal of the foreskin. It has been performed for many centuries for religious, social, and health reasons. Followers of the Jewish and Moslem faiths perform circumcisions for religious reasons. Today, however, circumcision is an emotionally charged issue. There are passionate advocates as well as die-hard critics. The current rate of circumcision among newborns in the United States is about 60 percent. The following chart summarizes some of the pros and cons cited by medical and lay literature.

PRO	CON
1. One of the few medical reasons to do a circumcision is the presence of a phimosis, a rare congenital condition of abnormal tightness and narrowing of the tip of the foreskin to the size of a pin hole. This can ob-	1. The foreskin is not some comical mistake. It protects the glans from urine, stool, and external irritation. It serves a sexual function by protecting the sensitive glans. True phimosis is extremely rare. The Na-

PENIS

struct the stream of urine. The urine may just dribble out, spray in all directions, or the foreskin may balloon from the pressure of the urine. Since urine can accumulate between the tight foreskin and glans and since it is hard to clean there properly, infections of the glans and foreskin develop. Phimosis never becomes wide enough to allow the foreskin to retract. This leads to difficulty in normal sexual development because erections are painful for adolescents and men. The treatment for phimosis is a circumcision.

tional Organization of Circumcision Resource Centers (NOCIRC) and the International Organization Against Circumcision Trauma (INTACT) are lay organizations that are trying to keep penises uncircumcised. No other animal species needs to be circumcised. Circumcision rates have fallen to 1 percent of newborn males in Britain, 10 percent in New Zealand, 40 percent in Canada. Few Asian or South American countries practice this ritual. It is a cosmetic procedure, like ear piercing and lip stretching. Studies have failed to demonstrate that circumcision in any way affects sexual performance or pleasure of either partner.

2. Several studies of large numbers of male babies in the 1970s and 1980s conclude that uncircumcised infants and children have a significantly higher incidence of urinary tract infections than circumcised males. Their conclusion is that removal of the foreskin facilitates genital hygiene

2. Proper hygiene reduces the incidence of penile inflammatory disorders in the young child and decreases the need for circumcision. The incidence of urinary tract infection in the uncircumcised child is low enough (about 1 percent) not to warrant routine circumcision of all male

PRO

and reduces contamination of the tip of the glans, thus reducing the chances of an ascending bladder or kidney infection. The most common bacterium isolated from the foreskin of adults is Group B streptococcus. It is one cause of severe neonatal infections.

3. The delicate foreskin is easily bruised and cut during sexual activities. This renders uncircumcised men more susceptible to sexually transmitted diseases like syphilis and herpes that spread via a break in the skin. Further, these foreskin abrasions predispose men to HIV infection by providing a site for transfer of infected cervical secretions. This puts uncircumcised men at a higher risk for contracting AIDS from both heterosexual and homosexual exposure than circumcised men.

4. Routine circumcision of newborns almost completely eliminates the possibility of cancer of the penis. Not only does cancer of the penis occur

CON

newborns. Most of the penile infections that do occur are not likely to progress to bladder or kidney infections. After circumcision, the tip of the penis is not covered and protected by the foreskin. Ammonia from urine-soaked diapers can irritate the glans.

3. In preventing the transmission of venereal diseases in general and of AIDS in particular, circumcision is not as effective as limiting the number of sexual contacts or using condoms properly. Even circumcised penises get sexually transmitted diseases. Variables like access to medical care, geographic location, hygiene, lifestyle, race, and socioeconomic factors play roles just as important in sexually transmitted diseases as circumcision.

4. The incidence of penile cancer is so low that routine, universal newborn circumcision is not indicated. Other variables (such as hygiene, family

PRO

CON

almost exclusively in un-circumcised men, but some doctors feel that cancer of the uterine cervix is less common in the female sexual partners of circumcised men.

history, sexual history, etc.) also are factors. Other more important elements are associated with cervical cancer in the female partner: age of first intercourse, number of sexual partners, possible viral transmission, family history, nutrition, and hygiene.

5. Circumcision is considered a relatively simple and safe procedure. The most common complications—infection and bleeding—are usually minor and preventable. Bleeding can be controlled with pressure or, rarely, with a suture. Good hygiene will control infection. Marking how much skin to take off before doing the procedure ensures that the correct amount of foreskin is removed.

5. Routine circumcision is not a simple procedure or one without peril. Excessive bleeding is the most frequent complication. Infections occur, just as after any surgical procedure. If insufficient skin is removed, the end ring of the foreskin may heal by contracting and thickening, thus producing a phimosis.

6. The infant's responses to the pain of circumcision are short, lasting only minutes. Use of a sweet-flavored pacifier seems to relieve pain and reduce crying.

6. Infants who are circumcised without anesthesia feel pain. Some doctors use a local anesthetic to deaden the nerves of the foreskin, but this too is not without risk (local blood clots, heart arrhythmias, etc.).

PRO

7. Routine newborn circumcision is a cost-efficient procedure because it results in a national saving by preventing penile cancer and eliminating the need for a later, more costly, circumcision for phimosis and infection.

8. Since the majority of males in the U.S. are still being circumcised, other boys want to "look like" the majority and like their fathers. It can be emotionally painful to be harassed about the appearance of one's genitals in the locker room.

CON

7. Because it is no longer considered a medical necessity, some health insurers and welfare programs refuse to pay or reimburse for a routine circumcision. Some medical economists feel that the cost of neonatal circumcision exceeds the benefits.

8. Fewer children are being circumcised now than several years ago. Only 60 percent of males are being circumcised now in the U.S., whereas 90 percent were circumcised in 1979.

It is wise to review a family's decision not to circumcise their baby boy at the routine two-week visit because the simple newborn procedure can still be done at this age without great risks if the parents have changed their minds.

Before any circumcision is done, the baby should be healthy, stable, and should have been examined by a doctor. He will determine whether there is a family history of hemophilia or other bleeding problems. Certain penile congenital anomalies (such as hypospadias, in which the urethral opening is in an abnormal location, and chordee, in which restrictive bands along the shaft of the penis do not let it extend to its full erect height) are contraindications to circumcision. The extra foreskin may be needed for future urological reconstructive surgery to repair these conditions.

Doctors are constantly weighing the risks versus the

benefits of certain drugs, procedures, lab tests, etc. The risks and benefits of a circumcision are too small to swing the vote universally either way, so it remains a decision to be made by the parents, not by the doctor. Their ultimate decision may hinge on nonmedical pros and cons.

The doctor doing the circumcision—or the *mohel*, ritual circumciser—offers advice about care of the penis after the circumcision. In general, the penis should be wiped gently with a soft cloth and warm water. Change the diapers frequently. If bleeding continues for a few hours, notify your doctor. A recently circumcised penis appears infected because it has some bright red areas and some patches of white, healing tissue. This is normal.

Penile Zipper Entrapment:

Penile zipper entrapment usually occurs when a young boy in a hurry, not paying attention to what he is doing, zips his fly before covering his penis with his underwear. The foreskin or shaft of the penis gets caught in the teeth of the zipper. This is both painful and frightening.

TIPS:

1. Apply a cold compress to the penis to relieve the pain while you help him.

2. With a pair of pliers or metal cutters, cut off the bottom end of the zipper. You may now be able to pry apart the zipper and release the penis.

3. Apply liberal amounts of mineral oil to the zipper and entrapped penile skin. With gentle traction, you may now be able to free the penis.

4. Wash the penis well in soapy warm water several times a day for the next four to five days.

5. Apply antibacterial ointment (e.g., Neosporin) to the damaged area four times a day. The boy may prefer to put the ointment on himself.

6. Give acetaminophen or ibuprofen for pain relief.

Pertussis

PERTUSSIS, also called whooping cough, is a dangerous childhood disease caused by a bacterium that produces thick tenacious mucus, which blocks the throat. As a result, spasms of coughing and choking, with redness of the face and bulging eyes, make it hard to breathe, eat, and drink. Immediately after the coughing attack comes the characteristic *whooping* sound as the child tries to draw in air through the swollen windpipes. Vomiting sometimes follows these spasms. The disease is very contagious and can last up to ten weeks. Humans are the only known hosts of the bacterium. It is spread by direct contact or coughing, and the incubation period is seven to fourteen days. About half of the babies with pertussis are so sick that they need to be hospitalized. One out of every 200 babies with the disease dies of it. In recent years, as many as 4200 cases have been reported yearly in the United States.

TIPS:

If you suspect your child has whooping cough:

1. Put him to bed. He may prefer an upright position.

2. Call your doctor. After examining the child, he may do a throat culture and treat with antibiotics.

3. Hospitalization is often necessary so that oxygen, intravenous fluids, and medicines can be administered and close observation maintained.

4. Encourage the child to drink extra fluids. It is more important for him to drink (especially clear liquids like water, tea, Jell-O, Gatorade, and broth) than it is for him to eat. Give him frequent sips rather than a lot at one time. Heavy meals may lead to vomiting.

5. Vigorous activity can induce coughing attacks. Try to keep the child entertained and quiet.

6. Do not smoke near the child.

7. Keep a cool-mist vaporizer in his room.

8. The best approach is prevention by immunizing against the disease with the DPT vaccine. See the entry on "Immunizations" on page 189.

Phenylketonuria

AMINO ACIDS are the chemical building blocks of the proteins in our bodies. Phenylketonuria (PKU) is an inherited disorder in which one of these amino acids—phenylalanine—accumulates in the body in abnormal amounts. This happens when there is a deficiency of the enzyme that normally breaks down phenylalanine. It occurs in 1 of 12,000 live births in the United States.

The legally required newborn screening test on blood taken from a baby's heel at two to three days after birth measures the amount of phenylalanine in the baby's blood. If a mother and her newborn are discharged from the hospital after just twenty-four to thirty-six hours, the baby may have to be brought to the office a few days later for this blood test. If the result is abnormal or borderline, the test should be repeated. If the diagnosis is confirmed, it is wise to measure all of the amino acids.

Although babies with this disorder appear normal at birth, the abnormal build-up of phenylalanine eventually damages the nervous system, causing developmental delays, mental retardation, seizures, autism, vomiting, hyperactivity, eczema, and a fair (or bleached) discoloration of hair and skin. If these children remain untreated, they develop a musty, pungent odor. As soon as the diagnosis is confirmed, the babies should be started on a formula low in phenylalanine, such as

Lofenalac or Phenyl-Free. Throughout their lives, these patients must be on a phenylalanine-restricted diet. Phenylalanine cannot be fully eliminated from the diet because a little is needed for normal growth. Some children can tolerate higher amounts of phenylalanine without problems when they reach adolescence. Blood tests at regular intervals will be needed to monitor the phenylalanine.

If treatment is begun by the time the baby is three weeks of age, the above complications can be avoided. Dietary control does not reverse the existing neurological problems, but it does prevent further damage. It will correct the skin rashes and depigmentation. Mothers with PKU who are not on dietary treatment throughout pregnancy have a higher incidence of giving birth to babies with birth defects, such as congenital heart disease and growth retardation.

PKU is inherited only if both parents carry the PKU gene. If there is a family history of PKU, genetic counseling should be obtained.

Pinworms

THE PINWORM is a common type of intestinal parasite that infects children in the United States. The condition is highly contagious and not necessarily associated with a dirty or nonhygienic environment, so it need not be a reason for embarrassment or disgrace.

The pinworm is white, thin, and small, less than one-half inch long. It looks like a small piece of white thread. The adult pinworm lives in the child's intestine and comes out at night to lay its eggs around the child's anus and buttocks. Since the pinworm is photophobic (afraid of light), it crawls back in during daylight. The tiny eggs cause local anal and vaginal itching and irritation. They are picked up by the child's fingers when he scratches and are transferred to the hands and mouths of playmates. Other eggs may drift into the air and be breathed in or swallowed in contaminated food. Dogs and cats do not carry or transmit pinworms. In severe infestations, some children complain of stomachaches and have poor appetites. Some have nightmares, and others grind their teeth. However, by far the greatest nuisance is the rectal itching. It may cause children to have difficulty in sleeping at night.

The Scotch tape test is used to help identify pinworms. Take a piece of clear (not opaque) Scotch tape and touch it to several areas around the child's rectum and surrounding skin. Do this early in the morning, so that the pinworms have had a chance to come out at night, but before the child gets out of bed, so that daylight does not chase the pinworms back in. Fold the Scotch tape so the nonsticky surface is exposed, place the tape in an envelope, and bring it to your pediatrician or local hospital lab on the same day. Even if the pinworms are not seen under a microscope their eggs can be identified. Occasionally, a parent can see the actual pinworms by shining a flashlight on the rectal area of an infected child in the dark, late at night.

Rarely, your doctor can determine the presence of pinworms on a routine blood count due to the presence of a certain type of white blood cells, called eosinophils.

TIPS:

1. Double-rinse sheets and pajamas.

2. Clean bed toys.

3. Cut fingernails and clean well. Wash the anus and genitals well each morning.

4. All family members should be checked and tested for pinworms.

5. Vermox (mebendazole) is a commonly used oral medicine against pinworms. Ninety-eight percent of this medicine is not absorbed by the body but travels through the intestinal tract, paralyzing the pinworms on its way. They will then be passed in the stool. The same dose—1 tablet given only once—is for children

and adults. All family members should be given it. The tablet may be chewed, swallowed whole, or crushed and mixed with food. Occasionally, your doctor may suggest a second dose two to three weeks later. Other medications are also available.

6. Be sure the child wears pajamas at night so that when he scratches, his hands won't pick up any eggs to reinfect him.

There are other types of worms a child can get through ingestion, from contact with other infected people, or from touching the contaminated feces of cats or dogs. Occasionally these cause unexplained fever and abdominal pain. If your child passes a worm, save it in a jar for identification. Otherwise, your doctor will ask you to obtain a stool specimen for inspection for ova and parasites. If necessary, special antiparasitic medicine will be prescribed.

Pityriasis Rosea

PITYRIASIS ROSEA (which means "rose-colored scale") is a common rash, thought to be viral in origin, that covers the trunk and extremities. It consists of a series of oval, raised, small (less than ½ inch), pink or light brown scaly lesions. The long axes of the oval lesions follow the normal skin lines on both sides of the body. This results in the typical "Christmas tree" distribution along the back, in which the lesions form interrupted or "dotted" lines that resemble branches of a pine tree. Another hallmark of pityriasis rosea is the "herald patch"—a single scaly, large (up to five inches in diameter) lesion that, in 50 to 70 percent of cases, occurs anywhere on the body approximately one to two weeks before the generalized rash appears. The herald patch may disappear before or during the generalized rash. The rash itself, which occurs equally in boys and girls, lasts anywhere from two to twelve weeks, and ranges from not at all itchy to very itchy. It is not contagious, so children may attend school, participate in all activities, and bathe as usual. Even close family contacts are unlikely to develop the disease.

Treatment is aimed at reducing the itching. Lubricating lotions, oral antihistamines, Aveeno oatmeal baths, or a topical steroid preparation will help. No treatment shortens the duration of the rash. Unless a secondary infection develops, there is no scarring. It is unlikely that the rash will recur in the same person.

Poisonings

CHILDREN ACT FAST . . . SO DO POISONS!

POISONINGS involve two million children under five years of age each year. Ninety-five percent occur in the home. Child safety closures have decreased the number and severity of childhood poisonings, as have containers that dispense certain products in nonlethal quantities. Some symptoms children manifest after ingesting a poison are loss of balance, irregular heartbeat, unusual breath odor, enlargement or shrinkage of the pupils of eyes, agitated behavior, burns around the mouth if the poison was corrosive, seizures (not associated with fever), and coma. Vomiting, cramps, and diarrhea are common symptoms of food poisoning.

TIPS:

1. Throw away all expired medications.

2. Ask the pharmacist to put only a small number of tablets in each of several bottles.

3. Keep all medications locked or in inaccessible places, such as *your* bathroom. Don't let your child watch you taking medicine. Always turn the light on to double-check a medicine when giving it to your child.

4. Use only child-resistant packaging and don't remove labels from any bottles.

5. Keep the local Poison Control Center telephone number accessible near several phones. You'll find it at the front of your phone book under "Emergency Numbers."

6. Keep a small bottle of ipecac in your home, but don't use it unless your doctor or the Poison Control Center tells you to. It is important to keep ipecac readily available because it is most effective if given within the first half-hour after the child ingested the poison. It induces vomiting by irritating the gastrointestinal tract. However, never try to make children vomit corrosive poisons, such as Drāno, bleach, oven cleaner, kerosene, turpentine, or gasoline. These can burn the esophagus and throat once again on their way up. Neutralize these with water while contacting the doctor. Likewise, syrup of ipecac should not be given to children who are drowsy, unconscious, or having seizures, or to children who have had certain stomach or esophagus surgeries. It should also not be used if the child swallowed a button battery or other small object that he could aspirate into his lungs when he vomits.

When ipecac is appropriate, use it the correct way:

Children 6–12 months: 2 teaspoons (10 ml or 10 cc)

1–12 years: 1 tablespoon (15 ml or 15 cc)

Adolescents: 2 tablespoons (30 ml or 30 cc)

Give 2 cups of water after each dose of ipecac. Some experts feel that having the child move and walk encourages the vomiting process. About 80 percent of children will vomit after 17 to 18 minutes. However, if 20 minutes pass without the child's vomiting, repeat the same dose. About 95 percent of children will vomit within 35 minutes of this second dose. Ipecac is available over the counter and lasts for several years without losing its effectiveness. If you do not have ipecac available, gag the child by placing your finger in the back of her throat.

7. Children should be tested periodically for lead poisoning. Refer to "Lead Poisoning" under "Safety Tips" on page 390.

8. Never put household cleaners in the same cabinets as food.

9. Never transfer leftover poisons to familiar empty food containers, like soda or milk containers, or empty cups.

10. Keep the jar, bottle, plant, berries, or can that contained the swallowed substance. Your doctor may need to have it tested. Bring the container to the phone so that you can read the exact name and contents to your doctor or Poison Control Center. If you are instructed to bring the child to the emergency room, bring the container with you. If possible, bring the child's vomitus as well. Drive carefully; you do not need to run red lights.

11. Never call medicine "candy."

12. Never run an automobile in an unventilated space, like a closed garage, for even a few minutes. Carbon monoxide has no smell and is invisible, but carbon monoxide poisoning can be lethal.

Aside from syrup of ipecac, your doctor may administer a slush of activated charcoal (by nasogastric tube, if necessary) to absorb the poison from the child's intestine. Some laxatives do the same. Sometimes antidotes are given to neutralize particular poisons. Blood and urine tests may be done. In some situations, hospitalization will be needed for observation, and, when necessary, to supply assistance for breathing, to administer intravenous fluids, and to follow neurological status. Sometimes the only treatment is to supply this supportive care until the poisonous material is used up by the body.

If the child swallows a small disc or button battery,

its location should be identified with x-rays. As noted above, do not give ipecac. If the object is lodged in the esophagus, it should be removed. If it is in the stomach and remains there for forty-eight hours, it should be removed. If it is beyond the stomach, and the child has no symptoms, just observe. Repeat the x-ray if the battery is not passed in the stool within five to seven days. If the child complains of abdominal pain or tenderness, the battery should be removed. The size, shape, and location of the swallowed article will determine whether it needs to be removed surgically or by a tube passed through the mouth into the stomach or intestine.

If a poison or corrosive chemical has spilled onto the child's skin or clothing, immediately remove the contaminated clothing. Flood the skin with plenty of water from a faucet or shower for fifteen minutes. Call your doctor or the Poison Control Center.

Before leaving this important topic, let's correct some myths. It is inappropriate to give vinegar or citric acid fruit juices to neutralize an alkali corrosive poison, like lye. The neutralizing reaction that occurs in the stomach causes heat to be formed, further worsening the burn injury. Similarly, sodium bicarbonate should not be given after an acid ingestion. The chemical reaction releases carbon dioxide in the stomach, distends it, and predisposes the stomach to perforation. The indiscriminate use of 4 percent whole milk to dilute a poison can actually increase the absorption of certain poisons, like camphor and gasoline. If you use any neutralizer, let it be water.

Remember, one moment is all it takes. . . . so take a moment to be poison-proof.

Polio

POLIOMYELITIS—polio, for short—is a serious viral infection of the spinal cord and nerves. It occurs only in humans. Although polio is rare today in the United States, there are many thousands of cases each year in other countries, so it is important to continue our immunization program against polio. Refer to the entry on "Immunizations" on page 189 for the recommended schedule of administration.

Polio starts like many other viral illnesses, with a fever, sore throat, headache, and muscle aches. Sometimes the illness stops with those typical viral symptoms without polio's even being suspected. In more serious cases, permanent paralysis develops. The incubation period is seven to twenty-one days. The legs are most commonly involved, making walking impossible. Paralysis can progress, calling for reliance on a respirator. Death can result from respiratory failure. The extent of the disease varies with each patient. It is spread by the fecal-oral and the respiratory routes. Antibiotics have no effect on this or any viral illness. The last epidemic in the United States occurred in 1979 among a group of people who had declined immunizations.

Returning to School and Day Care After Respiratory Infections

THERE ARE two main guidelines to follow when determining whether or not to send a child back to school after a respiratory illness:

1. The child should have no fever (i.e., temperature under 100° F rectally) for twenty-four hours.

2. The child should feel well enough to sit and concentrate in class, and any cough or cold symptoms should not be disruptive to the class.

It is not practical to rely on known incubation periods, or periods of time during which viruses are shed, because most children shed germs before they show the symptoms of their illnesses. Some illnesses shed viruses for weeks. If all children with runny noses stayed home, schools would have to close. Contact with respiratory infections simply cannot be avoided in a school or day care setting. Although it may be appropriate for your child to avoid gym and contact sports for a few days or weeks after some illnesses (e.g., flu, mono, pneumonia) until he gets his strength back, he can play with friends outside, attend parties and social events, and go on trips if he has had no fever for twenty-four hours. Keeping the child home at this stage of the illness will not prevent any complications.

Reye's Syndrome

REYE'S SYNDROME is a disease affecting children from infancy through the teen years, striking all races and sexes equally. It is a two-phased illness, because it is almost always associated with a previous viral infection, such as influenza or chickenpox. For a few days, the child seems to recover. Then, suddenly, there comes the second phase, consisting of violent vomiting, delirium, and even coma. These neurological symptoms can rapidly progress to death if treatment is not started early. A blood test drawn at the first sign of these abnormal symptoms will show a markedly abnormal liver. This aids in forming an early diagnosis. Reye's syndrome causes abnormal accumulations of fat in the liver and a severe increase of pressure in the brain.

The high incidence of this syndrome has decreased markedly, mostly due to awareness of the association between it and the use of aspirin by children with such viral illnesses as chickenpox and the flu. Aspirin is no longer recommended for fever-causing viral illnesses. Other terms for aspirin are acetylsalicylate, acetylsalicylic acid, salicylic acid, and salicylate. In 1974, 400 cases of Reye's syndrome were reported in the United States. In 1988, there were only 20 reported cases.

Treatment involves intensive care monitoring, intravenous fluids, and medications to control the brain pressure. The duration of the abnormal neurological symptoms is the best predictor of eventual outcome. Following a short course of mild symptoms, recovery can be complete. For more information on Reye's syndrome, call the Reye's Foundation at 1-800-233-7393.

A WARNING:

Pepto-Bismol contains aspirin among its ingredients. It should not be used if the child has chickenpox or flu.

Ringworm

RINGWORM is a fungal infection of the skin that typically produces an enlarging red ring of scaly, elevated, itchy tissue around a clear, normal-appearing center. When it occurs on the scalp, it usually makes the hair brittle and produces bald patches. The fungus can be transmitted through combs, brushes, hats, barrettes, and pillows. When ringworm is in the groin area, it is called "jock itch." It is spread by direct contact between people and can be caught from household pets or from soil. The fact that it forms one or several rings leads to the misnomer of "worm." Actually, it has nothing to do with worms. It may be confused with eczema or psoriasis when, as occasionally happens, there is no central clearing. The child may return to school after two days of treatment.

TIPS:

1. Your pediatrician will prescribe an antifungal cream or powder for the skin and an oral antifungal medicine for scalp lesions, because creams do not penetrate into the hair follicles to kill the fungus. Use the cream or powder for at least one week after the rash seems to have left. Antifungal shampoos also help cure ringworm of the scalp.

2. Have your child use separate towels and washcloths until the infection is gone. Wash hands well.

3. Have your veterinarian check your pet for ringworm.

Roseola

ROSEOLA, also called infant measles, sixth disease, and exanthem subitum, is a viral illness that can affect children between six months and two years of age. It has several unique features:

1. A very high fever (as high as 105° F) is typical for two to five days.

2. Although the child's parents and pediatrician are extremely concerned during these days, the child is unusually high spirited and does not seem very ill.

3. After the fever breaks, a rash develops, and parents and the pediatrician feel much better because now, in retrospect, they know the diagnosis is roseola. The rash consists of faint, nonitchy, red spots and bumps that first appear on the trunk but soon spread over the whole body. The rash fades over one to three days. Occasionally, swollen glands develop on the back of the neck.

4. It is not known how roseola is spread, but children who have it are considered contagious and should be kept indoors until they are fever-free for twenty-four hours. The incubation period is five to fifteen days.

5. Roseola is a benign disease, its only problems coming from the high fever.

6. There are no diagnostic tests for roseola.

7. Refer to the entry on "Fever" on page 134 for treatment.

Rubella

RUBELLA, also called German measles, is a contagious viral illness that is mild unless it is caught by a nonimmune pregnant woman in the first three months of her pregnancy. It is spread by coughing and sneezing, and it causes fever, swollen glands in the front and back of the neck, swollen and tender joints, tiredness, headache, and a rash. The rash, which lasts two to three days, starts on the head as flat or slightly raised red spots and spreads downward, covering the trunk in twenty-four hours. The incubation period is three weeks, and the patient gains lifelong immunity after contracting the disease. The contagious period is from one week before the rash until one week after its first appearance, so the child should not return to school until a week after the rash first shows up. Only rarely do serious complications, like encephalitis or bleeding tendencies, develop in the infected child. Since the disease is usually mild, the only way a definite diagnosis can be made is by doing blood tests to measure rubella antibodies during the illness and to document their increase four weeks later.

If a woman contracts rubella during the first month of her pregnancy, there is a 50 percent chance that the fetus will develop congenital anomalies. By the third month of pregnancy, the risk decreases to 10 percent, and it continues to drop throughout the pregnancy. The birth defects caused by rubella in a pregnant mother include heart disease, blindness, deafness, and learning disabilities. These babies are said to have the congenital rubella syndrome, and they can shed the rubella virus for months to years after birth, so they are a serious source of infection for other nonimmune children and adults, especially pregnant women. About one out of every ten women in the United States is not protected against rubella. If any pregnant woman is in contact with your child while he has rubella, notify her of his condition. If the pregnant woman is not immune, her doctor may administer a gamma globulin shot immediately. All nonimmune women who receive the rubella vaccine or who are exposed to rubella should avoid getting pregnant for three months. There is no evidence that rubella immunization of a child whose mother is in the early stages of pregnancy carries any risk of infection to the fetus. No woman who has rubella antibodies (because she had the illness or has received the vaccine) can develop rubella when pregnant, and the virus cannot affect her fetus, even if she is exposed to the virus while pregnant.

TIPS:

1. Treat the fever as described in the entry on "Fever" on page 134.

2. Encourage the child to drink extra fluids.

3. Oral and/or topical antihistamines will soothe itching, as will an Aveeno bath.

4. Antibotics do not help this or other viral illnesses.

5. For details of the rubella vaccine, refer to the entry on "Immunizations" on page 189.

Scabies

SCABIES is a highly contagious skin disease caused by a mite too small to be seen with the naked eye. It respects neither age, sex, nor socioeconomic status. It is transmitted by close personal contact, like crowded living conditions or shared beds. Since the mite cannot survive for more than three days away from human skin, scabies is only rarely caught from clothing or bedding. Despite the disease's contagious nature, it is not unusual to find a child with the condition in an otherwise unaffected family.

The most common symptom is a rash that itches intensely at night. Since small infants cannot effectively scratch, they may sleep fitfully and be cranky. The main lesions are burrows, caused by the burrowing mites. These burrows frequently get obscured by scratches and secondary impetigo. Lesions are most often found below the neck, in the webs of the fingers, armpits, waistlines, genitals, and around the nipples. In infants, the palms, soles, head, and neck are also affected. It is possible to catch scabies from animals. Since the rash develops anywhere from three to thirty days after exposure, children may infect others before it is apparent that they themselves are infected. This is why your pediatrician may recommend that the entire family be treated.

Two preparations for the treatment of scabies are Kwell lotion or cream and Elimite cream. Follow directions carefully, as the cream usually needs to be applied for several hours or overnight. If the child is a thumbsucker, cover his hand with a sock or other wrap to prevent him from ingesting the scabicide. Do not apply the medicine immediately after a hot bath, since the warmth increases absorption and the risk of toxicity (e.g., seizures). When using Kwell, you may repeat the treatment in one week. Because of its known toxicity, Kwell should not be used for children under six months of age or by pregnant women. Elimite can be used on children over two months of age.

Even if the insect is effectively killed, itching may persist for several weeks. Oral antihistamines (e.g., Benadryl) and topical anti-itching agents (including steroids) can help. Intensive efforts to decontaminate clothing and bedding are unnecessary and serve only to reinforce the incorrect notion that a household reservoir exists. Normal laundering and dry cleaning of clothes and bed linens are all that are necessary. Clothing that has not been in contact with human skin for three to four days cannot transmit scabies.

Parents should understand that having scabies does not imply poor hygiene. Frequent and overzealous bathing is not necessary, because bathing too often can dry out the skin and worsen itching. After repeated exposure to the mites, reinfections are usually milder. Children can return to day care or school the day after the first treatment has been completed.

Scoliosis

SCOLIOSIS is a curvature of the spine to the right or left. Although it usually develops at adolescence, it can be seen even in babies, though rarely. It is familial and is five to eight times more common in females than males. It can develop as a result of an injury or infection (e.g., polio) to the muscles or bones of the back or as a result of one leg's being shorter than the other. However, in the majority of cases, no cause is found. If it is detected early, its progression to an obvious deformity can be prevented. If it is left untreated, a "humpback" can form, and the patient can develop problems with breathing as the vertebrae and ribs literally squash the lungs.

Your child's doctor will test for scoliosis as part of the annual physical exam. Notify your pediatrician if you notice:

- One leg shorter than the other
- Shirts or pants hanging unevenly
- Uneven shoulders
- Uneven scapulae (wing bones) of the back
- Uneven hips

Some curves never increase, but others remain stable for years, only to increase rapidly during the adolescent growth spurt. If your doctor finds scoliosis, he will order x-rays and a consultation with an orthopedist. Mild cases will just require close observation, perhaps with some exercises. Moderate curves will require the child to wear a special back brace until she stops growing. In severe cases, surgical correction with insertion of a rod into the spine may be necessary.

Another cause of uneven shoulders is the child's common habit of carrying heavy items (especially bookbags) over the same shoulder every day. If your child must carry all those heavy books, have her alternate shoulders every day or use a backpack over both shoulders. For children or teenagers with scoliosis, consider the wise investment of buying or renting a second set of textbooks to keep at home so that she doesn't have to "shlep" these books back and forth each day. Many states have mandated school-screening programs for scoliosis for children between ten and eighteen years of age.

TIPS:

1. When your child is being examined for scoliosis, be sure her shoes are off and that she wears a gym outfit, a swimsuit, or other clothing so that her back and front can be viewed easily. If a curvature is detected by the school program, the child should be examined by her pediatrician. If scoliosis is detected in one child, be sure to have all siblings checked.

2. At the risk of sounding like a nagging parent, my best advice to the teenager with a slouching posture is "Be proud of every inch of height that you have." This simple philosophy will help to straighten out many backs.

Seizures

A SEIZURE, also called a fit or convulsion, occurs when the electrical impulses in the brain react abnormally to a problem area within the brain itself. The problem area can be an infection, a tumor, an injury due to trauma or poisons, or it can reflect a metabolic problem, such as low blood sugar. Some children experience an aura—a strange smell, a distortion of vision, or a stomachache—just before a convulsion starts. Frequently, no actual cause for the brain's reaction is found even with blood tests and x-rays. Epilepsy tends to run in families.

The child may cry at the start of the seizure, and he may urinate and defecate during the convulsion. Afterward, he may appear confused and sleepy. Sometimes, harmless breath-holding spells can have the dramatic features of true seizures, such as the child's turning blue, fainting, and experiencing shaking of the extremities. Tics, night terrors, and migraine headaches can also be confused with seizures. Various neurological tests (such as electroencephalograms, CAT scans, MRI's) help distinguish among these problems, each of which has a different prognosis.

Seizures Not Associated with Fever (Epilepsy):

Fewer than half of 1 percent of children have epileptic seizures—seizures not associated with fever. There are several different types of epileptic seizures, a few of which are described below.

Grand Mal Epilepsy: The child loses consciousness; the body stiffens; the eyes roll upward; the extremities and body twitch and jerk rhythmically; the teeth clench; there is frothing at the mouth.

Petit Mal Epilepsy: There are no dramatic convulsions. The child's eyes glaze over in a two- to three-second period of daydreaming. This can happen in the middle of a conversation or during any physical activity, such as bike riding. It may happen just once or twice or even hundreds of times a day. Petit mal is more subtle and harder to diagnose than grand mal. Academic performance can suffer.

Newborn Seizures: These may be due to infections, metabolic problems (such as low blood sugar or low calcium), hormone problems (such as thyroid abnormalities), withdrawal from alcohol or drugs acquired in utero, or congenital brain abnormalities.

Seizures Associated with Fever:

A febrile convulsion is a generalized seizure—resembling a grand mal type—due to a sudden rise in the child's temperature. It usually is short, lasting less than ten minutes. The height of the child's temperature does not determine the likelihood of a febrile convulsion. It can occur as the fever rises to 102° F or as it rises to 105° F. There is usually a history of febrile convulsions in the child's siblings, parents, or cousins. Two to four percent of all children under the age of five will have one febrile convulsion, but only a third of those will have a second convulsion.

Febrile convulsions do not fall under the category of epilepsy, and there is no connection between having febrile convulsions and developing epilepsy. Furthermore, although it is scary to watch any convulsion, a febrile convulsion does not cause brain damage or any other permanent neurological problem. This type of seizure rarely occurs once the child is over five.

The febrile convulsion is most likely to occur during the first twenty-four hours of the child's illness. It is impossible to prevent, because it takes an oral anticonvulsant, like phenobarbital, one to two weeks to reach a blood level that would obviate a convulsion. A child would have to take phenobarbital every day to prevent the febrile convulsion on that first day of illness. Although this is prescribed for children with recurrent febrile convulsions (and for children with epilepsy), it is not recommended for the child who has only one or two febrile seizures. Daily use of phenobarbital has been frowned upon because of poor compliance, behavioral side effects, and concerns about its effects on the IQ. Since Valium, taken orally, produces therapeutic blood levels in just one hour, recent studies have recommended its use as soon as the child susceptible to febrile convulsions develops a fever or at the first signs of illness. Only rarely is the convulsion the first sign of a more serious problem, like meningitis.

A comforting way to understand a febrile seizure is to consider it nothing more than an extreme chill. It is the body's way of saying, "Whoa! Slow down! This temperature is rising too quickly." Since heat leaves the body during the convulsion, the child's temperature is actually lower after a febrile convulsion than it would have been without the seizure. Therefore, a parent should be reassured that not only is the seizure not harmful, but that it may actually help the child deal with the fever.

TIPS:

1. Don't panic. Stay calm. The convulsion runs its course no matter what the parent does.

2. A convulsing child should be protected from harming his head. Hold him in your arms or turn him on his side with one cheek touching the floor. Pull his head backward to extend his neck. This ensures that his tongue won't roll backward and block his airway, and that he won't choke on his saliva. Don't try to put your finger or a foreign object into his mouth. This could cause injury to your finger or his teeth, or he could choke on the foreign object.

3. Loosen the clothing around his neck. Keep him lightly dressed so that he stays cool.

4. Note the time the seizure starts and ends. If the

seizure lasts for more than ten to fifteen minutes, call an ambulance or go to the nearest emergency room.

5. Call your doctor. The child may need to be evaluated to rule out certain illnesses and to assess his post-seizure neurological status.

6. If the seizure is caused by a fever, start sponge-bathing the child.

7. Once the child is alert and oriented, follow recommendations in the entry on "Fever" on page 134. However, if he is drowsy after the seizure—a condition called postictal drowsiness—you can let him rest or sleep. It is not harmful.

8. A child with grand mal or petit mal epilepsy may need to take certain drugs, called anticonvulsants, to control the condition. He will need supervision while swimming and bike riding. Thanks to these medicines, almost all of these children lead happy, normal, productive lives.

9. Schools and friends should be told about the condition so that they won't be frightened if a convulsion occurs in their presence.

10. Have a Medic Alert bracelet or necklace made for your child to wear at all times.

Sensitive Topics

WHAT AND how much should I tell my child about sex? How do I explain to him that his grandparent has died? How do I get him to stop cursing or using foul language without making him feel that he's a bad person? Should I tell my child that he's adopted? Now that my spouse and I are getting divorced, what should I tell the kids? What is the best way to tell my two-, three-, or four-year-old that I am pregnant, and that he can expect a young sibling—and some competition?

Questions like these are posed to pediatricians daily.

SENSITIVE TOPICS

Since each situation should be dealt with in its own way, it is difficult to formulate generalizations that will apply to all cases. There are, however, two practical suggestions that should always apply and will help you when discussing these topics with your children.

TIPS:

1. Always tell the truth. It is imperative that your child be given the simple facts *at home* by one or both of his parents. Otherwise, he will eventually learn partial truths, variations of the truth, or, even worse, complete falsehoods from friends, relatives, acquaintances, and possibly even strangers. This will lead to distrust and make him suspicious when the next topic is brought up. This does not mean you should subject him to long, detailed, and drawn-out lectures concerning sex, death, etc. Often, a short and simple (but truthful) explanation will suffice for the moment, which leads us to the second suggestion.

2. Always speak in a calm, relaxed, and non-threatening manner, even though your insides may be doing somersaults. If there is one goal you are trying to accomplish, it is *Always Make It Easy and Comfortable for Your Child to Ask His Next Question.* It may come in five minutes; it may not surface for five days. Regardless, the atmosphere that surrounds you while you're discussing these issues should be calm, comfortable, and conducive to your child's next question. Flare-ups, overreactions, and emotional demonstrations of frustration at having to repeat some answers several times all serve to stifle his healthy curiosity.

It requires much patience to discuss the simple and truthful facts of sensitive topics in such a relaxed manner. But these important discussions will lay the foundation for a close and trusting relationship in the future.

Separation Anxiety

SEPARATION anxiety is a common and normal occurrence in babies between six and fifteen months of age. A baby who until then has been very close to her grandparents or other caregivers may suddenly want only her mother, even to the exclusion of her father. Often there is no known traumatic event to trigger this separation anxiety, which can last from a few weeks to a few months. Sometimes the "special person" changes from the mother to the father or to a sibling. Usually, however, piercing cries start the minute the mother puts on her coat to leave or merely goes to a different room. This anxiety is the child's normal reaction as he realizes that there are "families" and "non-families." It is interesting to note that this fear of strangers is usually limited to adults. Remarkably, the child remains fascinated with other children.

One of the important ways to shorten the period of anxiety is to continue with any plans you have to leave, whether for a few minutes or a few hours. Once your baby learns that you always come back, she will feel a bit more secure about your leaving. Although she may test you over and over, you are allowed to have some free time alone or with your spouse, family, and friends to "clear your head." All other social obligations need not come to a halt. Of course, supply all the cuddling, loving, and reassurance while you are with that gorgeous child. Although separation anxiety can be just as stressful to the parent as it is to the child, the person who needs the most encouragement and reassurance is the relative or baby sitter who will be with the screaming child while you are gone. It is important for that person to read this so that she'll know that you and she are doing the right thing. It is imperative for the baby sitter to understand that the upset child is not commenting on the sitter's care or personality but, rather, is displaying the normal stage of separation anxiety. Teach your sitter the art of distracting the child, and be sure that favorite dolls and toys are handy. Finally, be sure to give the baby sitter an extra hug or tip for a job well done.

TIPS:

1. Don't prolong the agony. Your baby will pick up any negative and guilt-ridden vibrations you display on leaving. Keep smiling, give a quick kiss goodbye, reassure her that you will be back, and leave quickly, even if she cries. It will be easier for the baby sitter to distract her if you are not around. Don't keep coming back for one last kiss. If you follow this routine consistently, and in a loving atmosphere, the child will better adjust to your leaving.

2. Keep handy a special toy or "love object" for the baby to hold and cuddle. It is a good idea to rotate special love objects so that there is always a replacement if one gets lost or worn out. Prepare several sources of distraction to help the baby sitter.

3. Have a new baby sitter visit once or twice to play with the child while you are still home before you leave them alone together. Remind the sitter to approach the child gently and not too quickly. Many babies are intimidated by loud noises and dramatic gestures.

4. The child who is used to sitters at a young age (e.g., less than six months) tends to make the transition to day care more smoothly. The child who is accustomed to your coming and going will also have less separation anxiety when starting school. In today's climate, when both parents often have jobs and careers, a child may start school at a very young age. For some families it is appropriate and advantageous for the child to start day care as young as two years. A good and responsible day care center can stimulate a child just as well as some very busy parents. Refer to the entry on

"Caregivers and Day Care Centers" on page 46. Dealing with separation anxiety correctly from the start will set the tone for easier separation later on.

Sexual Development

MANY PROFESSIONALS in the same field of work communicate with each other through a coded language. Pediatricians use the Tanner scale to refer quickly and easily to the level of a child's or teenager's sexual development. Following is a summary of the Tanner stages.

Girls:

Tanner Stage I: The breasts are flat. There is no pubic hair.

Tanner Stage II: A small breast bud forms under the nipple. The nipple itself enlarges slightly. The outer surface of the vagina develops sparse growth of long, straight (or only slightly curly) hair.

Tanner Stage III: The breasts and nipples further enlarge, but the nipple, on lateral view, still is a continuous part of the breast elevation. The vaginal hair is darker, coarser, and more curled.

Tanner Stage IV: The nipple now forms its own secondary projection (bump) above the level of the breast. The pubic hair has filled in, forming the adult triangle, but does not extend onto the thighs.

Tanner Stage V: The breasts are those of an adult female. The nipple has recessed to the general contour of the breast. The pubic hair is adult in quantity and may extend onto the thighs.

The average age for a girl's height spurt is around twelve years, with the average onset of menses at twelve and a half, between Tanner stages II and IV. The correlation between menarche and height is as follows. A young woman usually stops growing in height within one to two years after her first period. It is especially important to relay this piece of information to the twelve- or thirteen-year-old preadolescent girl who, while undressing in the school locker room, inevitably worries if her development of secondary sexual characteristics is slower than that of her classmates. She should be reassured that those girls who already are fully developed and have periods will soon stop growing in height. She, however, still has years of growth ahead of her. It is also common for a very athletic girl to have delayed onset of menses and for her periods to be irregular. If a teenager has not had a period by the age of sixteen, it is appropriate to seek medical attention. Conversely, if the onset of puberty in a female occurs before eight years, medical attention should be obtained.

Boys:

Tanner Stage I: The penis, testes, and scrotum are of childhood size. There is no pubic hair.

Tanner Stage II: The penis does not enlarge, but the testes and scrotum do. There is sparse growth of long, straight (or slightly curly) pubic hair where the penis meets the abdomen.

Tanner Stage III: The penis enlarges in length. The scrotum grows and darkens, and the testes grow. The pubic hair is darker, coarser, and more curly.

Tanner Stage IV: The penis enlarges in length and the glans increases in breadth. The scrotum grows and darkens, and the testes grow. The pubic hair is adult in type but does not extend onto the thighs.

Tanner Stage V: The genitalia are adult in size and shape. The pubic hair is adult in type and extends onto the thighs.

The average age for a boy's height spurt is between thirteen and fifteen years. The average age of first ejaculation of semen occurs in early to mid puberty at about thirteen years, with wide variability. It usually precedes the pubertal growth spurt.

It is important for all preadolescent boys to know that those whose secondary sexual characteristics (see above Tanner stages, as well as shaving, changing of voice, sweating, and growing hair under the arms) are delayed have yet to enter their height spurt. As a rule, those classmates who now seem more developed will stop growing in height sooner than those who begin puberty later. Conversely, if the onset of puberty in a male occurs before nine years, medical attention should be obtained.

Few things are more frightening to the preadolescent male than noticing that he has a tender lump under one or both of his nipples. Quite a few teenage boys have come to my office worried that they are growing breasts. Rarely do I relieve my patients as much as when I reassure these young men that this is common and very normal. Three fourths of all normal fourteen-year-old boys develop palpable and sometimes tender breast tissue under one or both nipples. It sometimes swells due to injury, perhaps during contact sports. This physiological pubertal gynecomastia (breast enlargement) may resemble a flat button, a round marble, or a more visible enlargement. If it hurts, apply cold compresses and give acetaminophen or ibuprofen for pain. These "breast buds" usually regress after twelve to eighteen months. They are actually a healthy sign: the hormones are waking up. Since this is a benign condition, surgery is reserved for the very rare cases where the breast enlargement produces psychological problems. I always stress how proud I am of the boy that he brought this problem to his parents' attention and mine, and didn't remain secretive or modest about it. It is important to maintain open communication during this sensitive period, when so many changes take place.

Some drugs and hormones may enlarge male and female breast tissues. Among them are male and female hormones (e.g., birth control pills), steroids, digitalis, amphetamines, marijuana, and isoniazid (an antibacterial agent used in treating tuberculosis).

Sibling Rivalry

ALTHOUGH sibling rivalry is a continuous and dynamic process that occurs in all age groups, the jealousy is especially common for the one- to three-year-old when a new baby arrives. This "happy" event often produces aggressive behavior in the older child or results in his infantilization. He may want a bottle; he may want to breast feed; he may want to be held and carried around; or he may want to revert back to using diapers—just like the baby. After all, this older child, who has been the sole recipient of his parents' love and the center of their attention, must suddenly share their time with the baby. Some older siblings will resort to frequent "love taps" on the baby, increasing in physical force. Others find that misbehaving, whining, fretting, fussing, crying, and screaming will gain parental attention, however ill expressed.

TIPS:

1. It is important for parents to understand that sibling rivalry occurs in virtually every home. It is nothing to worry about as long as there is no significant verbal or physical abuse. The best way to change the behavior is to reward more mature and responsible actions displayed by the older sibling toward the baby. Encouraging words should be offered for good behavior, at first hourly and then daily.

2. Tell the older child the truth about your pregnancy and the expected arrival of the baby. It is appropriate to tell the older child about the pregnancy once the mother's physical changes become obvious. Let him help in preparing the baby's room, crib, toys, and clothes. If possible, put the new child in a separate room.

3. Tell the older child the truth about who will care for him while his mother is in the hospital.

4. Buy and wrap a few inexpensive gifts specifically for the older sibling. Store them in your entrance closet. When friends visit and bring a gift for the new baby, they sometimes forget to bring a present for the older child. Reach into the closet and give one of your prepared gifts to your friends. They can then give it to the older child. By doing this, you have accomplished two things. First, you have eliminated yet another potential source of jealousy—that the baby receives presents, but not the older sibling. Second, you have, in a polite and "pediatric" way, reminded your friends not to ignore the feelings of the older sibling.

5. Flip out the older child's baby picture album and show him how much fun and love he brought to the family when he was a baby.

6. Try to move an older child to his new bed and/or room long before the baby comes. This way, he won't feel that the baby is "kicking him out."

7. When the mother first comes home from the hospital, let someone else carry the new baby in while she spends a few minutes with the older child. Refer to the newborn as *"our* baby," not *"the* baby."

8. Start the older child in a playgroup, nursery school, or other daytime activity before the baby arrives. Once again, he won't feel that he is suddenly being kicked out by the baby, and you will have some time alone to take care of the baby and yourself.

9. Avoid starting to toilet train the older child in the few weeks before the baby is due. An initially successful

endeavor may be jeopardized when the older child sees all the attention the new baby is getting with diaper changes. After the older child has adjusted to the presence of the baby, you can initiate attempts at toilet training. At this point, praise him for age-appropriate behavior, such as using the toilet and feeding or dressing himself.

10. The usual advice received by parents is to give equal time to both children. This is simply impossible. More important than equal time is that the older child receive separate, individual parental attention. After my son was born, my older daughter and I would have frequent D and D days together—Daddy and Daughter days. We would be gone from morning to night doing age-appropriate activities. She is now seventeen years old, and we still cherish these days with each other.

11. Encourage older siblings to settle their arguments verbally (through negotiation and compromise, not name calling), and not physically. Try to stay out of the argument. Unless there is an obvious culprit, do not blame one child over the other. If the arguments accelerate, use time-out for both. For details, refer to Tip 2, on time-outs, in the entry on "Temper Tantrums" on page 325.

12. If an older sibling has a friend over to visit, the younger sibling should be provided with a friend or activity to keep him from intruding on the older children.

13. Tell your children that it is okay for them to be angry with each other. Both parents should set examples on how to settle disagreements peacefully.

14. Praise, compliment, and reward your children when they play together well and when they successfully solve a big disagreement.

Sinusitis

THE SINUS cavities are eight spaces, inside the bones of the front part of the head, that are connected to the inside of the nose. The sinuses serve many functions: they warm and humidify inhaled air, secrete mucus, capture and remove small foreign bodies, and impart resonance to the voice. Sinusitis is a bacterial infection of one or more of these cavities. Some sinuses (mastoid, ethmoid) are present at birth, but they are very small. Others (maxillary, sphenoid) first develop after birth, and still others (frontal) do not appear until the child is seven years of age. This is why sinusitis is uncommon in children under two. The older child or adolescent may have fever, greenish nasal discharge, bad breath, swelling or pain above or below the eyes—worsening if the child bends over with his head between his knees. In younger children, sinusitis can cause a persistent nighttime cough and can trigger an asthma attack. These children may also have fever, headache, and nasal congestion. Pressure, such as light tapping, over the involved sinuses causes pain.

In order to obtain a culture of the infected mucus in a sinus, the doctor must pass a needle through a nostril into the sinus. If this is necessary, it can be done by an ENT specialist. A helpful diagnostic test is a CAT scan of the sinuses, but it is expensive. A small but very bright light in a dark room can sometimes demonstrate differences when paired sinuses are illuminated. The side that does not transilluminate as well may contain fluid and be infected. Recurrent sinusitis can be due to blockage of the nasal passages by facial trauma, allergies, a foreign body, a tumor, infection, smoke, air pollution, low humidity, or diseases like cystic fibrosis and immune disorders. Barotrauma—discomfort caused by changes in barometric pressure—from swimming, diving, and flying may also bring about sinusitis.

Treatment includes oral antibiotics, which sometimes must be given for two to four weeks. Some doctors also advocate the use of oral decongestants as well as decongestant nose drops. However, nasal decongestants should never be used for more than four days at a time, because their prolonged use actually irritates the lining of the nose. Stop using them for one week, and then, if necessary, take another four-day course. A humidifier may supply symptomatic relief. Hot steam is of therapeutic benefit in that it may help to open up and drain the nasal passages. Use antihistamines only if the child also suffers from hay fever or other allergies. Otherwise, antihistamines can slow down the draining of mucus from the sinuses.

Adenoidectomy, with or without tonsillectomy, may improve the nasal passageway and eliminate a source of infection (tonsillitis and/or adenoiditis) in cases of recurrent sinusitis. Analgesics (ibuprofen, acetaminophen) may be helpful. For children who suffer from allergies, refer to the list of precautions in the entry on "Asthma" on page 14. Topical cromolyn sodium in spray form will also help these children. For children with more severe allergic problems, intranasal steroids may reduce the number and severity of sinusitis attacks. Rare complications of sinusitis include eye infections, meningitis, and brain abscesses.

Sinusitis is not contagious. Your child can return to school when she has been fever-free for twenty-four hours and feels better.

Sleeping and Bedtime Problems

Bedtime Routine:

BELIEVE IT or not, the half-hour before bedtime is probably the most important half-hour that you and your child will spend in a typical day. The bedtime rituals I recommend can be started by the time the baby is six months old and should be routine by one year. This half-hour is the time of day that, except for emergencies, should be reserved only for your child. These suggestions do not necessarily apply to daytime naps, but in the evening your child should receive a full half-hour of individual attention from one of his parents. Although parents may alternate these routines, both should always hug the child and kiss him good night.

TIPS:

1. Bedtime routines can best be established if daily events are set to occur at roughly the same time. The most important scheduled events are waking in the morning, going to sleep at night, napping, eating, and going outside for walks and playgroups.

2. Except for an emergency, don't deal with any household chores during this half-hour. Don't even answer the phone.

3. You can hold your child, play with him, sing to him, or enjoy any other interaction. Some parents start the bedtime ritual by bathing the child, changing him into pajamas, and brushing his teeth. Try to pick the same time every night. Don't cancel these rituals as a form of punishment for daytime misbehavior.

4. Don't be too stimulating, or your child might find

it hard to fall asleep. This is not the time for wrestling and horseplay. Put on relaxing music and let him take a favorite doll to bed once the half-hour begins. However, do not let him take his bottle to bed. If he starts to fall asleep while feeding at the breast or bottle during this half-hour, stop and put him in the crib to fall asleep. His last waking memory should be of the crib, not of the breast, bottle, his parent's arms, or a pacifier. (The pacifier should be completely discarded when the first teeth erupt.) This way he will learn to put himself back to sleep when he wakes up at night without needing his parents to put something back into his mouth or hold him in their arms.

5. Install a night light and leave the door slightly open.

6. A half-hour seems to be the right amount of time to cater to the child's nurturing and attention needs while not taking away too much time from your other responsibilities. However, most important, once this half-hour is over, give the child a hug and kiss, and leave the bedroom. If he cries, you can pat him gently for a minute, but you should leave while he is still awake. It is perfectly all right if he continues to cry for a period of time, because if you persist with this nightly regimen, he will soon learn the schedule and adapt to it.

If an infant in a crib continues crying, visit him after successively longer periods of time—first after five minutes have elapsed; then after another ten minutes; then after another fifteen minutes, etc. Use a watch so that you don't go back too soon. Stay only for a minute. Pat him gently; don't pick him up; don't stimulate him; don't turn on any bright lights. Once again, leave while he is still awake so that he doesn't feel you have to be present for him to fall back to sleep when he wakes up later at night.

If he is an older child in a bed and has a temper tantrum, protests about bedtime, or refuses to lie down, leave the room. If he leaves his bed, return him quickly to the bedroom without talking to him. (The only exception here is if he is toilet trained and needs to use the bathroom. In that case, let him take care of his toilet needs himself.) If he bangs on the door, tell him you must close his bedroom door, but that you will open it in a minute if he returns to bed. If he does, open the door. If he doesn't or if he tries to open the door, hold it closed. Locking the door should be avoided, as it is too scary for the child. If the screaming and pounding continue, open the door every ten to fifteen minutes, stating very quickly that you will keep it open if he lies down quietly. If he vomits from crying so hard, quickly change his clothes and sheets, and leave the room. Don't feel guilty! This vomiting won't hurt him, and you don't want him to use vomiting as a manipulative ploy.

This plan allows the child to learn that *he* is in control of whether the door is open or closed. If he stays in bed, the door is open. If he gets out of bed, the door is closed. Don't punish or spank him. Tell him that you want to support and help him through this tough problem. You should continue to reassure him through the closed door. When a difficult child ends up going to bed and staying there, reward him, the next morning, with an appropriate prize.

Both parents must be consistent and committed to these plans. The child will learn the rules only if both parents enforce them nightly. Be assured that your baby or older child will awaken in the morning happy and eager to see his parents, even though all of you may have had a terrible night's sleep. The training period outlined above will make these nights seem like distant and long-forgotten nightmares.

Eventually, the half-hour before bedtime will become the period when your child will confide his deepest emotions and secrets to you. He will discuss the events of his day during this half-hour, even though he may have been "too busy" to talk with you earlier in the day. Watching television together does not provide this close, personal interaction. This special half-hour will prove to be a most enjoyable and gratifying time for both you and your child.

Crying During the Night:

Refer to the entry on "Crying" on page 100.

Head Banging, Head Rolling, and Body Rocking:

Head banging, head rolling, and body rocking are common and normal in a child under three years of age. The rhythmical movements usually disappear within eighteen months of their onset. Like an adult swaying to music, a child rocking in bed or rolling his head from side to side is providing himself with a pleasurable, soothing, and comforting feeling. Although it is true that such behavior is also common in a child with obvious neurological and psychiatric disorders, if your child is developing normally, you have no reason to worry about a major problem just because he begins one of these rhythmic patterns.

Beyond three years of age, some children use such behavior to get attention. Others find that the distracting movements help them deal with anxiety about being alone or about some change and tension in their lives. Be assured that they will not injure themselves while head banging, although they may put a few dents in the crib, furniture, or walls.

TIPS:

1. Put a metronome in your child's room and set it to beat at the same tempo as your child's body rocking or head rolling. He may lie quietly as he concentrates on the ticking.

2. A child who rocks vigorously should sleep on a mattress in the middle of the floor (away from walls). This way, the entire crib won't rock back and forth.

3. Since these movements can be a sign that your child seeks extra attention, set aside extra time during

the day to be with him. The half-hour before bed is especially important. See first set of Tips in this chapter.

4. If the basis for the rocking motion appears to be emotional rather than self-soothing, then it is more important to deal with the emotional problem than to stop the rhythmic behavior. If you cannot determine the cause of the problem, seek professional help.

Naps:

Before discussing naps, let's review the normal amounts of daytime and nighttime sleep a child needs at different ages.

AGE	NIGHTTIME SLEEP	DAYTIME SLEEP
1 month old	9 hours	6 hours
6 months old	11 hours	3 hours
1 year old	11 hours	3 hours
2 years old	11 hours	2 hours
3 years old	11 hours	1 hour
4 years old	11 hours	——
6 years old	11 hours	——
10 years old	10 hours	——
13 years old	9 hours	——
18 years old	8 hours	——

A newborn baby sleeps 16 to 17 hours in each 24-hour period, but can't sleep for more than a few hours at a time. A six-month-old will take two separate one-to two-hour naps each day. A two-year-old will take one nap after lunch, lasting one to two hours. If a child of two or three still takes two naps a day, she may not get an adequate stretch of nighttime sleep. Children give up naps completely between three and six years, though they may benefit by just resting quietly during a fifteen-to thirty-minute "quiet time" after lunch.

Most adolescents do not get enough sleep. They could easily oversleep on schooldays and frequently sleep longer on weekends. When allowed to sleep as long as they like, teenagers average eight to nine hours of sleep per night.

During naptime, it is helpful to reduce any disturbing factors, such as lights and noise. Turn off all lights, and use opaque black-out shades on the windows. Curtains may help to muffle outside noise from traffic, trains, or airplanes. To drown out such intermittent distractions, it is helpful to supply a source of constant "white" noise, such as a vaporizer.

The last point regarding napping is that during the months of changing from two naps per day to one, and then from one nap per day to none, the daily nap schedule may vary. It is perfectly all right for your child to nap only every other day, every third day, or two days out of three. During the transitional stages, replace the naptime with a quiet, peaceful, restful period.

Nightmares and Night Terrors:

Children begin to dream after six months of age. Some children experience nightmares as early as eighteen months. Nightmares are frightening dreams followed by complete wakefulness. Night terrors are more extreme and frightening versions of nightmares. A child with night terrors may sit up screaming in panic or stand with his eyes wide open yet be unresponsive to his environment, not even recognizing his parents. He may scream about monsters, snakes, or scary situations. His heart may race; he may sweat; his pupils may be dilated; and he may seem to be looking right through his parents. He may say things that make no sense. During night terrors, the child may even push a parent away as if the parent is part of the dream. The episode may last for thirty minutes. In other words, the child awakens and cries *after* a nightmare but *during* a night terror. Although some children remember nightmares, they usually don't remember night terrors. Nightmares usually occur toward the end of the night, whereas night terrors occur during the first few hours after the child falls asleep. Even adults have nightmares, but night terrors usually stop by the time the child is ten or twelve years old.

A nightmare or night terror can be a response to a

high fever or to being overtired. It can be triggered by something the child may have seen in a movie or on television, especially just before bedtime. It is frequently difficult and tricky to figure out what could be frightening the child. Even an otherwise happy event, such as the arrival of a baby in the household, is anxiety-provoking to the older child.

TIPS:

1. When the child has a nightmare, turn on a light, put on some soft music, and hold him gently, speaking to him in a calming voice until the episode ends. Show your child that you are in control and will make sure that nothing bad happens. Don't raise your voice and scold him, as this may make him more hysterical. He may be reassured to learn that you too have nightmares and that they are a normal occurrence. If he comes to your bedroom, hold and hug him, and then return him to his bed, but never close his door if he is afraid.

2. If it is a night terror, let the episode finish by itself. Don't shake him, shout at him, or try to wake him. Keep a night light on in his room and perhaps play some soft music. An alternative is to install a dimmer on his light switch and gradually lower the brightness. Speak slowly, calmly, and reassuringly. Give him his favorite toy for security. Although the disturbed parent may find it hard to go back to sleep, the child will usually sleep quite easily after the night terror is over.

3. During the day, interpret his nightmare or night terror in a positive way, and install a happy ending to the dream and into his subconscious for the future. Suggest a magic weapon that overcomes the bad person or event, and draw pictures depicting the happier ending. If wild running, with its potential for injury, is part of the night terror, the child may be safer sleeping on the first level of the house or in a finished basement. Guard the windows.

4. Violent or horror movies should be avoided by children under thirteen years of age. Between thirteen and seventeen years, each child's sensitivity must be considered. Check if scary movies are to be shown at slumber or Halloween parties.

5. As is true of many social and emotional problems, the severity is measured by the degree to which the episodes interfere with the child's normal social and learning environment. I frequently ask parents, "Is it affecting the child outside your front door?" In other words, is the current problem (in this instance, nightmares) interfering with his socializing or with his academic performance? If the aberrant behavior is limited to the confines of the child's own home, it is rarely necessary to seek professional psychological help. However, if it does affect his sociability and make him insist on sticking close to home, or if the episodes increase in frequency (more than once per week) or in duration (lasting more than a half-hour), then your pediatrician may prescribe a mild sedative while consultation and treatment with a child psychologist takes place.

6. Don't forget to prepare baby sitters for these episodes. Explain to them what a night terror is so that they do not overreact.

Sleeping in Parents' Bed:

Many parents find it easier to give in to their child's desires to sleep in the parents' bed rather than argue or cause nighttime disturbances. Some parents actually prefer to have their child in bed with them. In general, this is not a good idea and can cause problems. It is a difficult habit to break, so it is better not to start it. Here are a few reasons to avoid sharing your bed with your child.

• People sleep better alone in bed. The movements of one person during the night force the other person in the same bed to wake up frequently or to change stages of sleep. As a result, neither person sleeps well.

• Your child should not rely on this arrangement to be a happy, secure, and independent person. Sleeping alone is important for normal psychological development.

• Allowing your child to sleep between the parents may let him feel too powerful and in control. These mixed signals worry the child, who needs to know that his parents are in control.

• Sharing a parent's bed is not a long-term solution for any sleep problems the child may be having.

• The time will soon come when the parents want to be alone in bed. This is a no-win situation. The child doesn't understand why he suddenly is being kicked out, and the parents feel guilty for the sudden change in sleeping arrangements. As each month passes, the habit becomes harder to break.

• If the parent is single or the spouse is out of town or just not yet ready for bed, the child may feel that he is replacing the missing partner. He may feel that he is responsible for the separation. When a single parent begins a new relationship, or when the spouse is ready for bed, the child will resent being displaced by the "intruder."

• If your child needs to be with you in your bed, it will be hard for you to leave him with a baby sitter.

TIPS:

1. If your child has been sleeping with you, clearly state that he is too old to continue this habit and that, starting tonight, he will sleep in his own room.

2. If he comes into your bed at night, return him immediately to his own bed without any pleasant conversation. If he tries to leave his room again, temporarily close his door. Tell him you will open it only if he stays in bed. If you are a sound sleeper, put a loud bell on your doorknob to wake you if he comes back in. It is all right if he stays in his room and plays or reads and doesn't fall asleep. However, he must learn not to interrupt other people's sleep.

3. Expect some crying, but continue to be firm and

consistent. Both parents must agree and be committed to this plan.

4. Praise and reward your child in the morning if he stayed in his own bed all night.

5. If living conditions, such as cramped quarters or visiting someone's home or a motel, require the child to share your bedroom, give him his own corner of the room. Place his cot or mattress, together with his toys, in that corner. Put his decorations on the nearby wall for him to see. Place some type of separation (curtain, luggage, dresser) between your bed and his corner.

Sleepwalking:

Sleepwalking is a problem inherited by 10 to 15 percent of normal children. It usually occurs within two hours of bedtime. Calm sleepwalking can start as early as when the child learns to crawl or walk. Agitated sleepwalking occurs from middle childhood through adolescence. Most episodes last about fifteen minutes.

TIPS:

1. Talk quietly and calmly. Do not try to wake him.

2. Since your child may be looking for the bathroom, gently lead him there before bringing him back to his bedroom.

3. Protect him from serious accidents by putting gates on stairs and locks, beyond his reach on all outside doors. He should not sleep on the top of a bunk bed. Keep floors and stairs uncluttered. Be sure hallways are lit.

4. Make sure that he gets enough sleep by keeping to a reasonable daily schedule.

5. Put a bell on his door so that you will know when he sleepwalks.

6. For several nights, note how long it takes him to start sleepwalking. Then wake him fifteen minutes before the time you expect him to sleepwalk. Keep him up for five minutes. Wake him like this for seven nights in a

row. Whenever the sleepwalking returns, repeat the procedure for seven nights in a row.

Sore Throat (Pharyngitis) and Tonsillitis

A SORE THROAT is one of the most common reasons children come to the pediatrician. About 90 percent of sore throats are due to viral infections, like the common cold or the flu. These viral sore throats can be mild, with only a slightly red throat, or severe, with pus (whitish exudate) on the back of the throat, and can be accompanied by swollen glands of the neck. Hoarseness and "pink eye" together with a sore throat suggest a viral cause.

Strep Throat and Tonsillitis:

Group A beta-hemolytic streptococci are the bacteria that cause "strep throat." This condition is usually associated with a fever, a severely painful throat, headache, and "feeling bad." However, sometimes children with strep throat have only a slight fever, minimal sore throat, and occasional vomiting or abdominal pain. The throat may be only slightly red or may be very inflamed, with pus. There may be red spots on the palate and swollen glands in the front of the neck. If the glands in the back of the neck are swollen, this could indicate infectious mononucleosis. It is very unusual for a child under one year of age to have a strep throat.

The tonsils are clumps of pink tissue on the sides of the back of the throat. They grow in size during childhood but usually shrink from adolescence into adulthood. Tonsillitis means infection of the tonsils, and, as with the throat, the infection can be caused by either viruses or strep bacteria. One virus that infects the tonsils is the Epstein-Barr virus, which causes infectious mononucleosis.

By the way, most kids hate to have the doctor gag them with a tongue depressor to examine their throats. They're perfectly willing to open their mouths wide and say "Ehh" (which works better than "Aahh") if the doctor won't use a tongue depressor. Practice this at home and mention it to your pediatrician before he examines your child. Another reason to practice at home is that most parents who have never looked at their child's throat almost always think that the throat is red. Practicing while your child is well will help you appreciate the normal pink color.

One cannot distinguish a viral sore throat from a strep sore throat by simply examining the throat. Although viral infections are usually milder than strep infections, there are far too many exceptions to rely on this generalization. The classic way to differentiate between the two is to have your pediatrician take a throat culture. A throat swab (similar to a Q-Tip) is thoroughly rubbed along the inflamed area of the throat and tonsils (if they are present). The swab is then smeared on sheep blood mixed with gelatin lying in a plastic container, and the container is placed in an incubator. After one to two days, this container is checked for the growth of group A beta-hemolytic streptococci. Rapid strep tests are available in some offices; the throat swab is mixed with certain chemicals and a positive reaction means the child has strep. The rapid strep tests are not quite as accurate as the regular throat cultures, but they are helpful and reliable in certain situations.

A viral sore throat lasts a few days, usually resolves on its own, and is not as serious as a strep throat because a viral infection does not cause the same serious complications that strep does. (See below.) This is fortunate, because there is no antibiotic that fights a viral sore throat. Symptomatic relief is obtained with acetaminophen, ibuprofen, throat lozenges or spray, a half-strength mouthwash (half mouthwash plus half water) used for gargling, a lot of fluids—warm or cold, whichever the child prefers. This is a good time for yogurt, ice pops, ice cream, or milk shakes because they are soothing and easy to swallow. If it hurts your child to swallow, don't force her to eat solids. Try pureeing her food. A child should not be given an antibiotic for a viral illness because she may experience the antibiotic's side effects—diarrhea, rashes, vaginitis, swollen joints—without any of its benefits.

For strep throats, penicillin (or erythromycin for children allergic to penicillin) is the drug of choice. If it is administered by mouth, the antibiotic must be taken for ten days, even though the child will feel better in a few days. Otherwise there may be a relapse. Another option is the intramuscular shot of penicillin (not available for erythromycin), which replaces the ten-day oral course.

Many pediatricians currently feel that it is not necessary to do a routine follow-up throat culture if the child is completely well after the ten days of oral medicine (or ten days after the shot). If, however, the child complains of a sore throat at that time, many pediatricians would repeat the culture. Since this "policy" is controversial, check with your own pediatrician. It is important that no antibiotic be taken by a child with a sore throat until a throat culture is done. Even 1 dose before the culture can affect the outcome. Never use leftover antibiotics from siblings or friends. If clinically indicated, an antibiotic can be started overnight, once the throat culture is done, until the results are available. Delaying treatment by one or two days, though, will not increase the child's risk of developing the complications of strep outlined below.

If a child gets frequent strep throats, a throat swab should be sent to the laboratory for more definitive identification of the type of strep. In addition, the entire family, all household members, and a teenager's boyfriend or girlfriend should be cultured to see if they are strep "carriers." This means that they have streptococci bacteria in their throats but are not sick. That is, they do not develop complications from strep, but they can infect others. The child who gets sick recurrently may be cured if the household carrier is treated.

Another reason for recurrence of strep infection is that the tonsils, which usually fight infection because they are similar to lymph glands, ironically sometimes *cause* infection by harboring the strep bacteria deep in their own tissues. Once the penicillin is stopped, the "hiding" strep return to the surface of the tonsils, and the symptoms come back. Sometimes another antibiotic is prescribed, or the penicillin (or erythromycin) will be given for a lengthened course of treatment—up to four to six weeks. If this fails to eradicate the strep, and there are no household carriers, then the tonsils may have to be surgically removed.

The child with a sore throat may return to school if she has no fever (less than 100° F) for at least twenty-four hours, and if she feels well enough to sit and concentrate, and her cough will not be disruptive to the class.

When a strep throat is accompanied by a rough, slightly itchy, sandpaper-like rash of the abdomen, chest, armpits, and groin, the child has scarlet fever. Another distinct characteristic of the rash is that it does not affect the area around the mouth. This rash, caused by a certain toxin that is present in some strep bacteria, is not contagious and will fade within a week. The skin on the fingertips as well as the areas of skin where the rash was most prominent may then peel. Your child may return to school after a bout of scarlet fever if she is fever-free for twenty-four hours and feels well. Scarlet fever got a bad reputation because in the era before antibiotics it could lead to the more serious complications of strep infections. (See below.) Today, however, there is no difference in the seriousness of a strep infection with or without the rash of scarlet fever. The treatment is the same for both.

The most important complications of group A beta-hemolytic strep infections are rheumatic fever, rheumatic heart disease, glomerulonephritis (an infection of the kidneys), and Sydenham chorea (see below).

Rheumatic Fever and Rheumatic Heart Disease:

These rare complications of untreated strep infections occur when the strep bacteria stimulate the formation of antibodies against some of the body's own organs, including the heart, joints, brain, and skin. It usually starts within one to two weeks of the strep throat. Heart involvement (carditis) occurs in 50 percent of children with rheumatic fever and results in cardiac rhythm problems, damage to the heart's valves, and heart failure. Joint involvement results in arthritis, which can affect more than one joint. Brain involvement results in chorea—the involuntary, purposeless movements of the arms and legs. Skin involvement results in the development of nodules (bumps under the skin), commonly of the legs. Children with one episode of rheumatic fever are at a greater risk for a second episode. They are therefore put on long-term prophylactic antibiotics to prevent future strep infections.

Acute, Poststreptococcal Glomerulonephritis:

This rare complication of treated and untreated strep infections develops in a way similar to rheumatic fever, but the antibodies attack the filtering part of the kidneys. Blood will leak into the urine, turning it dark brown; high blood pressure and headaches may develop; swelling of the face, ankles, and wrists may be present. Although the high blood pressure is usually self-limiting, antihypertensive medications are sometimes needed. This kidney problem is usually short-lived and heals completely in most children.

Sydenham Chorea:

Sydenham chorea is the only neurological complication of strep infections, and it shows up much later (even several months after the strep infection) than the above manifestations. It occurs alone and in fewer than 10 percent of cases of rheumatic fever. The three main features of Sydenham chorea are:

- chorea—uncoordinated and uncontrollable writhing movements
- decreased muscle tone
- extreme mood swings

The movements may be subtle and difficult to detect, but a deterioration of handwriting can be a clue. From one to all four extremities may be involved, as may the facial muscles. Feeding, dressing, and walking may be difficult, and speech may be affected. The jerky movements increase with stress and decrease during sleep. The chorea may last for several months or one to two years. Treatment consists of daily penicillin until adulthood to prevent the cardiac problems of rheumatic fever. Sedatives to control the clumsy movements are also of benefit to some children.

Other Causes of Sore Throats Are:

- Diphtheria
- Infectious mononucleosis
- Dry air at home, especially in children with large adenoids and allergies who breathe through their mouths. A humidifier or vaporizer will help this problem.
- A scratch or burn by a foreign object, such as hot pizza or soup, a small toy, a chicken bone or a fish bone, or a caustic material, like cleaner or bleach
- Environmental irritants, such as cigarette smoke, industrial soot, dust, and chemicals
- Allergies, such as pollen or molds
- Voice abuse, such as yelling or loud and prolonged singing

Tonsillectomy

Before we leave the important topic of sore throats, let's review the reasons to have a tonsillectomy. Times have changed. When I was a child, my tonsils were removed simply because my sister was having hers taken out. Today we are a lot more medically and academically selective in our choice of children who need tonsillectomies, because we now know that the tonsils serve the useful purpose of making antibodies to fight upper respiratory infections. They also help to confine infections to the throat rather than spreading to the neck or into the bloodstream.

One reason to perform a tonsillectomy, as noted, is recurrent (five or six bouts per year) streptococcal infections of the tonsils which do not respond to long-term antibiotics. Parents should not confuse pus on the tonsils with debris of food, which sometimes gets lodged in the crypts or pits of the tonsils. This white debris will come out by itself eventually and does not cause pain. A second indication for tonsillectomy is a peritonsillar abscess—a serious infection, consisting of a walled-off abscess near the tonsil and soft palate. After the infection is brought under control with intravenous antibiotics and drainage of the abscess, the tonsils are usually removed, because this type of infection can recur. A third indication for tonsillectomy is sleep apnea—interruption of breathing while the child sleeps. Just because tonsils are large, they do not have to be removed. But if they or the adenoids are so large that they actually touch each other and block the windpipe and the back of the throat, the child may stop breathing for a few moments. If your child snores, has large tonsils, and has moments of not breathing during sleep, she may require surgical removal of the tonsils and adenoids. This child will also have muffled speech without any nasal resonance. Some doctors also recommend removal of large tonsils and adenoids if they block the eustachian tube, resulting in recurrent ear infections.

The tonsils should not be removed for frequent sore throats caused by viruses. Since the viruses infect the entire throat, removal of the tonsils will not prevent these infections. Most children stop having tonsillitis when they are around ten; the tonsils start to shrink, and resistance to infection becomes stronger.

Stitches

FOR ALL abrasions, scratches, wounds, and cuts, follow the first-aid measures in the entry on "Bites and Stings" on page 27. Whether stitches will be needed for a given cut depends on many factors: length and depth of the cut, location on the body (facial cuts will be stitched more readily than cuts elsewhere), cause of the cut, shape of the cut. The amount of bleeding usually has little to do with whether a cut needs stitches. Sometimes small cuts produce a lot of bleeding. Smaller cuts or abrasions can be sealed and covered with Band-Aids, butterfly bandages, or Steri-Strips—small adhesive tapes that can be cut to the size of the wound. These draw together the edges of the wound to promote healing with minimal scarring. However, stitches are usually needed for the following:

- A cut with jagged edges
- A cut where there is a gap or hole
- A cut longer than a half-inch
- A cut on the face

Ideally, a cut should be stitched within two or three hours to decrease infection. It *must* be stitched within twelve hours, or infection is likely to set in. Remember to review the child's tetanus immunization status. (The inside of the mouth heals well, and a cut on that surface usually will not need stitches, but this should be decided on an individual basis.)

Stomachaches

THE WORD *stomachache* and the phrase *abdominal pain* are used interchangeably by lay people and doctors. All children have stomachaches at one time or another, sometimes because they've eaten too much too fast, sometimes because they have constipation or "gas." However, a stomachache can also be the tip of a more serious iceberg. Some indications that a stomachache is possibly serious are vomiting, pain that wakes a sleeping child, blood in the stool, pain with urination, the child's refusing to walk upright or walk at all, pain in the scrotum or groin, weight loss, a recent injury to the abdomen or back, the abdomen's appearing swollen and feeling hard. Sometimes the abdominal pain reflects an infection in another part of the body, such as a sore throat, an ear infection, or pneumonia. Even coughing from the common cold can cause a stomachache.

One of the dilemmas faced by the parents and pediatrician of a child with a stomachache is how much of a work-up (x-rays, blood tests, stool cultures, consultations, etc.) to obtain. We don't want to miss a serious problem, even though 99 percent of stomachaches are psychosomatic. The disorders that cause *recurrent* abdominal pain and require immediate treatment are urinary tract problems, which can readily be diagnosed through a urinalysis and urine culture, and inflammatory bowel disease, gastroenteritis (stomach flu), gastroesophageal reflux, and lactose intolerance, which soon make their presence known with worsening symptoms. Therefore, if the abdominal pain is recurrent, we have the luxury of doing the work-up in an organized and deliberate pace. A time-honored pediatric observation is that the longer the recurrent abdominal pain remains confined to the area around the bellybutton, the more likely it is to be psychosomatic in origin. The remainder of this entry will deal with the above symptoms, some of the more common diseases associated with them, and practical tips on dealing with them.

Appendicitis:

The appendix is a small tubular cul-de-sac that protrudes from the large intestine in the lower right side of the abdomen. It has no known function, and a person can do well without one. When its opening becomes blocked, as it may with fecal material, bacteria will grow inside and the appendix will swell. Typically, the abdominal pain starts around the bellybutton and moves to the lower right side after a few hours. However, up to 20 percent of children will complain of pain on the left side of the abdomen. There is often a low-grade fever, a loss of appetite, vomiting, but only rarely is there diarrhea. The abdomen will feel hard when pressed, and the right leg may be kept in a bent position. The child will not want to move and will find it hard to sleep. Appendicitis requires surgical removal of the appendix before it bursts and causes serious complications. A burst appendix could spill pus throughout the abdomen, causing peritonitis, a potentially fatal infection.

If you suspect that your child has appendicitis, do not give him laxatives, because they can cause the inflamed appendix to burst. As a matter of fact, don't give him anything to eat or drink until your doctor examines him. If emergency surgery is necessary, it will call for general anesthesia, which must be given on an empty stomach.

Although it can occur in babies, appendicitis is rare in infants under one year of age. Many hospitals allow parents to accompany their children into the preparation or "pre-op" room before surgery, as well as into the recovery room after surgery. It is reassuring for these frightened kids to see a familiar face. When children undergo abdominal surgery for other reasons, the appendix is usually removed prophylactically. Finally, it should be kept in mind that persistent right or left lower abdominal pain in a female could also represent ovarian problems.

Diarrhea:

Refer to the entry on "Diarrhea" on page 112. Diarrhea refers to an increase in the frequency of the child's stools. If the stool is looser than normal, but there are only one or two stools per day and the child is happy and playful, this is not true diarrhea. If the diarrhea is accompanied by vomiting and fever, it could be a symptom of a stomach virus (viral gastroenteritis) or food poisoning (bacterial gastroenteritis). Diarrhea can also be part of other illnesses, like influenza, an ear infection, cystic fibrosis, lactose intolerance, and celiac disease. Parasites, which can be acquired when one travels to a foreign country, are another cause of diarrhea. Stress, such as problems in school or with one's parents, is an important component of irritable bowel syndrome, another cause of diarrhea. As noted below, diarrhea is a major problem in inflammatory bowel disease. Some medicines, such as certain antibiotics, can cause diarrhea. Untreated diarrhea can result in water loss and dehydration. Signs of dehydration are lack of tears, decreased urine output, sunken fontanelle, lethargy, dryness of the mouth, and a tendency for the skin to remain "tented" when it is pinched. The entry on "Diarrhea" discusses appropriate dietary management. Check with your pediatrician before giving your child an antidiarrhea medicine.

Food Poisoning:

Within two to twenty-four hours of eating a food contaminated with certain bacteria, a child will undergo vomiting, fever, diarrhea with blood and/or mucus, and muscular weakness. Some bacteria release toxins that irritate the lining of the intestine. Among the more common are salmonella, shigella, staphylococci, and E. coli. Honey has been dropped from most pediatricians' "recommended" list because some batches of honey were tainted with bacteria that cause botulism.

Certain chemicals, insecticides, and plants are also causes of food poisoning. Treat the fever and diarrhea as outlined in the entry on "Diarrhea." Tell your doctor about your suspicions and list what the child ate. Save and bring to your doctor, hospital, or local Poison Control Center any food, plant, or chemical that you suspect your child ate. Refer to the entry on "Poisonings" on page 260. Many cases of food poisoning can be treated at home, though some children will require hospitalization for intravenous fluids and medications.

Gastroesophageal Reflux:

In the world of healthy newborns and babies, there are spitters and nonspitters. Those of us who have spitters may thrill our dry cleaners with our frequent business, but the babies remain happy and grow normally. Spitting should not be confused with true vomiting. Refer to the section on "Vomiting" on page 314 later in this chapter. However, if the spitting is so frequent and severe that the infant doesn't gain weight normally, he is said to have gastroesophageal reflux. For unknown reasons, the normal narrowing of the base of the esophagus, which keeps food down in the stomach of most children, is not present in these babies. As a result, even the slightest movement lets the food come right back up the esophagus and out of the baby's mouth. The baby's rolling around and crawling can trigger the spitting up. Sometimes this food goes back down the "wrong pipe" (i.e., the trachea) and enters the bronchi and lungs, and that can cause lung infections and wheezing. Recurrent vomiting can also cause bleeding and abnormal narrowing of the esophagus. A change of formula does not help this condition, because all liquids reflux. (Formula intolerance is usually associated with severe vomiting, diarrhea, weight loss, and rashes.) The problem often corrects itself by the time the baby is a year old. Until that time, try thickening the feedings with cereal (by adding 1 to 2 tablespoons of cereal to every 4 ounces of formula in the bottle) to help gravity keep the food down in the stomach. The holes in a normal nipple will have to be enlarged for these feedings. The child should be kept upright in an infant seat, frontpack, or backpack for up to forty-five minutes after each feeding. I know how much fun it is to tickle, jiggle, and play with a contented baby after she has fed, but if she has G-E reflux . . . don't! Food stays down better if the child is put to sleep on her stomach, with the head of the crib or mattress raised slightly (up to 30 degrees). When you change the baby's diapers, keep her head and shoulders elevated by resting them on folded towels. Don't close the diapers too tight, or they will put pressure on the stomach. Occasionally, medications to strengthen the bottom of the esophagus and hasten the rate of stomach emptying are used.

Inflammatory Bowel Disease (Crohn's Disease and Ulcerative Colitis):

Inflammatory bowel disease is a chronic condition in which the intestinal tract is inflamed for unknown reasons. Stress aggravates but does not cause the disease. Ulcerative colitis involves inflammation of the large intestine, and Crohn's disease involves both the small and large intestine. Symptoms are abdominal pain, loss of appetite, weight loss, failure to grow, depression, intermittent fever, bloody diarrhea, rashes, joint pains, clubbing (swelling and bluish discoloration) of the fingertips, and chronic infections around the rectum. These symptoms may be mild or severe enough to require hospitalization. X-rays are usually abnormal, and blood tests may show that the liver is inflamed. Pediatric gastroenterologists will supervise treatment with good nutrition and anti-inflammatory medicines, reserving surgery for the severest cases.

Intussusception and Other Causes of Acute Abdomen:

Intussusception is an emergency condition in which a piece of intestine suddenly slips into another piece of intestine, like a telescope. These interlocked intestines swell, causing an obstruction. It is more common in boys than in girls, and usually occurs when the child is less than two years of age. The child will suddenly scream, vomit, turn pale, pull his legs up to his stomach, and may get a fever. The spasms may occur, on and off, for a few hours. Soon, he will pass stools mixed with blood and mucus, classically described as "currant jelly" stools. A barium enema is diagnostic and, in many cases, therapeutic, because the entering barium sometimes pushes out the telescoped piece of intestine. If it doesn't work, surgery will be necessary. A similar condition is volvulus, in which a piece of intestine actually loops and twists around itself. The resulting obstruction requires surgical correction. Other common causes of abdominal pain that indicate the need for surgery are inguinal hernias and torsion (twisting) of the testicles.

Irritable Bowel Syndrome:

Irritable bowel syndrome is a condition in which abdominal pain and diarrhea and/or constipation are responses to life's stresses and emotions, even happy ones. All x-rays, cultures, and blood tests are normal. The child usually does not wake from sleep with pain. She has a good appetite and grows normally. Antispasmodic medication and psychotherapy may be needed if symptoms are severe.

One practical tip to distinguish between emotion-based, functional, or "psychosomatic" abdominal pain and an acute or "surgical" abdomen is to notice whether the child's eyes are open or closed while you press on his abdomen. A child with an acute abdomen will watch very carefully every move the examiner makes. His eyes will be wide open, "pleading" with the examiner to leave his belly alone. The child with functional pain will close his eyes more easily. This test is not foolproof; it's just another clinical tool.

Lactose Intolerance:

Lactose is a sugar found in milk and dairy products. Lactase is an intestinal enzyme that breaks down the lactose sugar so that it is more easily absorbed into the body. People who are born with an inability to make a normal amount of lactase, and people who make less lactase as they age, are "lactose intolerant." Some viral illnesses irritate the lining of the intestine and wipe out the lactase. Although the lactase reappears in a few days, the temporary disappearance leaves the child lactose intolerant for that time. The lactose sugar then goes through the intestine undigested and produces excessive hydrogen gas. Within one to two hours, this results in burping, flatus, vomiting, diarrhea, abdominal pain, nausea, and sometimes headaches. The condition can be diagnosed by a lactose breath test, an office test done by many gastroenterologists. Treatment calls for the use of milk and dairy products with only small amounts of lactose, such as Lactaid milk. In addition, lactase capsules or drops can be taken to help with digestion of foods with lactose. This is not an all-or-none phenomenon. Some people make 25 percent of the normal amount of lactase, some make 50 percent, and others make 75 percent, so the amount of lactose in milk and dairy products that can be tolerated varies from person to person. A program of gradually increasing the intake of milk and dairy products will help determine how much lactose can be ingested without causing problems.

Pyloric Stenosis:

The pylorus is a tube of muscle at the end of the stomach. It initially contracts to prevent food from leaving the stomach, and then relaxes to allow the food to pass through to the intestines. In pyloric stenosis, this muscular tube is too thick, so the passageway for food is too narrow. The cause is unknown, and it is more common in firstborn males than in other babies. During the first month of life, breast milk, formula, and water manage to slip through the narrowed pylorus without causing many problems. After about a month, however, the stomach tries to push the increasing amounts of food through the thickened and narrowed pylorus with decreasing success. The powerful stomach muscles force the food back up the esophagus until it shoots out of the baby's mouth. This projectile vomitus can reach as far as six feet from the body. Even clear liquids (water, tea, Pedialyte) will be vomited. Since this is a "mechanical" problem, due to the narrowed pylorus, changing formulas will not help, but if the condition is left untreated, dehydration and weight loss can follow. Sometimes your doctor can actually feel the thickened pylorus while examining the child's abdomen; it is approximately the size of an olive. Ultrasounds and x-rays for which barium is swallowed will show the thickened pylorus. Pyloric stenosis is cured with a surgical procedure in the hospital.

Vomiting:

Vomiting is the violent expulsion of stomach contents. If a baby's vomiting is recurrently projectile, it could be due to pyloric stenosis (see above). Vomiting also occurs because of other conditions, such as viral and bacterial gastroenteritis, the flu, an ear infection, bronchitis, meningitis, food poisoning, appendicitis, and even the common cold. Motion sickness and head trauma are common causes of vomiting. Refer to the respective entries for details and tips. Vomiting, if untreated, can lead to dehydration and serious salt imbalance.

TIPS:

1. When the pediatrician says that it is safe for the child to drink, give frequent sips of clear liquids, not a lot at one time. Appropriate clear liquids are water, tea, clear juice, Pedialyte (or Lytren or Ricelyte) for a baby under one year of age, but breast feeding in smaller quantities than usual is usually safe. The older child should receive water, tea, Jell-O, Gatorade (or a comparable electrolyte drink), clear broth, 7-Up, Sprite, ginger ale, and ice pops (not fruit juice pops). Slide the stick of the ice pop through the X in the plastic lid of a soda or juice cup; the upside-down rim will catch most of the

drips. Avoid milk and dairy products. It is best to offer small amounts (1 to 3 teaspoons) every ten minutes. The older child who has gone twelve to twenty-four hours without vomiting can be started on the BRAT diet. (Refer to the entry on "Diarrhea" on page 112 for details of this diet.) Remember, if appendicitis is a possibility, you should give no fluid until the child is examined by your doctor.

2. Keep a bedpan or small garbage can (lined with a plastic bag) near the child's bed so that he doesn't have to run to the bathroom to vomit.

3. A cool compress on his forehead can be comforting.

4. Refer to the entry on "Fever" on page 134. Sponge-bathe with room-temperature water. If the child is vomiting the medicine that lowers fever, try the suppository form of acetaminophen. However, this too should be avoided if appendicitis is a possibility.

5. Your doctor may prescribe an antiemetic medicine (orally, rectally, or by injection) if the vomiting persists.

6. If a child vomits medicines that are to be taken daily, such as antibiotics, antipyretics, or most cough medicines, and the vomiting occurs within a half-hour of his taking the medicine, these medicines can be repeated once. If the vomiting recurs, or you are just not sure what to do, call your doctor.

Stool Color

I AM OFTEN asked what color a baby's stool should be. The following list should help answer many questions.

• Yellow, green, and brown are all normal for a baby.

• Many harmless (and some harmful) items can

color the baby's stools if they are ingested. Red may come fron red gelatin, red licorice, beets, red medicines, tomato or fruit juices, or Kool-Aid.

• Since red or black may also represent bleeding, notify your pediatrician immediately if you see either of these colors. A simple test on the stool can distinguish between a serious bleeding problem and a harmless food discoloration.

• Black may also come from iron drops or pills, as well as foods with a high iron content, Pepto-Bismol, spinach, grape juice, black licorice, or materials with lead (such as peeled paint).

• Yellow or white may come from antacids.

• Green may come from spinach, Gatorade, or lime gelatin.

Stuttering

STUTTERING, also called speech dysfluency or stammering, is common, especially in boys in the two- to three-year age group. Many specialists believe that the child's mind is thinking faster than his mouth can work; he knows what he wants to say but is too excited to get it out in time. The phase commonly lasts for two to three months. This type of speech dysfluency occurs in 90 percent of children. True stuttering (see below) occurs in only 1 percent.

Stuttering is considered severe if the child has trouble with more than 10 percent of his speech or if the difficulty persists after five years of age. True stuttering is four times more common in boys than in girls, and is often accompanied by facial grimacing or tics. A speech and language pathologist will help to develop an appropriate plan for the child.

TIPS:

1. Provide a calm, relaxing, and reassuring environment. Don't correct the child's speech and don't finish his sentences. Don't force the child to slow down, and discourage others from doing those things. Such well-intended actions merely call attention to the stuttering. Sometimes the hardest action of all is to do absolutely nothing.

2. Have the child read books to you, recite nursery rhymes, and sing simple songs. The parent should speak slowly and carefully.

Teeth

FOR SIGNS, symptoms, and treatment of eruptions of new teeth, refer to the entry on "Teething" on page 321. Those pages also cover the usual sequence of eruption of the primary or baby teeth. It is important to emphasize that the time of the appearance of baby teeth is not a neurological or developmental milestone. It is completely hereditary. Yet another old wives' tale is the belief that the later the teeth come in, the stronger they are, but the quality of the child's teeth is only determined by heredity, not time of eruption. It is important to remember that whoever finds the first tooth must buy the baby's first pair of shoes . . . another old wives' tale!

There are thirty-two permanent teeth, the first of which are called six-year molars; they usually appear at age six or seven. During the next six years, the primary teeth fall out and are replaced by permanent teeth. Four additional molars will emerge at the end of this period. Sometimes a permanent tooth makes its appearance before the baby tooth falls out, so two teeth occupy the same spot, one behind the other. Don't worry. The baby tooth will soon fall out, or you can have it removed by the dentist. Finally, the last molars, called wisdom teeth, emerge when the young adult is between seventeen and twenty-one years old.

Tooth decay and the common cold are the most common disorders of mankind. A cavity is a hole caused by erosion in the enamel or surface of a tooth. Good dental care, improved diets, and the use of fluoride have all helped to fight tooth decay. An adequate daily supply of fluoride can reduce the number of cavities by 50 to 80 percent. When fluoride is incorporated into the enamel of the teeth as they are being formed, the teeth become harder and more resistant to decay. After the baby teeth appear, their outer surfaces acquire fluoride from water, chewable fluoride tablets, fluoride rinses, and fluoride toothpastes. However, in communities that do not have fluoride in the water, you can get fluoride *into* the enamel by administering fluoride orally as soon as the newborn period. Since the teeth are just being formed, this fluoride will be concentrated in the enamel, helping the teeth resist cavities. Even after teeth erupt, orally ingested fluoride strengthens the enamel from the inside.

Many communities have naturally occurring fluoride in their water and others add a controlled amount of fluoride to the local water supply. If your water is not fluoridated, you can obtain fluoride drops or tablets (or vitamins with added fluoride) by prescription from your pediatrician at your baby's first office visit. The mother's drinking fluoridated water or taking fluoride supplements during pregnancy has not proven to protect the child's teeth. Breast milk and formulas contain only trace (and therefore insufficient) amounts of fluoride. It is wise to maintain the child's fluoride supplements until he is fifteen or sixteen, because enamel continues to form until then. After that age, fluoride toothpastes and rinses are sufficient to minimize tooth decay.

Fluorosis is a condition caused by excessive fluoride intake, i.e., above the recommended dose, for a prolonged period of time. The teeth may become spotted, pitted, and stained. Do not exceed the prescribed daily dose. The occasional swallowing of fluoride toothpaste, however, does not contribute significantly to fluoride intake, so it is not a cause of worry. Staining of the teeth also results from the use of certain antibiotics (e.g., tetracycline) at too young an age. Tetracycline should not be given to children under the age of eight.

"When should my child start brushing her teeth?" Let me answer this question by asking another. Have you ever wondered why dogs don't get cavities? (I'm sure you've been up nights worrying about this.) Well, one reason is that they have spaces between their teeth, so their tongues can clean the teeth well after they've eaten. Babies, too, have spaces between their teeth, so food does not tend to accumulate there. That means that young children don't require daily brushing until they are two years old, when the teeth become more crowded. Until then, just wipe the teeth with a soft washcloth. Children love to imitate their parents, so let them watch you brush your teeth. This way you can better supervise their brushing technique. One cute trick is to let your child brush your teeth while you brush hers. It's messy but fun!

The child should make his first dental visit when he is around three. It is a good idea to "play dentist" at home to familiarize your child with what will happen. Avoid using negative words like *hurt* or *shot*. Answer questions honestly but not too specifically. Pediatric dentists have their own special ways of explaining procedures to kids.

It is normal for x-rays to be taken periodically, and as long as the child wears a lead apron, there is no health hazard from this relatively low level of radiation when it is administered intermittently.

When your child's permanent molars erupt, consider protecting them with sealants—clear plastic coatings applied to the chewing surfaces of the teeth. These form a barrier that keeps food and bacteria out of tiny grooves in the teeth, and are nearly 100 percent effective in preventing decay in the molars.

A well-balanced diet keeps teeth healthy. Calcium is important for proper development of teeth and bones, and babies get calcium through breast milk or formula during the first months of life. Subsequent good sources of calcium are yogurt, cheese, ice cream, milk, sardines, green leafy vegetables, and dried beans. Suggestions for older kids: add a slice of cheese to sandwiches, shred cheese into salads, serve macaroni and cheese, serve creamed vegetables and soups. Lactose-intolerant children can use Lactaid milk and dairy products. All children over two years of age should use low-fat milk and dairy products.

For information on bottle mouth syndrome and how to prevent the dental malocclusion it can cause, refer to the entry on "Bottle Mouth Syndrome" on page 34. The pacifier should be stopped when the baby is six months of age or as soon as the first tooth erupts. The bottle should be stopped when he is between twelve and fifteen months. Never put your baby to bed with a bottle.

A baby tooth does not need to be replaced if it gets knocked out accidentally. If a permanent tooth is knocked out, it should be replaced quickly (preferably within an hour). Wash the tooth gently under running water, put it in a clean container, and cover the tooth with milk. An older child can simply keep it between his lower lip and gums while you seek dental assistance. Likewise, if any tooth is loosened, chipped, or shoved into the gums, have a dentist check the condition and the viability of the tooth. Sometimes dental appliances, such as splints, will be applied to give the tooth a chance to reattach well.

Teething

WE'RE TOLD that Adam and Eve had many advantages, but their chief one was that they were created with teeth. They never went through the painful process of teething.

There is a wide range of time for the first tooth to erupt. The average is six months, but some children get their first tooth at one year of age, and some babies are born with what are termed "natal teeth." There is no correct pattern or order of eruption, but the following represents the usual sequence:

• The bottom central incisors (middle two teeth) come first.

• The upper four central and lateral incisors follow at an average of one tooth per month.

• The bottom two lateral incisors.

• Then at roughly twelve to fifteen months, the four first molars.

• The four canines (also called eyeteeth).

• Then, the four second molars.

You must be aware, however, that there are other patterns of appearance that are perfectly normal. Sometimes the gums appear bruised and bluish and may bleed a little when a tooth erupts. This is harmless and will stop on its own.

The nerves from the teeth and gums enter the brain in the same area as the nerves from the ears. Occasionally the brain misinterprets the pain from teething as pain coming from the ear; this is an example of referred pain. Because of it, some babies will pull at their ears, bang the side of their heads, or pull the surrounding hair. That's all due to teething. Sometimes teething is associated with a low-grade fever,

TEETHING

and it can be difficult for a parent to distinguish between teething and an ear infection. One tip is that if the fever is higher that 102° F, it is not due to teething.

Although a belief cherished by academicians is that teething is not associated with low-grade fevers, runny noses, loose stools, irritability, or waking up more than usual, I am convinced that these professionals must examine books instead of children. Most busy pediatricians have noticed the frequent simultaneous occurrence of these side effects as well as an increase in drooling and a desire to chew on things. Besides, if both of my grandmothers say that teething causes these problems, then it must be true.

Some babies have no problems at all while cutting teeth; others have a difficult time with some teeth. Many of us remember from our wisdom teeth that the process was a painful one. I am certain that it is for some babies, too.

For those babies who seem to be in pain from teething, there are three levels of treatment.

TIPS:

Level 1. Try over-the-counter topical analgesics such as Anbesol, Orajel, Num-Zit. If they help, stick with them as needed. If not, proceed to level 2.

Level 2. Whiskey. Yes, that's right, this old-wives' tale is true! Although the American Academy of Pediatrics has declared alcohol off-limits, nevertheless if it is used only topically and applied to the gums no more than twice a day, it will not be absorbed systemically. But—and it's a big but—if alcoholism exists in your family, you should never have any alcohol in your home. For those people, and for those whose babies are not helped by whiskey, proceed to level 3.

Level 3. Call your pediatrician for prescription topical analgesics, such as viscous Xylocaine or paregoric.

Always remember at any level:

- Stay with the weakest effective analgesic.
- You can administer Tylenol, if needed, in addition to the topical medicines.
- Massage the gums with a hard, cold object, like a teething ring or a frozen bagel.

Television

THE AVERAGE American child watches television for twenty to thirty hours per week. For some, this represents more time than they spend in school. For the first time in history, children are born into a symbolic world that does not originate with parents, religion, or school, and requires no literacy. It is incumbent on the parents, therefore, that they not allow television to become a substitute role model. It is our joy and responsibility to set an appropriate moral example for our children and to teach them to improve their vocabulary. Don't allow television to become a baby sitter. It is perfectly all right to share some television time with your child and to use it as an excellent source of news, politics, geography, and science. It allows children to see different lifestyles and cultures. But it is necessary to put restrictions on both time and program content. As the child gets older, peer pressure enters into the picture; the child is encouraged to view more shows. The operative sentence here should be "Each family has its own rules."

Most parents assume that daytime shows, especially cartoons, are all safe for a child's viewing. In truth, some children become very frightened—to the point of having nightmares—because of the violent activities displayed on some cartoons. A cartoon character may bore holes in people's heads. Other characters may assume the shape of containers they are shoved into. It is hard for many young children to separate fantasy from reality when it comes to these depictions of violence, so carefully screen all programs you allow your child to view.

Let me illustrate this point with a fascinating case history. A three-year-old boy who had been toilet trained for over six months became constipated for two months. He would hold in his stool for four to five days and then move his bowels only while standing up, wearing a diaper. He adamantly refused to sit on the toilet. His physical and neurological exams were normal. With medication, he returned to his regular daily bowel movement. However, he persisted in moving his bowels only while standing up. Finally, he gave in to his mother's persistent questions and told her that he had seen a television commercial in which a toilet bowl turned into a monster, with the seat cover making a chomping movement. The image scared him so much that he wouldn't sit on the toilet for fear that it would "get him." Many viewers complained about this commercial, but it was not discontinued until the advertiser's contract expired.

Similarly, violent or horror movies and video games should be avoided by children under thirteen. Between thirteen and seventeen, each child's sensitivity must be considered. Check to see whether scary movies are to be shown at slumber or Halloween parties. Video games aren't all bad, because the necessary interaction between child and machine promotes memory, sequencing, planning strategies, eye-and-hand coordination, and imagination. Still, screen carefully and encourage your child to play video games with other children.

Some other problems with television are:

• The portrayal of teenagers on TV is distorted and overemphasizes their sexuality and their crises.

• TV has become increasingly sexual, more by innuendo than by explicitness.

• Alcohol is always present on TV, yet the true effects of alcohol are rarely depicted.

• TV is overpopulated with doctors, lawyers, and policemen, and portrays few blue-collar workers to teenagers who are struggling with their own career plans.

• Obese people are rarely shown on television.

• TV advertising directly influences the family's food purchases and the snacking behavior of children.

• The frequent use of food in TV programs provides a message that food should be used for activities other than the satisfaction of hunger.

• There is a direct relationship between obesity and the time spent viewing TV. Children watching TV are not participating in more energy-intensive activities, and then tend to eat more of the high-calorie foods advertised on TV. Eating while watching TV is an additional source of excess calories.

One question often asked is whether the child is exposed to dangerous radiation from all these hours of viewing. In a nutshell, the answer is no. According to the Food and Drug Administration's Center for Devices and Radiological Health, no measurable radiation emissions have been detected in TV sets made since 1984. The FDA established standards for acceptable emissions in 1970, and TV sets made from 1974 to 1980 had emissions well below the suggested ceiling.

Temper Tantrums

TEMPER tantrums frequently occur in children between one and three years old because this is the age when kids know what they want and what they are feeling, but they don't yet have the facility to express their desires in words. Consequently, they act out their frustration and anger. In addition, at this age they first discover that they are able to refuse other people's requests. As their vocabulary and verbal ability grow, their temper tantrums will lessen. Aggression in younger children can be channeled to more productive endeavors as they grow up, and they will usually be successful adults.

Temper tantrums come in all different sizes, shapes, and degrees. If they are dealt with appropriately, they will be given up after no more than a year. The following list of tips is specifically for those actions which are socially not acceptable, such as hitting, kicking, and biting.

TIPS:

1. Stay calm. Don't let the child see that you're upset. Don't take the child's negative response personally and don't assume it is meant as disrespect. The response is meant to express independence, not to annoy you. Merely say that you see how upset the child is, so you will leave him alone until he cools off. Tell him to come to you when he wants to talk. Then ignore the tantrum and walk away. Even if he holds his breath and turns blue, he won't harm himself; a natural reflex will make him breathe even against his will. Don't slap him or throw water on him. He'll come out of it himself. Just make sure that his immediate environment is "child-proof" and free of sharp objects. Give him a little time to recover, and after the tantrum, be friendly and return the atmosphere to normal.

2. If his temper tantrum involves socially unacceptable behavior, then use time-out as the intervention of choice. Time-out consists of isolating a child in a boring place immediately after he has misbehaved. It allows the child to calm down and think about what he has done. It is more effective than spanking, scolding, and shouting, which engender poor self-esteem. There are no negative side effects or emotional scars from the appropriate use of time-out. It also allows the parent or caregiver to have her own time-out for reassessing her emotions and preparing a game plan, instead of resorting to punishment she may later regret. Be sure your child's baby sitter and all caregivers learn this technique. Time-out teaches children who exhibit aggressive or violent behavior, like hitting, biting, or kicking, to solve their problems peacefully and in a controlled state of mind. Parents who use such techniques are excellent role models for their children.

Since younger children usually respond to a stern face and an authoritative voice, time-out is rarely needed before the child is eighteen months old, at which point the technique can establish who is "the boss." It is frequently needed for children between two and five years, and occasionally for those between six and twelve. Adolescents can be grounded from social activities with peers, which is a form of time-out.

The child should be sent to a quiet spot, like a corner or facing a blank wall. He should not be able to watch television or see other people. The quiet spot can be in the same room as a parent only if the child has real separation anxiety. However, the parents should not look at or talk to the child. It is preferable for the child to sit in a high-backed chair with side arms so that he has physical boundaries. The limit on distractions will enable him to think about his misconduct. Avoid using rocking chairs, which can tip over, or chairs on wheels. If a chair is not available, he can stand or sit in the corner. If he misbehaves in the car, the parent can pull over and have the child sit on the floor in the back seat while the other occupants step out and enjoy the surroundings.

Use the formula of one minute of time-out per year of life, with a maximum of ten minutes. In other words, a three-year-old gets three minutes. Keep on hand the kind of egg timer that ticks continuously and rings when the time is up. Place it near the child but out of reach. It will prevent a power struggle between the child and parent as to when time-out is over. Take the timer along on trips and vacations.

TEMPER TANTRUMS

A protesting child needs to be gently led or carried to the time-out corner. The parent shouldn't spank or acknowledge these protests, but should clearly and simply state what the child did wrong. Tantrums during time-out should be ignored, just like tantrums outside time-out. If the child vomits while in time-out, the parent should quickly clean him without offering comforting words. If the child leaves too early, the parent should take him back quickly and the timer should be reset from the beginning. Dangerous objects, like scissors and knives, and valuable objects, like jewelry and vases, should be moved to a distance far from a time-out area. If a child claims to enjoy time-out, he is probably saying that to upset the parent. The parent should walk away without changing the strategy or technique.

An out-of-control child may need to be held in time-out by the parent. The parent should place him in the chair and hold him by the shoulders from behind so that the child can't see her. If the child agrees to stay, the parent can let go. When used correctly, this approach eliminates escape attempts within one week of initiating time-outs. It is not reasonable to expect a child to be quiet during a time-out until he is at least three years old. As a last resort, a screaming child can be put in a bedroom while the door is held shut for a maximum of three to five minutes. The need to hold the door closed will also stop after a few times.

As an alternative to time-out, the child over five years of age can be grounded—deprived of the use of television, stereo, video games, toys, telephone, and from playing outside or having friends over.

If you have never used time-out, first explain it and demonstrate it to your child in a quiet, loving manner. Tell him it will replace yelling and spanking. For the first two or three days, a parent may need to use time-outs ten to fifteen times each day to get an aggressive toddler's attention. If it is used repeatedly, consistently, and correctly, the child's behavior will improve. Most undesirable behavior will show a marked reduction within two weeks. Occasionally, referral to a child psychologist may be appropriate.

Once the time-out is over, parents should not apologize or feel guilty. They should treat the child normally and give him a clean slate. As a matter of fact, time-outs should be offset by positive reinforcements later the same day. One way to do this is to give two time-ins for every time-out. A time-in is a brief (one to two minutes), positive, close parental interaction, such as hugging and playing. It is most effective when it is done right after the child does something good.

3. Never allow the child's temper tantrums to succeed. Once the tantrum is over, he still must do whatever you originally said he should do. Conversely, if there was something you said he could not do, after the tantrum he still cannot do it. If you show that these tantrums never succeed, they will stop sooner.

4. Set limits. Be firm but loving. Although the child (and teenager) won't admit it, he needs and wants his parents to set limits and rules in his own home. Every child needs the feelings of security that, in his own home, his parents are the bosses. Each toddler will constantly test, in a healthy way, the limits his parents set. For example, a child may repeatedly approach a plant or delicate piece of furniture he has previously been warned to stay away from. The parents or caregivers must *consistently* be firm and strong in their disciplinary conviction. This discipline will be learned by the child if it is taught consistently.

5. Don't hit, kick, pull hair, bite the child back, or wash his mouth with soap as a disciplinary measure "to show him what it feels like." This merely teaches the child to deal with his out-of-control emotions in socially unacceptable physical ways. Remember, a parent is the primary model for the child in dealing with his anger. Verbalize your child's feelings for him. Say, "I know that you're angry. You want to hit your brother, but we cannot hit other people." Allow him to release his emotions by punching the pillow or teddy bear.

Although spanking succeeds in getting a child's attention in the short run, it also teaches the unfortunate lesson that big people can get away with hitting little people. Repeated spanking loses its effectiveness. Even those disciplinarians who believe that a rare spanking can be effective agree that a parent must abide by the following rules:

Never use paddles or belts, and never hit on the face. It is demeaning and dangerous. If necessary, spank only once, with an open hand, through clothing. Hitting more than once may dissipate your anger, but it won't teach the child anything. Never spank when you have lost your control or when you are drunk. Parents who do so need counseling themselves. Never allow caregivers and teachers to spank your child. A teacher of mine once said that in order to be effective, a spanking should be like a treat—unexpected and rare.

6. Temper tantrums may happen in public places and can be very embarrassing. Simply pick the child up and remove him to your car or other safe and quiet environment. Every parent of a former two-year-old will understand and sympathize with your situation.

7. Offer the child two or three acceptable choices for the activity at hand. This gives the child a greater feeling of self-control and lessens his feeling of being overwhelmed. For example, instead of arguing over whether he should get dressed, make getting dressed a "given," and allow him to choose from two or three appropriate outfits. In addition, allow him to choose whether to put his shirt or pants on first. Other examples: instead of arguing over whether he is to take a bath, make that a given, and let him choose which toys to take into the tub and which soap and shampoo to use. Let him choose which fruit to eat for a snack and which cereal to eat for breakfast. The more you let him feel that he is in control, the more cooperative he will become.

8. Screen carefully any television shows the child

watches, including cartoons. After parents, TV characters are next to serve as role models. Their aggressive
behavior must be of concern to all parents.

9. Give your child the opportunity to adjust to what
you think will soon be a situation that could trigger a
temper tantrum. That is, say to him, "In ten minutes, it
will be time for your bath." Then, "In five more minutes, it will be time for your bath." This gimmick helps
to decompress potential outbursts.

10. If a child reacts in an appropriate and surprisingly
mature manner to a potentially volatile situation, such
as sharing a favorite toy, reward him. A hug or a kiss or
just a few encouraging words about his grown-up behavior will go a long way to improve his conduct. The
old adage applies to this situation: "You catch more
flies with honey than with vinegar."

11. A child sometimes experiments with actions like
hitting, pinching, scratching, pulling hair, biting, kicking, and throwing things. If he does any of these in a
day care setting, the parents of the other children may
want him expelled. Although a child may learn to bite
by nibbling his parents in a playful manner when he is
teething, the same thing done in another child's home
may result in his being asked not to return. Occasionally, children are aggressive because they receive spank-
ings at home or witness the abuse of a parent or sibling.
Although parents at first may think biting, pulling hair,
or hitting is cute, the action eventually becomes a game
to the child. He learns to bite when he is frustrated,
angry, and when he wants to intimidate others. It is
very important to interrupt this primitive behavior at an
early stage.

12. Interrupt aggressive behavior with a sharp *"No!"*
Use an unfriendly voice and look the child straight in
the face. But never call your child a "bad boy." He
simply may have done a "bad thing."

13. Never laugh when your child bites or kicks, and
never treat such actions as a game. Never give in to his

demands just because he bites. Put him down immediately and walk away.

14. Give special attention to the victim. Pick up the injured child and give him extra sympathy.

15. Adolescent rebellion represents a difficult problem. After all, one of the main accomplishments of adolescence is that the teenager becomes psychologically independent of his parents. Peer pressure encourages different dress, talk, and actions. At the same time, teenagers try to develop a more mature relationship with their parents. The transition is characterized by a certain amount of normal rebellion, defiance, and discontent. Labile emotions and frequent mood swings are expected. To encourage the more grown-up aspects of this new relationship, parents should treat their teenagers as adult friends. Take advantage of shared activities, like shopping, driving, playing ball, cooking, and eating together, as times for relaxed, mature conversation. Since it is essential to reinforce that the parent is still the boss, the adolescent can be grounded from the use of television, telephone, stereo, and a car. If a teenager breaks something, she should pay for its repair or replacement or do extra chores to pay it off. She should clean up the messes she makes. Although some talking back is normal as adolescents express their anger, name-calling is not acceptable. Leave the room and apply grounding instead of getting into a shouting match.

16. If all else fails, you may need to try consultation and counseling for your child and yourself with a child psychologist. Remember, positive reinforcement by showing your approval for your child's good behavior is the most powerful way to obtain desired results.

Before leaving this important topic, let me offer a particular philosophical approach to temper tantrums. Tantrums can be looked upon as an important, positive, and valuable experience of childhood if they are dealt with appropriately. Through them, the child learns that there are certain things he can and cannot do. There are limits to his actions, and the parent is the boss. The child also learns that it is permissible to get angry and to express that anger. He discovers that these feelings soon will pass. The parent who keeps this in mind will be able to cope more successfully with temper tantrums.

Testes

Undescended Testes:

THE TESTES are the glands where sperm and male sex hormones are made. They are formed in the embryo in the abdomen and descend into the scrotum shortly before birth. They remain in the scrotum throughout life, away from the internal heat of the body, which could harm the sperm at puberty. Occasionally, one testis or both will fail to descend by birth. If they have not descended by the time the boy is one year old, a urologist should be consulted. He may recommend surgery to bring the testes down, because spontaneous descent does not occur after the first year. The use of hormone shots to try to bring down undescended testes is advocated by some doctors. (The advantages and disadvantages of each mode of therapy should be discussed on an individual basis.) Another reason to bring down the testes is that a testicular tumor, though very rare, is much harder to detect early if the testes remain in the abdomen. The incidence of testicular cancer is slightly higher in undescended testes.

Sometimes the normal testes retract into the abdomen when they are touched by another person or when the environment is cold. They will shortly return to their normal position.

Rarely, at surgery or during the work-up prior to surgery, it is found that the "undescended" testis in fact never actually developed. A male can function sexually and be fertile even with one testis. A prosthetic testicle can be inserted into the older child's scrotum for cosmetic and psychological benefit.

Torsion:

Acute pain and swelling of the scrotum, which develops a bluish or reddish discoloration, is a pediatric emergency. It can indicate a torsion, or twisting, of the testis. Sometimes there is a precipitating trauma, like a fall. A urologist should be consulted immediately. Sometimes the swelling is due to an inguinal (groin) hernia, which extends down into the scrotum. This too will require surgical repair. A hydrocele (painless collection of fluid above the testis) usually resolves spontaneously by the time the boy is one year old.

(*Testis* is the Latin word for "witness." The relationship between the testis and a witness can be traced to Roman law, under which only those who had testes were admitted as witnesses—that is, were allowed to "testify"—in court. This may have been sexist, but it's true.)

Tetanus

TETANUS, or lockjaw, is a serious disease caused by a bacterium often found in dirt, gravel, rusty metal, human and animal waste, and even house dust. The bacterium enters the body through a cut or wound and then causes the muscles of the body to go into spasms. The jaw muscles usually "lock" first, making it impossible for the child to swallow. The first muscle spasms may be delayed by occurring months after the wound is sustained. Irritability, neck stiffness, and fever also develop. Tetanus kills three out of every ten people who get it, but almost no cases occur in children because of the success of the tetanus vaccine. This vaccine should also be given to adults every ten years to help them maintain immunity.

TIPS:

If your child sustains a cut:

1. Clean all wounds thoroughly.

2. If the wound is large or needs stitches, make sure that the last tetanus booster was given within the past five years. Smaller cuts and wounds are protected by a booster for ten years. If your child is not up-to-date with his tetanus shots, he may require a second shot of human antitetanus immune globulin for immediate protection and should also get the regular tetanus booster shot at the time that care is provided for the wound. This is most effective if administered right after the injury, but the shot can be helpful if given within forty-eight hours of the trauma.

3. If tetanus develops, the child will need hospitalization for observation, intravenous fluids, antibiotics, and antitoxin. He should be placed in a quiet, dark, intensive care environment with minimal stimulation.

4. Sedation and muscle relaxants, like Valium, may be needed to control spasms.

5. For details about the tetanus vaccine, refer to the entry on "Immunizations" on page 189.

Things to Prepare Before the Baby Comes

The Nursery:

THE BABY's room should be away from the kitchen and other noisy areas. A southern exposure is ideal; a room facing east will need opaque black-out shades to keep out morning light. Window treatments are an easy and inexpensive way to add stimulating color to a room. Another money saver is unfinished furniture, painted to match the walls.

Basic furniture requirements are crib; changing area or table; comfortable chair or rocker for feeding; small table near the rocker; good sources of light; hamper for dirty clothes; large diaper pail; a variety of storage bins. Some suggestions for storage are wheeled stacking bins; baskets and plastic crates (for diapering supplies now, toys later); bookcases with adjustable shelves (for folded clothing, books, and soft toys); peg racks or hooks mounted on walls; rolling under-the-bed storage containers; a chest of drawers (sometimes it will have the changing table as its top). Be sure that area rugs have nonskid pads beneath them and that electrical cords are all behind furniture. All electrical outlets should have safety plugs. A smoke detector should be in the nursery or right near it. Windows should have locks and guards; pull cords for blinds and shades should be tied up, less than twelve inches long, out of reach of older children. Refer to the entry on "Cribs" on page 96.

Clothing:

• Diapers—A newborn may need to be changed up to ten times a day for the first month or so. If you choose cloth diapers, you'll need about four dozen. You'll need half this amount if you also use disposable diapers or if you have a diaper service. Plan on using about 300 to 350 disposable diapers in the first month.

Cloth and disposable diapers cause a similar rate of diaper rashes. Disposable diapers are convenient and are better at preventing leakage of urine and watery stools, but they are more expensive and less "ecologically friendly" than cloth diapers. Some parents compromise and use cloth diapers during the day at home and disposable diapers at night and when traveling. You can wash cloth diapers yourself, or you can make use of a diaper service, which picks up its cloth diapers from your home and provides a clean batch of sterilized diapers weekly.

• 6 cotton undershirts (with snaps or ties, rather than pullovers, to make it easier to dress and undress the infant)

• 3 gowns

• 3 stretch suits

• 4 pairs of waterproof underpants if you are using cloth diapers

• 8 safety pins if you are using cloth diapers. However, newer cloth diapers come with Velcro fasteners

• Sweater set and hat

• Blanket sleeper

• Booties or socks

Bed and Bath:

• 6 washcloths

• 2 or 3 hooded bath towels

• Bathinette or portable baby bath with sponge linings. A kitchen sink can serve this purpose initially, but watch out for hard surfaces and sharp edges. Be sure not to turn on the hot water, which could cause a burn. Until the umbilical cord falls off, keep the water level below the cord. Most children can use a regular bathtub by the time they are six to twelve months of age.

• Brush and comb

• Infant nail scissors

• Soap or liquid bath cleanser, shampoo, baby bath oil, baby powder, cotton swabs, moist towelettes

• 2 or 3 crib blankets. Refer to the entry on "Cribs" on page 96.

• 6 fitted crib sheets

• 2 flannelette-coated waterproof sheets

• 2 quilted crib pads

• Comforter or quilt

Feeding Equipment:

- If you are breast feeding, at least 2 bottles. Refer to the entry on "Breast Milk Versus Formula" on page 36.
- If you are bottle feeding, at least 8 bottles
- Extra nipples and caps
- Bottle brush and nipple brush
- Baby dishes and utensils
- 4 or more bibs

Basic needs:

- Infant seat with a safety strap
- Pacifier
- Rectal thermometer
- Vaseline
- Toys and mobiles
- Car seat
- Carriage or umbrella stroller
- Front or back baby carrier, preferably with a head support. Carrying a five- or six-month-old in front can give some parents a backache.
- Insulated bag for diapers and bottles
- Humidifier, preferably a cool-mist one.
- Nasal suction bulb (aspirator), with a small, clear plastic tip that can be removed for cleaning
- Automatic swing, especially for colicky babies. They come in windup-spring, pendulum-driven, or battery-powered models.
- Playpen, which can be used regularly by a baby of three to four months
- Gates for stairways without doors

Medications:

- Acetaminophen (Tylenol, Tempra, Panadol) drops
- Syrup of ipecac
- For the older child, have a decongestant, antihista-

mine cough medicine, eardrops for pain, and decongestant nosedrops.

Phone numbers:

For baby sitters, keep an emergency list next to the phone. It should contain:

- Your pediatrician's number
- The number where you and your spouse can be reached
- The address and telephone number of your own home
- The name and phone number of a neighbor or relative
- The local police and fire department number, usually 911.

Thumbsucking

ALTHOUGH some adults cringe at the sight of a child sucking her thumb, they would do well to put this "problem" into perspective. Thumbsucking can soothe a baby who is hurt, bored, or upset. Studies have shown that some babies start sucking their thumbs in utero and continue after birth to comfort themselves. Thumbsucking does not mean that the child is insecure, maladjusted, deprived of loving attention, or has emotional problems.

Many pediatric dentists agree that they would rather have the one- to three-year-old suck her thumb than her bottle, because the child can munch down hard on her bottle, causing malocclusion and "buck teeth." The thumb has bones and nerves, so she can't bite too hard on it. Tooth-related problems can be worse in prolonged bottle feeders than for thumbsuckers. All agree, however, that if thumbsucking persists beyond four years of age, the child may then incur dental problems as well as teasing from other children. A thumbsucker who is five to seven years of age, which is when permanent teeth erupt, may develop an overbite or a gap in the bottom teeth and in the upper teeth.

So, if your child sucks her thumb when she is under four, ignore it or distract her with a toy, without even mentioning the thumbsucking. Only 20 percent of thumbsuckers are still at it by the time they're four or five. The habit tends to linger if there is a power struggle between the parent and child. Your first goal in helping the four-year-old thumbsucker, then, is to gain her cooperation and her desire to stop. Show her pictures of children with buck teeth and with spaces in their teeth. Show her the red, wrinkled, and irritated thumb. Her cooperation may follow the comments, disapproving glances, and rejection by other children.

If she agrees to try to stop, have her put a Band-Aid or fingernail polish on her own thumb as a reminder. Most important, praise her for the minutes, hours, and days that she does *not* suck her thumb—especially after situations in which she previously would have sucked. This sounds easy, but it is hard to remind yourself continually to praise her throughout your busy day. Still, it works! A reward at the end of a day without thumbsucking will not only help her feel good about her accomplishment but will also remind you to praise her again. Some suggestions for rewards are sticker charts or an extra story at the end of the day. One cute idea is to make a dot-to-dot diagram of a desired toy. If the child goes an entire day without sucking, two dots are connected. When all the dots are connected, the child receives the toy.

In some children over four, I have had success with a bitter-tasting solution called Stop-Zit. Apply it to the thumb (or whichever fingers your child sucks) in the morning, at bedtime, and throughout the day when thumbsucking is observed. After a successful week, gradually decrease its use, but repeat the program if thumbsucking recurs. Don't use Stop-Zit as a punishment. Try to rely on the reward system. Once again, your child's cooperation is essential.

Thumbsucking during sleep is involuntary and is best approached once the child has achieved daytime control. Put a glove, finger cot, mitten, splint, tape, or other creative covering on her finger with her cooperation.

Pediatric dentists have removable or fixed appliances that help the seven- or eight-year-old child who wants to stop thumbsucking. A behavioral modification program devised by a child or adolescent psychologist is reserved for the teenager who has unsuccessfully tried to break herself of this habit.

SOME IMPORTANT "DON'TS":

1. Don't pull her thumb out of her mouth while you tell her how unhappy you are with the habit.

2. Don't call her a baby.

3. Don't slap her hand, criticize, ridicule, or punish her.

4. Don't make thumbsucking a showdown between you and the child. You will lose, because the thumb belongs to her.

5. Don't allow her to use a pacifier after her baby teeth erupt. If the two- to four-year-old suddenly has the pacifier taken away, she may start to use her thumb as a substitute pacifier. (This does not happen with a six-month-old.) Remember that there is no proof that thumbsucking leads to nail biting.

Thyroid

THE THYROID gland is located in the front of the neck, under the Adam's apple. It uses iodine from our diets to make thyroid hormone, which is necessary for normal growth and development. When the thyroid gland is affected by infection, tumors, iodine deficiency, or an autoimmune disease, either too much hormone (hyperthyroidism) or too little (hypothyroidism) hormone is produced. Hyperthyroidism causes enlargement of the gland (goiter), irritability, nervousness, rapid heartbeats, tremors, fatigue, intolerance to heat, weight loss despite an increased appetite, decline in school performance, insomnia, and bulging eyes. Hypothyroidism causes slow growth, weight gain despite decreased appetite, constipation, intolerance to cold, and delayed onset of puberty.

Babies born without a thyroid gland or with a nonfunctioning one have congenital hypothyroidism; they have no thyroid hormone. This happens twice as often in girls as in boys. The pituitary gland (master gland of the body) produces the thyroid-stimulating hormone in increasing amounts to stimulate the thyroid gland to make thyroid hormone. In congenital hypothyroidism, there is a large amount of thyroid-stimulating hormone but no thyroid hormone, since the gland is absent or not working right. Such an infant may have a large tongue (which can interfere with breathing), feeding problems, lethargy, constipation, a hoarse voice, lower than normal temperature, and prolongation of neonatal jaundice. One early clue of hypothyroidism is a larger than normal soft spot (fontanelle) on the head. Children with hypothyroidism grow at a slow rate and can develop severe neurological problems, including mental retardation.

Since these catastrophic events can be prevented if the disease is diagnosed early, blood-screening testing of newborns for congenital hypothyroidism by heel stick has been legally required since the mid 1970s. The problem occurs in 1 out of 5000 live births in the United States. Both thyroid hormone and thyroid-stimulating hormone can be measured with this test. If the results are strongly indicative of congenital hypothyroidism, a pediatric endocrinologist should be consulted immediately. If the results are questionable, a repeat specimen will be needed, because slightly abnormal results are sometimes obtained on normal babies. About 10 percent of babies with congenital hypothyroidism will be missed with this screening process due to errors in processing the samples or because the hormone abnormalities were not clearly evident in the newborn period. Retesting of any infant with the above symptoms should be done even though the baby was screened as a newborn. Other factors that can skew the results of the newborn screening test are a newborn's illness, prematurity, maternal exposure to antithyroid medicine, and poor maternal and neonatal nutrition.

Treatment with daily oral thyroid hormone starting in the first three months of life will prevent the mental retardation and other complications of hypothyroidism. Treatment may continue for the rest of the patient's life, or, in some cases, until he reaches his full adult height.

Older, healthy children may first develop hypothyroidism through thyroiditis, an autoimmune disease in which the body makes antibodies against its own thyroid gland. These children may experience constipation, fatigue, and intolerance to cold, but they do not suffer the neurological problems of babies. Thyroid tumors and diseases of the pituitary gland can also cause hypothyroidism. Once again, treatment involves oral thyroid hormone replacement.

Any enlargement or swelling in the front of the neck should be evaluated by your child's doctor. Hyperthyroidism (overreactive thyroid) is less common, but a tumor of the thyroid may produce too much thyroid hormone, and medication or surgery may be needed.

Toilet Training

TOILET TRAINING is the quintessential example of a goal that can be achieved in many ways.

Since most kids train for bowel movements between two and four years of age, it usually does not pay to start toilet training until twenty-one months at the earliest. There seems to be a correlation between speaking well (e.g., using intelligible phrases) and toilet training. Therefore, if your child is not yet speaking in phrases, consider delaying her toilet training a bit. If she complains when her diaper is wet or soiled, she's indicating that she's ready. She should also have the dexterity to pull her pants up and down by herself.

The most important aspect of training is your attitude. Don't get frustrated! If it works, great. If it doesn't work, that's okay, too. Sometimes children successfully train for a short period, a few days or weeks, but are not yet neurologically or socially mature enough to sustain the training. Likewise, nighttime control may not be achieved until months after daytime control. If nighttime control is delayed, don't berate your child and don't feel that you have failed. It's all right. Patience and kind persistence will help your child develop normal training habits.

Imitative behavior plays an important role in toilet training, especially for urinary control. Dad, bring your son to the bathroom and demonstrate appropriate pride when he tries to imitate you. It is also helpful to "toilet train" a doll that wets. The doll is given water and carried to the potty. As it "urinates" in the potty, have your child praise the doll for being successful.

When your child is sitting on a potty, her feet should always rest on something solid, for support and comfort. It also helps her develop the necessary intra-abdominal pressure. Therefore, if the potty sits on

344

the toilet, have a stool nearby for her to rest her feet on.

Compromise is the operative word; encourage the process of toilet training but don't force the issue. A time-honored method is to pick one day a month, preferably a day when you have more time than usual, to pursue toilet training. There is a reflex in all of us called the gastro-colic reflex; it's the urge to have a bowel movement shortly after eating a meal. It is as if the gastrointestinal tract is "clearing the way" for more food. Children, too, have this reflex. So have your child sit on the potty for fifteen to twenty minutes after each meal on that day. Be creative. Read to her, play games, tell stories. If she is successful, reward her with a hug, kiss, or a present, like a crayon. Keep a new box of crayons handy, and give her one crayon for each success on the potty. This way, she will be rewarded, but you won't go broke! One pediatrician suggests the following formula for rewards:

- One M&M if the child tries to use the potty.
- Two M&M's if she pees.
- Three M&M's if she poops.

If the reward works, do the same thing the next day and the next. If it doesn't, don't try again for another month. But rest assured; one of these months, without your changing the method, it will work. "Why?" you may ask, since you did nothing different. Because she was ready!

Daytime control of urine and stool is easier and usually isn't achieved at the same time as nighttime control. Only a few newly trained children will be dry at night. "Accidents," especially bed-wetting at night, are common, possibly even hereditary. When a new baby arrives it is common for an older sibling to infantilize his behavior even to the extent of untoilet-training himself. Moving to a new home or having an ill family member are emotional traumas that can also cause accidents. The older sibling will get much more attention by having his diaper changed than by going to the potty by himself. Speak to your doctor if these accidents persist beyond the age of six. Refer to the entries on "Bed-wetting" on page 22 and "Constipation" on page 80. Since asking parents for help in going to the potty is an easy way to get attention, many children will have dry runs.

Teach your daughter to wipe from front to back to keep bacteria from the bowel movement away from the vagina. Demonstrate to all children proper hand-washing hygiene after wiping. A small stepstool may be necessary to help your child reach the sink on her own.

Tongue

"Black" tongue:

A black-looking tongue, sometimes with hairy projections along its surface, can appear during prolonged antibiotic therapy. When the antibiotic is stopped, the black color and hairy texture disappear. Also, oral medications that contain bismuth (e.g., Pepto-Bismol) may cause a black tongue. This, too, is reversible.

"Geographic" Tongue:

Approximately 10 percent of children have smooth, sharply demarcated red patches on their tongues in "maplike" configurations. These patches, which are not tender, move along the surface of the tongue to different positions. Sometimes they disappear, only to return later. The cause is unknown. No treatment, other than reassurance, is needed.

Tongue-Tie

A SHORTENED frenulum—tongue-tie—is of no functional significance if a newborn is able to maintain an adequate sucking seal around a nipple (breast or bottle) and feed well. This small piece of tissue under the tongue, which sometimes does not allow the tongue to protrude outside the mouth, should not cause any speech problems later on if the tongue can move well enough to maintain a strong suck. If sucking does cause problems, the newborn's frenulum may have to be cut. However, the need for this procedure is very rare, though it was done more frequently in previous generations. Since there is always the risk of bleeding or infection, don't let your relatives make you feel guilty that you didn't have the baby's "tongue-tie" snipped. Let them call your pediatrician.

Torticollis (Wryneck)

TORTICOLLIS is a twisting of the neck to one side in an unnatural position. There are two types, acquired and congenital.

Acquired:

Acquired torticollis can follow strenuous play or other physical activity, an upper respiratory infection or abscess, a trauma, or it can be an unusual reaction to some drugs. Usually only the muscles are involved, such as after "sleeping wrong." The child will hold her head to one side because it hurts to turn it. The neck muscles never rest, as they are always working to hold up the head. However, if she lies down with her head completely flat, she will experience some relief. The bed supports the head, so the neck muscles can relax.

The condition should not be confused with the "stiff neck" of meningitis, when the child is unable to bend her head forward. The child can't touch her chin to her chest in meningitis, but she can in torticollis. Meningitis also usually causes headaches, fevers, extreme irritability, or listlessness. The child with torticollis can walk and talk normally and does not look sick.

Discuss your child's condition with your pediatrician. If the condition is particularly severe or lasts for more than three days, x-rays may be necessary to rule out any involvement of the bones in the neck.

Treatment consists of bed rest with the child's head flat, acetaminophen or ibuprofen for pain relief, and warm compresses to the neck. If the pain is severe, a cervical collar may be recommended.

Congenital:

The head tilting of congenital torticollis is usually discovered in the first month or two, because there is a lump in the neck muscle on the side opposite where the chin is pointing. This lump is a fibroma, a mass of thick connective tissue that develops in utero or during birth trauma. It is associated with breech and forceps deliveries and is more common in females.

Although the lump goes away by the time the baby is three or four months old, the head tilting can persist. Excellent results can be obtained with stretching exercises. Position the child in the crib so that she has to turn her head the way she doesn't want to in order to look at a favorite toy or into the room. Surgical correction is only rarely needed if conservative measures are unsuccessful by the time the child is two years of age. Any asymmetry of the skull and face will disappear as long as corrective measures are taken during childhood.

Toys

TOYS ARE such an important part of our children's lives that they merit special attention. The numbers are staggering. Retail toy sales in the United States are estimated at $9 billion. Nearly 150 million new toy cars alone are produced each year worldwide. (My nurse thinks they are all in her son's closet.) Over 150,000 different toys are produced each year by over 1500 toy manufacturers. The Consumer Product Safety Commission has set mandatory safety standards for electric toys, toys with sharp points and edges, toys with small parts, and paint in toys (no lead). However, the federal government has only limited control. It is up to the manufacturer to comply with the requirements. The bottom line is that the responsibility for choosing safe toys rests with parents.

Toys should not come apart into pieces that can be swallowed. A good rule of thumb is that every piece should be larger than the hole in the cardboard tube of a roll of toilet paper.

Plastic does not show up on x-rays. The Mattel Toy Company has developed a plastic compound that contains barium sulfate, which does show up on x-rays and so will greatly help to reduce problems associated with an aspirated plastic part. Uninflated balloons can be aspirated, and so can torn-off pieces of the plastic lining of disposable diapers. Some dolls, like Cabbage Patch Kids, come with their own disposable diapers, so be careful.

Even noise from some toys can be harmful. Noise levels above 100 decibels can damage hearing. The labels on rolls of caps for toy guns state that they should not be used closer than 12 inches to the ear. Battery-operated toys are safer than electrical ones because they cannot cause burns and electric shocks. Avoid toys with sharp or protruding parts like metal axles surrounded by soft rubber or plastic. If the child falls on one of these, the axle could inflict a penetrating wound. Strings on pull toys should be less than 12 inches long so that they cannot form potentially strangulating loops.

One of the great dilemmas for a parent is to buy a toy appropriate for an older child and then keep it away from the younger sibling. Among my most frequent pieces of advice to parents is, "Think like a kid! Think of the possible mischief you could get into with this toy." By doing so, you can avoid many problems for your child.

Following is a list of appropriate toys for various age groups:

Infancy to 1 year old:

- Blocks made of plastic
- Music boxes or animals
- Rattles
- Soft, washable animals, dolls, balls
- Suspended, bright, moving objects, kept out of reach
- Play boards that attach to the crib
- Floating bath toys
- Squeeze toys
- Highchair toys with suction-cup bases

1 to 2 years old:

- Blocks made of wood
- Cloth or plastic books with large pictures
- Sturdy dolls
- Push-and-pull toys
- Toy telephones
- Toys with openings of different shapes and blocks of different shapes to go in them

2 to 5 years old (preschool):

- Books
- Blocks
- Crayons, clay, nontoxic fingerpaints
- Hammer and bench
- Housekeeping toys
- Large stringing beads
- Outdoor toys, swings, sandbox, slide
- Playhouse, rocking horse
- Tricycles, wagons
- Wooden puzzles graded according to age

5 to 9 years old:

- Books
- Card and board games
- Doctor and nurse kits, policeman's hat and badge, cowboy hat
- Hand puppets
- Tea party utensils
- Balls
- Bicycles
- Crafts, music and rhythmic toys
- Electric trains
- Jump rope
- Roller skates, ice skates, skis
- Sports equipment—lightweight bat, baseball glove, etc.
- Construction sets
- Doll clothes, feeding sets, furniture
- Walkie-talkie
- Magnifying glass, binoculars
- Scrapbooks
- Coloring books
- Makeup kits

- Yo-yo
- Kite
- Model airplane kits, graded in difficulty
- Ping-Pong set
- Computer games
- Small remote-control vehicles

10 to 14 years old (preteen):

- Books
- Computers
- Hobby collections, Erector sets with engines, chemistry set
- Microscopes
- Table and board games
- Outdoor sports equipment

Finally, remember that hinged toy chests can be dangerous. A safety hinge or lid support devices should be used so that a lid cannot slam down. The hinge (a ratchet) should allow the lid to be kept open in any position. In some chests, it may be safer to remove the lid completely. In addition, be sure the toy chest has ventilated openings to prevent suffocation in case your child does crawl into it. The toy chest, just like all of your child's furniture, should have rounded or padded edges and corners.

Tuberculosis

TUBERCULOSIS is a bacterial disease that affects the lungs, kidneys, lymph glands, and covering of the brain. It is spread by coughing and sneezing. Pasteurization of milk has eliminated the spread from infected cattle. Children under three years of age are particularly susceptible to the spread of TB bacteria throughout their bodies.

When a healthy child becomes infected by TB bacteria, the body's immune system forms a strong wall around this first lesion, in the lung, inhibiting its spread. If the child does not get reinfected, he may never be sick from that first exposure. However, this quiet infection can be reactivated by certain drugs, such as steroids. If the child is sick or malnourished, that lesion will break out of its confining shell and spread to other parts of the body. The child then may lose his appetite and experience weight loss. He may develop a chronic, productive cough, fever, lethargy, and headaches. Swelling of the lymph nodes in areas surrounding the lungs and neck will cause coughing, wheezing, recurrent pneumonia, difficulty in swallowing, and swelling of an extremity because of blockage of the normal blood return. If the nerves of the voice box are compressed, hoarseness will develop. Night sweats occur when the fever abates during sleep.

Whereas it takes only one or two days to grow strep bacteria from a throat culture in a petri dish, tuberculosis bacteria are very slow-growing. They can take up to three weeks to show up, so diagnoses most frequently rely on skin tests. These skin tests (Tine and Mantoux tests), implanted on the forearm, help to determine whether the child has been infected with the tuberculosis bacterium. All children should have one of these skin tests yearly or every two to three years, according to the locally recommended immunization schedule. Children known to have been in contact with a person who has active TB should be given a skin test at some time between six weeks and three months after the exposure. The period from infection to positive skin test is six weeks.

After the skin test, the child may wash, swim, and engage in all usual activities. If the injection site turns red, lumpy, or bumpy after two to three days, return to the office to have the swelling measured. A positive test does not necessarily mean that the child has active tuberculosis. A chest x-ray (and, on rare occasions, cultures of the child's sputum and/or stomach juices) will help determine this. If those lab tests are normal, it may still be that a quiet infection (see above) exists. Even a newly diagnosed quiet infection should be treated with medication.

Drugs, rest, and a well-balanced diet are the mainstays of treatment for active TB. Children with TB can attend day care and school if they have been receiving chemotherapy for two to four weeks and their symptoms have disappeared. The drug of choice for both quiet infections and active TB is isoniazid. It is taken orally and is generally tolerated well. Rifampin is another antituberculosis medication. It is important to remember that rifampin can cause an orange discoloration of the patient's tears, urine, and saliva. It is scary unless you are prepared for it. Several other drugs are used—some individually, some in combination. The medicines are taken for several months, frequently for up to a year. If the cough has disappeared and the patient with active TB has been on medication for two to four weeks, he is not contagious.

Some situations that prevent a child from showing a positive response to the skin test are: being less than six months old; having a concurrent severe illness, such as cancer or chronic renal disease; taking certain medicines (e.g., steroids); and being malnourished. On the other hand, false positive results can occur following repeated TB skin testing or after immunization with BCG (a bacterium called Bacillus Calmette-Guérin). The BCG vaccine was developed to reduce the incidence of tuberculosis, and is used in developing countries where there is a high incidence of TB. However, since BCG is a weakened strain of the tuberculosis bacterium, subsequent skin tests may be positive from the BCG, and not from a new infection of tuberculosis. It is therefore not routinely used in the United States. The false-positive reaction after the BCG vaccine measures less than 1 centimeter in diameter. If the skin test reaction is greater than 1.5 centimeters, one can assume that a new tuberculosis infection has occurred. By ten years after the BCG administration, this false-positive reaction disappears, and the skin test can be read as if BCG had never been given.

Twins

SINCE THE topic of twins, by definition, involves numbers, let's start with some statistics. The overall incidence of twins in the United States is 1 in 80 births. Black Americans have twins at a rate of 1 in 77 births, and white Americans at 1 in 88 births. Triplets are born in 1 of 10,000 births. The odds of a woman having two sets of identical twins are 1 in 70,000, but a mother of fraternal (nonidentical) twins has three times the chance of having a second set of fraternal twins as the general population. Women between thirty-five and thirty-nine years of age have a ten times greater chance of having twins than teenage mothers, and women who take fertility drugs have an increased chance of having fraternal twins. Fraternal twins are three times as common as identical twins. A third of all fraternal twins are the same sex. Ten to 20 percent of all multiple pregnancies are first discovered at birth.

Identical twins result when a fertilized egg splits after conception. These twins are genetically alike, with the same chromosomes, same sex, identical blood types, and same hair and eye color. However, each twin has unique personality traits, even though both may demonstrate similar interest patterns, attitudes, and feelings. Identical twins do not have identical teeth, birthmarks, or fingerprints, and often grow to slightly different heights and weights.

Fraternal twins result from two fertilized eggs and are as similar or different as other brothers and sisters. They may or may not be of the same sex. Their social development can be as different as single-born siblings. Although female fraternal twins have a slightly increased chance of giving birth to fraternal twins (1 in

60 births), male fraternal twins do not have an increased chance of fathering twin children. Similarly, sisters and daughters of fraternal twins have a slightly higher rate of bearing twins than the general population. Brothers and sons of fraternal twins do not. The incidence of identical twins is unrelated to any of these genetic influences.

Siamese twins receive their name from Chang and Eng, who were conjoined twins from Siam (now Thailand). Siamese twins result from the relatively late and incomplete separation of identical twins in utero.

Examination of the placenta or placentas is helpful, but not a foolproof method of determining whether twins of the same sex are fraternal or identical. Detailed blood typing, tissue typing, and DNA analysis are more reliable.

Some early problems encountered by twins are premature birth, respiratory distress (more common in the second baby or Twin B), intrauterine growth retardation, and twin-twin transfusions, in which one twin receives more blood than the other and is larger in size. Noticeable differences in size of identical twins usually even out by the time the babies are six to twelve months old. Hip dislocations are common, due to uterine crowding.

Recent research indicates that 20 to 40 percent of all twin gestations are resorbed by the body during pregnancy; that is, the body reclaims the tissue of one fetus and absorbs it. The one remaining from these "vanishing twins" is born as a singleton.

Practical tips on the day-to-day handling and management of twins are best obtained from *Twins* magazine and from the Mothers of Twins clubs. There are national and local branches of these clubs, whose function it is to share the trials and joys of raising twins, triplets, and more. Aside from providing practical solutions to problems—what is the best stroller, or what is the best way to breast feed twins, etc.—they also have parties for the children, parents, and grandparents; speakers; sessions to discuss helpful hints; and newsletters loaded with practical advice. Most of these clubs have libraries with books about twins for the parents as well as for the twins and their siblings to help them better understand and enjoy each other. Of course, most local libraries also have excellent resource and "how to" books about twins. Some examples are:

And Then There Were Two – Twins Mothers' Club

Care of Twin Children: A Common Sense Guide for Parents – R. Theroux

Two of Everything But Me – Marion B. West

When it comes to preparing for twins, expectant parents often ask whether they should get two of everything—a double stroller, an extra-large changing table, two highchairs, two cribs, etc. Most parents of twins would answer yes. By feeding, changing, and walking the twins at the same time, these parents can devise a schedule that will allow them to attend to and care for the other aspects and responsibilities of their lives. Mothers can actually breast feed the twins simultaneously, change diapers at the same time, and put the twins to sleep together—even in the same crib at first.

It is appropriate to *end* this chapter with the following startling revelation. During their first month of life, a set of twins needs between 400 and 500 diapers.

Umbilicus (Bellybutton)

Umbilical Cord Care:

WHEN THE umbilical cord is cut, shortly after delivery, the remaining stump can act as a portal of entry for infection, so the nurse will treat it with an antiseptic agent, such as the purple triple-dye. The stump will dry, shrivel up, and fall off at any time up to one month of age. While it is still attached, it is best to sponge-bathe the baby with a washcloth, trying to keep the umbilical cord dry. This helps to prevent the introduction of infection and to speed up the falling-off process. Rubbing alcohol should be applied twice a day to the base of the stump until it falls off. This, too, acts as a drying and antiseptic agent. Folding the diaper lower than the umbilical cord also helps to keep the cord clean and dry.

Once the cord falls off, the baby can be bathed in a regular bath and get her bellybutton wet. It is common for the bellybutton to ooze a little blood, on and off, for one to two weeks after the cord falls off.

If, at any time, the skin around the cord gets red or swollen, or develops a green or yellow discharge with a foul odor, notify your pediatrician. This could represent an infection.

Sometimes, a small piece of umbilical cord remains in place after most of it falls off. This little piece of soft, pinkish tissue is called an umbilical granuloma. Your pediatrician may cauterize it with a stick of silver nitrate, which will turn the granuloma white and then brown. This procedure will help the tissue to dry more quickly and fall off sooner. Contrary to an unusual old wives' tale, it is not recommended that you save and carry around the fallen umbilical cord for good luck!

The way in which the umbilical cord is cut and clamped has nothing to do with whether the baby will develop an "inny" or an "outy." The shape of a child's bellybutton is determined by heredity. Many "outies" in newborns become "innies" as the child grows.

Umbilical Hernia:

An umbilical hernia is a bulge under the skin of the bellybutton due to a weakness in the underlying muscle wall. To better understand this, look at a playground filled with children. You will notice that those kids less than three or four years have potbellies (even those who are thin). Those who are five and over have flat abdomens. This is because the muscles on either side of the abdomen do not fully join and close in the midline until the child is about four, so many children have protrusions through the weakened midline of the abdomen for the first year or two. This umbilical hernia should be easily reducible (pushed back) with gentle pressure. It will, however, tend to bulge more when the child cries or coughs. Strapping it with a belly band or taping it flat with a coin is ineffective. Surgery for umbilical hernias is rarely needed and is reserved for the unusual situation of (1) symptoms like abdominal pain or vomiting, (2) persistence of this hernia beyond eight years of age, at which point it could become a cosmetic concern for the child.

An umbilical hernia is not to be confused with an inguinal hernia, which is also a bulge due to muscle weakness, but it is located in the lower right or left groin area and may extend into a boy's scrotum or a girl's labia. This type of hernia is usually not present at birth but can develop at any age. An inguinal hernia usually does not resolve spontaneously and therefore will require surgical repair.

Urinary Problems

Urinary Tract Infection (UTI)

Females:

Pain or burning on urination is more common in girls than in boys. It is usually due to a bacterial infection ascending from the vagina. If the vagina is irritated and the urine is normal, the condition is called vaginitis. Refer to the entry on "Vagina" on page 366 for the causes and care of vaginitis. When only the bladder is involved, it is called cystitis. When the kidneys are involved, it is called pyelonephritis.

Newborns and infants with UTI's may have fever, jaundice, irritability, vomiting, diarrhea, and poor appetites. Older children may complain of pain on urination, may need to urinate frequently, may wet their beds, and may feel the urgent need to rush to the bathroom. They may have fever, lower abdominal pain, and lower back pain. The diagnosis is made by analyzing the urine—a urinalysis—for white blood cells, red blood cells, and certain chemicals. All should be absent from a normal urine or be present in only very small quantities. In addition, a urine culture should be done once the child's vagina has been thoroughly cleaned. If the child is not yet toilet trained, a plastic urine-collection bag can be placed over the well-cleaned genital and perineal area. Remove the bag immediately after the child voids. If the urine is collected at home, pour it into a sterile jar and take it to the office or lab as soon as possible—certainly the same day. If this method of urine collection is unsuccessful or thought to be unreliable, a thin tube, called a catheter, can be passed up the urethra (the small opening through which the urine comes out) two or three inches until it reaches the bladder. Although there is some discomfort when the catheter enters the sensitive urethra, the procedure is not painful. The catheterization will eliminate the chance that the urine will be contaminated by the surrounding vaginal skin as it comes out. In the newborn, another procedure—a suprapubic tap—can be performed. A sterile needle is inserted through the cleaned skin of the lower abdomen, and when the tip of the needle enters the bladder, urine is drawn back into a syringe.

In all these instances, the urine should normally prove sterile; i.e., free of bacteria. But if a significant amount of bacteria grows from the removed and cultured urine over the next twenty-four to forty-eight hours, then the child has a bacterial urinary tract infection. It is imperative to use great care when collecting these urine specimens to make sure that the grown bacteria do not represent contamination from surrounding skin or stool. It is also necessary to rely on these urine cultures for diagnosis because, although white blood cells, red blood cells, and abnormal chemicals in the initial urinalyses do suggest the presence of a bacterial UTI, they could also be present for other reasons. Red and white blood cells might show up in abnormal amounts in the urine because of trauma, vaginitis, kidney disease, and viral UTI's.

Treatment for a bacterial UTI consists of a seven- to fourteen-day course of antibiotics. Most urine cultures indicate "sensitivities"; that is, they reflect which antibiotics the grown bacteria are most sensitive to. Rather than wait the one to three days it takes to learn these sensitivities, your doctor may start an antibiotic that usually works against the bacteria that cause UTI's. (The antibiotic cannot be administered before the urine is taken for culture, or it could affect the outcome.) This antibiotic can be continued, stopped, or changed, depending on the results of the urine culture and its sensitivities. Some doctors will order a second urine culture three days after the antibiotic has been started and a third culture once the child has been completely off antibiotics for three or four days. Both of these cultures should be sterile.

To help relieve the pain on urination, another medicine, pyridium, can be given for two days along with the antibiotic. Pyridium quickly supplies a topical analgesic effect to the lining of the urinary tract. It also relieves the feelings of urinary urgency and frequency associated with infections, trauma, and surgery. It is important for the child and parent to know that pyridium turns the urine orange or red, because this phenomenon is scary if it is not anticipated.

Some girls have internal physical abnormalities of the bladder, ureters, or kidneys that can contribute to the recurrence of UTI's. One example is vesicoureteral reflux. When a normal bladder contracts, it forces all the urine out of the body through the urethra. Urine does not normally leave the bladder by going back up the ureters toward the kidneys. But this vesicoureteral reflux does occur when there is an abnormality at the junction of the ureters and bladder. The "refluxed" urine returns to the bladder, where it stays between voidings. Bacteria can grow in it, and when the infected urine is refluxed again, it can infect and scar the kidneys, leading to serious health problems, like high blood pressure and kidney failure. Therefore, all girls who have had two or three UTI's should undergo radiologic and/or sonogram studies to rule out internal anatomical problems. If the child is less than one year old, these tests should be done after the first UTI. If no abnormalities exist, the UTI's merely represent a nuisance. If physical abnormalities do exist, they will have to be dealt with by urological surgery or daily low-dose antibiotics given prophylactically. Urine cultures and x-rays should be repeated periodically to monitor the status of the reflux.

Many cases of mild reflux (in which urine backs up only partway through the ureter toward the kidney) resolve spontaneously as the child grows. At this point, the daily prophylactic antibiotics can be stopped. If the reflux is severe (and urine backs up all the way to the kidney) or if a moderate reflux does not resolve by itself, surgery will be needed to prevent the complications of recurrent infections.

Sexually transmitted diseases can mimic the symptoms of a UTI. The diagnosis is made from a culture of the vaginal discharge.

Males:

Although boys have a lower incidence of UTI's than girls, a larger percentage of boys will have the infections as a result of internal physical abnormalities. Therefore, boys should have radiologic and/or sonogram evaluations of their urinary tract after their first UTI, regardless of their age. Refer to the entry on "Penis" on page 248 for the relationship of circumcision to UTI's. The same problems of vesicoureteral reflux that occur in girls also occur in boys. The symptoms are the same as for girls, as is the need to obtain accurate urine cultures. Treatment, again, involves antibiotics and/or surgery. Sexually transmitted diseases can be diagnosed by culturing the penile discharge.

TIPS:

1. Give acetaminophen for pain relief.

2. Encourage the child to drink extra fluids. This dilutes the urine, making it less painful for the child to urinate.

3. Avoid bubble baths. Wash off soap and shampoo thoroughly. It is best to shampoo your child's hair at the end of the bath so that she won't sit in the soapy water, which can irritate the vagina. Keep the bath time less than fifteen minutes, and have the child urinate after the bath.

4. Be sure your daughter wipes her vagina from front to back after urinating or defecating. Refer to the section on "Vaginitis" in the entry on "Vagina" on page 366.

5. Until medical attention is obtained, it may hurt less if she urinates while sitting in a warm bath.

6. Always finish all of the prescribed antibiotic even if the child is feeling better. Stopping prematurely could cause the remaining bacteria to grow and reinfect the urine.

Blood in Urine:

Hematuria means blood in the urine. It is categorized as either *gross* (not because it looks disgusting, but because "gross" also means "observable") when the urine is obviously red or dark in color, or *microscopic* when the urine looks normal but blood is seen under the microscope as part of the urinalysis. Gross hematuria can result from trauma, urinary tract infection, and kidney disease. However, the urine can also appear red for other reasons, with no blood in it at all. The child's eating beets or drinking dye in colored fruit drinks and medicines can turn it red. When the body's muscles are broken down by disease or injury, a protein called myoglobin enters the urine from the damaged muscle, and it turns the urine red. Hepatitis causes a bilirubin-like pigment to enter the urine, making it dark. In each of these examples, a microscopic examination of the discolored urine will not reveal red blood cells.

If red blood cells are seen on the initial urinalysis, but the urine culture is sterile, the doctor may order tests to rule out kidney, ureter, and bladder disease as the source of the blood in the urine. If these too are negative, the child has a viral UTI, and, as with all viral infections, antibiotics will not help. The viral cystitis infection will leave on its own in less than a week.

Any injury to the penis, bladder, ureters, and kidneys can cause gross or microscopic hematuria. Sports injuries, car accidents, and rough horseplay can injure a child's back (and kidneys) or abdomen (and bladder). X-rays and/or sonograms will help to reveal where the bleeding is.

Acute poststreptococcal glomerulonephritis is a kidney disease due to a strep infection of the throat or skin. It can cause blood in the urine. Refer to the entry on "Sore Throat (Pharyngitis) and Tonsillitis" on page 299.

Some children have too much calcium in their urine because of a poorly functioning "filter" in the kidneys. This excess calcium may form crystals and stones in the urine, which irritate the inner lining of the ureters and bladder, causing bleeding and pain. Drinking extra fluids to dilute the urine and taking diuretic medicines are helpful.

Sugar in Urine:

Refer to the entry on "Diabetes" on page 107.

Bed-wetting:

Refer to the entry on "Bed-wetting" on page 22.

Frequent Urination:

Frequent urination can be a normal, temporary response to increased fluid intake. It may also indicate a urinary tract infection, the irritative effect of blood in the urine, diabetes mellitus, diabetes insipidis, stress, and an obsessive-compulsive psychological disorder.

Frequent urination is a desired effect or side effect of some medicines (diuretics, caffeine, etc.).

Strong Urinary Odors:

Urine can smell strong if the child is not drinking enough or has lost water through diarrhea. The concentrated urine will have an odor like ammonia. Infected urines also smell "funny." Some medications, especially antibiotics, give the urine their own smell. Some foods, like asparagus, cause strange urine odors. Some metabolic diseases, such as diabetes and disorders of the normal metabolism of amino acids, create distinctive urine odors.

Changes in Urine Color:

Red: See "Blood in Urine," above.

Orange: The antibiotic rifampin and the urinary tract pain reliever pyridium turn the urine orange.

Blue or **Green:** Some blue or green vegetable dyes used in cake frosting turn the urine the same color as the dye.

Black: Some pinworm medicines and rhubarb can turn the urine black.

Cloudy: If urine is allowed to sit in an office before being tested or is refrigerated overnight for testing the next day, normal crystals will form, giving the urine a cloudy appearance. The crystals will dissolve and the normal color return when the urine is warmed up. A urinary tract infection may also make the urine appear cloudy.

Vagina

THE THIN walls of the vagina in a prepubertal girl do not offer much protection, due to the low amount of estrogen. This sets up the vagina and surrounding skin for local irritation. As urine irritates the sore skin, urination will be painful. Likewise, the moist and closed environment in a diaper encourages the development of inflammation of the vagina, or vaginitis. Following is a list of common causes of vaginitis, with practical tips on how to cure them and avoid them.

TIPS:

1. Be sure that the child or her caregiver wipes from front to back—i.e. from vagina to anus. Otherwise, bacteria from stool may enter the vagina and cause vaginitis.

2. Try a change of laundry detergents or soaps. Some children become sensitive to the same chemicals they earlier could tolerate without difficulty. Change to a mild, unscented soap, and be sure to wash off thoroughly all soaps and shampoos after the child's bath. Shampoo her hair as the last part of the bath. Also, because some alcohol-containing wipes and many bubble baths irritate vaginas, avoid them if they cause symptoms.

3. Use white cotton panties. Avoid nonbreathing materials like nylon and Dacron. The dye in some panties may irritate an already sore vagina.

4. If your child has finished swimming for the time being, have her change into dry clothes. Don't let her sit around the pool or at the beach in a wet bathing suit for long periods. Be sure she is cleaned well after playing in a sandbox.

5. To help air-dry the skin, let your daughter sleep in

a nightgown without panties. During the day avoid tight-fitting clothes, especially jeans.

6. A vaginal discharge associated with rectal itching may be due to pinworms. See that entry on page 257.

7. A foul odor with a bloody or purulent discharge from the vagina may indicate the presence of a foreign body. Although girls are naturally curious about their vaginas, and some masturbate frequently, it is not common to find a foreign body as a cause of vaginitis. However, an item as innocent as toilet paper is a foreign body if it remains in the vagina. Unless the foreign body is easily accessible, do not try to remove it by yourself. Bring it to the attention of your doctor.

8. A mucousy, clear discharge may develop, intermittently, a year or two before a girl's first period. This is normal, and shows that the young lady's hormones are "waking up" in her body.

9. A common type of diaper rash and vaginitis is due to a *Candida* fungal infection. This frequently occurs with the use of antibiotics, and your doctor can prescribe an antifungal ointment. Some babies have a similar mouth infection called thrush. This requires an oral antifungal medicine, which your doctor will prescribe.

10. If episodes of vaginitis recur frequently, consider the possibility of sexual abuse. Refer to the entry on "Child Abuse" on page 58 for signs that a parent should look for.

11. Your pediatrician may want to obtain a urinalysis to rule out diabetes, and a urine culture to rule out urinary tract infection.

12. If your daughter does get vaginitis, encourage her to take a "sitz bath" in the morning and again at night. Add 2 tablespoons of white vinegar to her regular bath water and have her sit in the tub for five to ten minutes. In addition, if she feels a burning sensation when she urinates, have her urinate in a bathtub full of lukewarm, soothing water; that may be less painful. En-

courage her to drink a lot so that the urine won't be concentrated. A diluted urine won't burn so much.

13. Sometimes a newborn girl actually has a "period" a few days after birth as her mother's hormones leave her system. Similarly, a newborn boy's and girl's breasts are enlarged due to the mother's hormones. These diminish over the first few months of life. Many newborn girls normally have a mucousy white discharge, on and off, for a few weeks. Wipe it away gently with a cotton ball and lukewarm water.

14. Many baby girls have their labia minora (inner vaginal lips) stuck together. If they have no trouble urinating and no pain, there is no need to do anything. This condition, called labial adhesions, disappears by itself when the labia separate as the children grow. Forcibly separating them does not work, as they will only rejoin. If, however, adhesions do cause symptoms, your doctor will prescribe a cream that will gently separate the lips.

15. Those girls who are too "busy" to spend time on a toilet may not completely empty their bladders. The remaining urine may later dribble out, causing irritation and pain. Insist that your child take her time in the bathroom.

16. Finally, sexually transmitted diseases, such as gonorrhea and syphilis, as well as some illnesses accompanied by rashes, such as chickenpox and scarlet fever, are notorious for producing vaginal irritations. Each of these vaginal infections requires medical attention. A sitz bath with Aveeno several times a day is soothing.

Vitamins

Babies:

A NEWBORN's immature liver and intestines cannot make vitamin K, which is necessary for normal clotting of the blood. Therefore, all newborns should receive an injection of vitamin K shortly after birth.

Breast milk contains all the other necessary vitamins and minerals, except for vitamin D and fluoride. Refer to the section on "Fluoride" in the entry on "Teeth" on page 317. Nursing babies should receive supplemental vitamin D, usually given in a preparation that also contains vitamins A and C. If the water is not fluoridated, fluoride can be added to the preparations too.

Commercial formulas with iron contain all of the baby's vitamin and mineral needs, except for fluoride. The baby will need fluoride supplements only if the water supply is not fluoridated. Although added vitamins can be stopped after the child is one year old, fluoride should be continued until he is fourteen to fifteen.

Children over One Year of Age:

Most American children do not need vitamin or mineral supplements in their diets. A typical American diet, with food from each of the major food groups, contains more vitamins than a growing child needs. Refer to the section on "Food Groups" in the entry on "Eating Habits and Picky Eaters" on page 122. Extra vitamins are merely voided with the urine. Common sources of vitamins are:

Vitamin A: Milk, butter, margarine, cheese, eggs, liver, carrots, yellow and green vegetables, tomatoes, many fruits. Vitamin A is needed for healthy eyes, bones, teeth, and skin.

Vitamin B Complex: Cereals, pasta, bread, nuts, peanuts, milk products, meats, many vegetables. The B vitamins maintain healthy skin, eyes, and nervous system and prevent anemias.

Vitamin C: Oranges, orange juice, grapefruit, tomatoes, potatoes, leafy green vegetables like cabbage and broccoli, pineapples, berries, melons. Vitamin C maintains healthy skin and promotes good wound healing. It is added to infant formulas but is absent from cow's milk.

Vitamin D: Nearly all cow's milk sold in the United States is fortified with vitamin D. Fish in the diet and exposure to sunshine are good sources of vitamin D. It is needed to maintain strong bones and teeth.

Vitamin E: Green leafy vegetables, nuts. Premature infants need vitamin E to prevent the development of anemia. It is given as oral drops.

Vitamin K: Vitamin K is made in the intestines of normal, healthy children. It is also found in many different foods, especially green leafy vegetables. Vitamin K promotes the normal clotting of blood and is needed to maintain healthy bones.

Some children do need supplemental vitamins. These include children who have problems with intestinal absorption; children with cystic fibrosis; allergic children on highly restricted diets; premature babies; and babies who were born with low birth weights. The benefits of extra vitamin C for normal children are controversial. There are so many anecdotes and stories about how extra vitamin C has helped a given child or a certain family fight off infections, like the common cold, that I have no objections to its use. I can't formally and scientifically recommend and prescribe extra vitamin C as the ultimate cure for the common cold, but, frankly, it doesn't matter because it can't hurt.

Walkers

ABOUT ONE million walkers are sold yearly in the United States and used for infants as young as five and six months of age. Infants sitting in a walker should be able to touch the floor with their feet in order to move around. Problems to be aware of:

Tipping over: This can occur when the walker is moving between different surfaces, such as floor to rug, over a door threshold, on a carpet with high shag, or on tiles of even slightly varying heights. To help prevent tipping over, buy a walker with a wheel base that is wider at the bottom than at the top. Choose a model that locks in place if one wheel is not on a level surface. Use the walker only on smooth surfaces, and make sure that all doors are closed and stairways are guarded. Although some people feel that babies who use walkers learn to walk later than babies who don't use walkers, this has not been my experience. Nevertheless, walkers should be used only with the cautions included in this chapter.

Falling down stairs: Gates should guard all stairways. Do not allow your child to use a walker near curbs and swimming pools.

Entrapping fingers: This is less of a problem on new models. It used to occur when children were lifted into or out of the walkers. Protective devices consisting of covers over accessible coil springs, protective spaces between scissoring components, and locking devices to prevent frame collapse have all been devised to prevent these entrapment problems.

Using the walker as a baby sitter: Never ignore the child or leave him unattended.

Warts

WARTS ARE caused by viruses that can spread anywhere on the body as well as onto other people. They can grow singly or in groups, have the same color as the skin, and are commonly found on the hands, knees, and feet. The incubation period is from one to eight months. If ignored, they usually go away, but that can take up to two years. The best treatment is to leave them alone. Although they are of cosmetic concern to some children, they cause medical problems only if they bleed recurrently, get infected, or irritate fingers when the child is, say, writing. Some immunity to wart infections develops in adulthood. Warts are *not* cancerous.

TIPS:

1. Keep the skin clean and dry. Don't allow your child to pick, chew, or bite the warts, because these actions could infect the warts and make them spread.

2. Apply over-the-counter wart-remover medicine after softening the wart with warm water and then putting Vaseline on the surrounding tissue so that the acid solution does not destroy normal skin. Follow instructions carefully. Afterward, cover the area with a Band-Aid. Don't use these medicines on the face or genitals; they could scar the skin. They can be used on the skin of children over one year old, but be sure to close all medicines tightly and store them out of children's reach.

3. If these medicines don't help, your doctor may use a heated electrical needle to burn off the wart after he has anesthetized the area. This procedure is called electrocautery.

4. Liquid nitrogen or laser treatments are also used by dermatologists to remove warts.

5. Warts on the bottom of the feet, called plantar

warts, are particularly troublesome. They grow into the foot because the child steps on them. As a result, they may impinge on nearby nerves, bone, or surrounding tissues, resulting in pain. Electrical, chemical, laser, or surgical treatment will be needed to remove plantar warts. Be sure your child wears coverings on his feet at swimming pools, showers, and gyms.

SAFETY TIPS:

Airplane Safety

AN INTERESTING reflection of our times is that many children have been on airplanes more times than they have been on subways. Since air travel has become so common, here are some practical tips to keep in mind while traveling with children.

TIPS:

1. If your child suffers from motion sickness, sit as close to the wings of the plane as possible. Refer to the entry on "Motion Sickness" on page 230.

2. The ears equilibrate internal pressure with external pressure when we swallow, not just when we suck. That's why our ears "pop" and feel better after we drink during ascent or descent. Chewing gum or sucking a candy, therefore, does not help the child's ear unless he swallows. It is a good idea to breast- or bottle-feed a baby as the plane goes up or down. A toddler or older child should have a box of juice (or a thermos) handy to sip from, with a straw, when the plane climbs and descends. Once the plane is level, this is less of a problem. It is wise not to give the child anything to drink for an hour before the flight and for an hour before the descent so that he'll be thirsty enough to sip his drink during those times. Another maneuver is to hold the child's nostrils closed and have him try to exhale forcibly.

3. If your child has recently had an upper respiratory infection or an ear infection, your pediatrician may prescribe a decongestant for the day of the flight.

4. If your child is to have his own seat on the plane,

bring his car seat for him to use on the flight and during your travels.

5. If, during the flight, it becomes necessary to use an oxygen mask, put yours on first so that the child won't be afraid to wear his. He will then use imitative behavior and feel better about putting the mask on his own face.

6. Air-sickness bags make good disposable containers for dirty diapers or other soiled items.

7. It may be wise to take a lightweight collapsible stroller on the plane. Most models fit in the overhead storage compartments.

8. Liquid medicines, especially insulin, may freeze if they are stored in the hold of an airplane, so carry such medicines with you on the plane.

9. The best way to avoid jet lag is to adapt and conform to the time period you are in. If it is nighttime, try to sleep. If it is daytime, try to stay awake. Do your best to have your child's schedule follow the same pattern.

SAFETY TIPS:

Bicycle Safety

THE MAJORITY of children's bicycle accidents don't involve cars. They are falls or collisions with other bicycles or people. The following tips will reduce your child's risk of serious head injury by 85 percent.

TIPS:

1. Be sure your child is wearing appropriate protective gear, such as a helmet and elbow and knee pads. The helmet should have adjustable shock-absorbent pads inside to ensure a proper fit. If the helmet does not

already have a reflecting trim border for nighttime use, add reflecting decals.

2. The seat should be adjusted so that your child's feet can rest on the ground while he is still sitting. Resist the temptation to save money by buying a bike he will "grow into." Young children should have bikes with foot brakes, because they frequently are not strong enough to use hand brakes.

3. Children under ten years of age should never ride bikes on the road, even when just crossing it. A new rider should stay on sidewalks, bike paths, and driveways. It is safest to ride single file.

4. Never let your child carry friends in his bicycle basket.

5. If he must ride at night, be sure he is wearing brightly colored clothes, and see that the bicycle has reflecting decals. The bicycle should also have a headlight and a flashing taillight.

6. Check the air pressure in the bike's tires periodically.

7. Don't let your child ride while wearing loose pants or a long coat. If necessary, put clips or rubber bands around the bottoms of pants to keep them from getting caught in the chains.

8. Don't let your child ride his bike in the rain. The brakes won't work as well, and car drivers are less likely to see the bicyclist.

9. In your community try to establish barriers and bicycle paths to separate the bicyclists from car traffic and pedestrians.

10. Adults who carry children on their bicycles should use a rear-mounted child seat with safety straps and side panels. The child, even as a passenger, must wear a helmet.

11. Since many accidents occur when the child riding a bike breaks a traffic law, teach him the following rules of the road:

• Stop at all intersections. These are where most car-bike collisions occur.

• Ride with the traffic. Riding on the wrong side of the road increases the risk of collision eleven times. With wrong-way riding, the biker ends up at a place in the intersection where car drivers often do not see them. Second, motorists tend not to search in front of them for oncoming bicycles. Third, an oncoming bicycle can't be seen by a car driver coming around a curve in the road.

• Obey all traffic signs, stop signs, and lights.

• Use hand signals.

• Walk—do not ride—bikes across intersections.

• Do not wear headphones of any type. It is important to hear all traffic sounds.

All above tips and rules also apply to skateboards, roller skates, Rollerblades, and minibikes. Skateboards should never be hitched to a car, bicycle, or truck. Children under five years of age have proportionately large heads which make them prone to head injuries and they lack the coordination needed to master roller skates and skateboards.

SAFETY TIPS:

Calling the Doctor

WHENEVER you call your doctor, it is a good idea to keep in mind the following points.

1. State your child's name, age, and his recent weight.

2. Know when the current problem started.

3. Don't rely on feeling the child's forehead to determine the height of a fever. Take the temperature before you call.

4. State clearly any known medical conditions (diabetes, congenital heart disease, etc.).

5. State any known allergies to medicines.

6. If the child is currently on any medicines, have the bottle(s) nearby so that you can give the name, directions, doses, and expiration dates as needed.

7. Be familiar with the phone numbers and hours of a few local drugstores.

8. Always have pen and paper handy to jot down any directions your doctor may give.

SAFETY TIPS:

Car Safety

ANY BOOK on pediatrics would not be complete unless it contained pointers on how to avoid the number one cause of death in all pediatric and adolescent age groups—car accidents. Motor vehicle accidents kill and cripple more children in America each year than cancer, child abuse, respiratory diseases, suicide, and crib death . . . combined! Therefore, the ABC of well baby care is *A*utomotive *B*aby *C*are. To illustrate this point: the body of a six-month-old child (weighing approximately sixteen pounds) traveling in a car going thirty miles per hour obtains a force of seven hundred pounds during a collision. This is comparable to the force of falling out a third-story window. The obvious way to prevent injuries from such accidents is to encourage the use of car seats. Another advantage of car seats is that they keep children in their places, allowing the driver to pay better attention to the road. It is now the law in every state that infants and children must ride buckled up in car seats or seat belts.

Other forms of transportation should always be considered. There are ten times as many deaths per passenger mile in cars than in buses, and twenty times as many deaths per passenger mile in cars than in trains or planes.

Half of all car deaths occur in collisions with trees, telephone and utility poles, and other rigid objects a few inches or feet from the roadside. There are no trees or poles along the runways of airports, and roads and highways should be made similarly safe.

There are many different makes and styles of car seats, with new models coming out all the time. There are three basic types:

1. Infant car seats, which all face the rear. These are not the infant seats used to feed a baby at home.

2. Convertible seats, which can be used to face rear or front.

3. Booster seats, which are front-facing.

A good source of up-to-date information on state-of-the-art car seats is the Consumer Products Safety Commission (1-800-424-9393), or write for the Shopping Guide from the American Academy of Pediatrics, 141 Northwest Point Road, P.O. Box 927, Elk Grove Village, Illinois 60009. It will supply the answers to many questions, such as: When do I turn the car seat around from rear-facing to front-facing? How do I best secure this car seat in my car?

Air bags are great lifesavers. However, a rear-facing car seat should never be used in the front seat of a car with a passenger-side air bag. In an accident, the rapidly inflating air bag could push the infant into the back of the front seat and cause injuries.

For most models it is safest to keep the car seat in the middle of the backseat of your car. Your newborn infant should be placed in a car seat during his very first ride home from the hospital and every ride thereafter. Use two blankets or towels between the side of the car seat and the baby's head and shoulders to help prop and secure him. If the infant's head flops forward, tilt the seat back a little and wedge padding under the base of the seat. The natural parental urge to hold and cuddle the baby in your arms or lap in the car will not protect the baby adequately. If you should be involved in a collision, your reflex action will make you thrust your arms forward and out to protect yourself from hitting the dashboard or seat in front. The baby would then go flying forward.

TIPS:

1. Don't allow a baby or child to ride on an adult's lap.

2. Don't allow adults to ride unrestrained in the car. Passengers riding loose endanger the lives of those who are wearing restraints.

3. Do use a rear-facing car seat until the baby is one year old or 26 inches tall or weighs 20 pounds. Your car seat manual will supply specific recommendations. Use the car seat belt to keep the car seat in place at all times, even when the child is not in it. That way, it won't move around and harm other passengers.

4. Do keep your child in a car seat until he weighs at least 40 pounds. Again, refer to the car seat manual.

5. Do switch to a regular lap belt once the car seat has been outgrown. The lap belt should be placed over the child's hip bones, not across the abdomen. Seat belts that lock only on impact are inadequate, because they do not hold the seats in place around sharp turns or on big bumps. However, do not add the shoulder harness until the child is 55 inches tall. Otherwise, the belt may fall across his neck. Never share a seat belt with your child. In an accident, he could be crushed by your body.

6. Don't use any car seat that was made before January 1, 1981. Those made earlier do not meet today's strict crash standards.

7. Do teach your child to get out of the car on the

sidewalk side, even on quiet streets. Never open the door to let him out in the street.

8. If you rent a car in another city, rent a car seat too.

9. In hot weather, check all metal parts of the car seat and straps before putting your child in. Hot metal strips could burn his skin. Vinyl seats can get hot, too, so cover them with a cloth towel or a blanket.

10. Those children who grow up protected by car seats and seat belts will be the safe buckled-up drivers of tomorrow. Likewise, children will learn and adopt bad habits from their parents. Alcohol is a factor in half of all car accidents involving teenagers. Set a good example. Don't drink and drive. Give frequent praise for proper conduct while your child is riding in a car and while your teenager is driving the car.

Safety tips:

Giving and Taking Medications

THIS CHAPTER will offer some practical tips on one of mankind's most difficult feats: giving children medicines. Every pediatrician and each of the families he cares for has a bunch of "tricks of the trade" for administering oral or injectable medicines, as well as eyedrops, nosedrops, eardrops, and nebulized medicines. Here are just a few:

Oral:

DOSES

  1 cc = 1 ml
  5 cc = 1 teaspoon
15 cc = 3 teaspoons = 1 tablespoon
30 cc = 2 tablespoons = 1 ounce

Since we have different sizes of "teaspoons" in our homes, get a 5 cc syringe and be sure that your "medicine teaspoon" measures 5 cc. (Some "dessert teaspoons" are smaller and some are larger than 5 cc.)

Ask your doctor to familiarize you with the prescribed medicine. Should it be taken before, during, or after meals? What are the side effects? How often and for how long should the medicine be taken?

All children should be upright when taking oral medications so that they don't choke. It is easier to give a baby his medicine in a dropper or syringe than in a spoon. Wrapping a baby inside a blanket will prevent his arms from flailing at you while you give him medicine.

Liquid medicines and tablets (whole or crushed) can be mixed with a food that has a strong, sweet taste. Although applesauce is often suggested as something to make medicine palatable, I find that it is too bland and doesn't mask the taste or texture of many medicines. You may have more success with jelly, yogurt, regular milk, ice cream, chocolate milk, or a spoonful of chocolate syrup. Use only a small amount of drink so that you're sure he gets all the medicine. Erythromycin, a very important and effective antibiotic, is notorious for causing stomach upsets. Giving it after a meal or snack (i.e., not on an empty stomach) and putting it in one of the items suggested above will help. If most oral medicines are vomited within a half-hour after they are taken, they can be given one more time. If they are vomited again, or if you are not sure what to do, call your doctor.

Eyedrops:

Refer to Tip 2 in the section on "Pink Eye" in the chapter on "Eyes" on page 129. Eyedrops should be at room temperature. First clean away any discharge by wiping with a moist cotton ball from near the nose outward across the eye. A baby can be placed in a "papoose"; wrap his arms against his body inside a blanket. Since eye infections spread easily, it is usually necessary to treat both eyes. Have your baby or child lie down or bend his head back. With his eyes open or closed, drop a little puddle of eyedrops in each corner where the eyes meet the nose. When he opens his eyes, enough drops will go in, even though some trickle down his cheeks. Never let the dropper touch the eyes, or it will pick up and transfer the infection elsewhere or into the bottle. Check the directions carefully.

Eardrops:

They should be at room temperature. Have the child lie down with the head turned so that the ear to be treated is up. Drop in the prescribed amount of drops, and have the child lie there for one minute. Then do the other side. A small wad of cotton can be placed outside the ear canal for five minutes to prevent the ear drops from running out.

Nosedrops:

They should be at room temperature. Use a "papoose" if necessary. (See above under "Eyedrops.") Tilt the child's head backward and give the prescribed dose. Decongestant nosedrops should never be used for more than four days in a row. Otherwise, they irritate the nose, actually producing more secretions.

Intramuscular Injections:

When a shot has to be given in a child's leg, it will be less painful (and the pain will last a shorter period of time) if the leg muscle is relaxed rather than tense. One way to make it relax is to have the child wiggle his toes while he's getting the shot. The maneuver will also serve as a distraction from the shot.

Inhaler:

There has been a recent surge in the use of inhalers or "puffers" by children and adolescents with asthma and other respiratory problems. Be sure that you and your child are familiar and comfortable with the proper use of an inhaler. If you have any questions, let your doctor demonstrate its appropriate use. Be sure the child . . .

• Shakes the inhaler before each use.

• Breathes out to expel as much air as possible from the lungs.

• Puts the mouthpiece in his mouth and pushes down on the canister while he breathes in slowly, inhaling through his mouth only. If necessary, pinch the nose closed.

• Holds his breath as long as possible, and then breathes out.

• Waits one minute if two puffs are prescribed, shakes the inhaler again, and repeats.

• Cleans the inhaler daily.

Many allergists and pulmonary specialists recommend the use of "spacers" with inhalers. (See Tip 1 in the entry on "Asthma" on page 14.) With inhalers alone, 65 percent of the medicine reaches the lungs. With a spacer, 95 percent of the dose reaches the lungs. The tube goes between the child's mouth and the inhaler and fills up with the medicine after the inhaler is pushed down. The child can then breathe in the medicine from the spacer at a more relaxed pace.

Nebulizer:

A nebulizer changes a liquid medicine into a mist, which the child then breathes in through a mask. A portable nebulizer can be bought for home use (under a doctor's supervision) for a child with recurrent respiratory problems. It can be used for a child who is too young to master the mechanics of an inhaler.

SAFETY TIPS:

Halloween and Party Precautions

THE FOLLOWING list of practical tips and safety precautions applies to Halloween as well as all parties your child attends.

TIPS:

1. All costumes should be flame-resistant and loose enough to allow the child to wear warm undergarments when walking outside. The masks should be easy to look through (especially when crossing streets) and easy to breathe through.

2. All facial paints, glitters, and makeup should be nontoxic. Children with many allergies and sensitive skin should avoid these products.

3. Neon glow tubes contain a chemical that can irritate the skin and eyes. Teach your children not to break or crush these tubes.

4. Children should not eat anything until their parents inspect all treats for torn or unsealed wrapping. Fruits should be washed and cut open to be checked for foreign objects. Likewise, homemade treats from strangers should be discarded. It is not recommended that you arrange to x-ray candies or other treats. X-rays are expensive and do not guarantee that many poisons will be detected. Notify police of any suspicious treats or harmful objects found in food.

5. Children should "trick or treat" only at homes of friends or people they know.

6. Leave on your outside lights for all children to see where they're going. Your pets should be kept far from the front door so that they don't scare other children.

7. Consider a neighborhood party as a safe alternative to "trick or treating."

SAFETY TIPS:

Injury Prevention: Six Basic Tips

ALL CHILDREN should live in an environment that contains the following six basic injury-prevention items, whether at home, in a playgroup, in camp, or at school.

1. Currently approved child car seats.

2. Smoke detectors and fire extinguishers. There should be at least one fire extinguisher for each story of the house. Everyone, including older children, should be taught how to use the extinguisher.

3. Safe hot water temperatures at the tap. Maximum hot water temperature should be 120° F (48° C).

4. Window and stairway guards or gates.

5. One-ounce bottles of syrup of ipecac to induce vomiting. Have the telephone numbers of the child's pediatrician and the local Poison Control Center immediately available. Use safety caps on all medicines and keep the containers out of the reach of climbing children. Throw away expired medicines.

6. Safety plugs for all unused electrical outlets.

Kitchen Safety

THE KITCHEN is potentially the most dangerous room for a child. Think of the possible sources of trauma—sharp instruments, boiling water, heavy utensils, etc. To spot hazards you might otherwise overlook, get down on your hands and knees and look at the kitchen from a toddler's perspective. Use the following list of practical tips as a guide to babyproof this central room of every home.

TIPS:

1. Keep hot pots and pans on *rear* burners, with all handles facing inward. Don't wear loose sleeves while cooking over a stove.

2. Keep cups of hot coffee or tea away from counter ends and table edges.

3. Mount irons on the walls and keep them there. Be sure the electrical cord is out of reach. If appliances must be kept on a counter, place them near an outlet so that there is no extra slack in the cord. Coil any excess cord and bind it.

4. All sharp knives, forks, and other instruments should be stored in drawers or cabinets that have childproof closures.

5. Be sure your pet's bowls are cleaned and put out of reach after use.

6. The kitchen is the ideal place for a playpen; you and your child can see each other while he remains safely enclosed.

7. Don't use tablecloths on the kitchen table. Every toddler is eager to demonstrate the magic trick he can do by pulling the edge of the tablecloth.

8. Keep a fire extinguisher in the kitchen. Keep

nearby a folding fire ladder that hooks over a window-sill. Be sure matches are stored out of a child's reach.

9. Keep lids on garbage cans closed to discourage garbage exploration by the inquisitive child. Install a cover on the garbage disposal switch.

10. Always keep the following items locked in a storage area: Drāno, products with lye, antifreeze, gasoline, kerosene, paint, paint thinner, turpentine, weed killers, pesticides, power tools. Never put poisonous items into unmarked containers or beverage bottles.

11. When you go to the fridge, use this as an opportunity to teach your child about the need to keep certain foods refrigerated to prevent food poisoning.

12. Teach safety points about blenders, food processors, microwaves, grills, and even about not poking a fork or other metal into a plugged-in toaster. Don't you yourself use a knife or fork to remove toast from a toaster even if the toaster is unplugged. Children also should be taught not to wash electric gadgets while they are plugged in.

13. Be very careful if you use a microwave to warm up a bottle. Although the outside of the bottle may feel lukewarm or "just right," the inside could be scaldingly hot. Babies have burned their palates this way. Therefore, either warm the bottle up by placing it under a hot water tap for two to three minutes, or put it in a dish of hot water. Regardless, always test the temperature of the milk itself before giving it to the baby; you can place a few drops on your wrist.

14. Don't drink any hot beverage while the baby is in your arms.

15. Don't let a toddler play with plastic bags or try to blow up balloons. He could suffocate and choke. Remember that the serrated cutting edges on plastic wrap boxes are very sharp and could easily cut the child.

16. Have emergency phone numbers, including that of the Poison Control Center, near the kitchen phone.

17. Install safety gates at the top and bottom of stairs.

18. Keep bowls of nuts, popcorn, candy, and other smooth round objects away from young children, who could choke on them.

19. Keep house plants out of reach. Know the names of your plants so that if your child ever eats part of one, you'll be able to notify the Poison Control Center.

20. Be sure that all throw rugs have nonskid backing so that you and your child don't slip.

21. Put covers on heating ducts and radiators, with openings small enough to prevent little fingers from touching the hot parts. Space heaters and stoves should have guards to prevent burns.

22. Install antiscald devices on all faucets; they will shut off the flow if the water gets too hot (over 120° F or 48° C).

23. Move chairs away from windows, which should have properly installed window guards, especially if you live on the second floor or higher.

24. Tie up any excess cord from curtains and blinds so that no cord is longer than twelve inches.

25. Children should use paper or plastic cups in the kitchen, and *everyone* should use them in the bathroom for drinking (and gargling). Glass can break on tile or other hard surfaces, and broken glass is a particular danger in the bathroom, where people are frequently barefoot.

26. Since children like to hide in closets, be sure that all closet doors can be opened from the inside.

27. All furniture should have rounded corners and blunt edges. Padded corner and edge protectors should cover furniture with sharp edges.

SAFETY TIPS:

Lead Poisoning

LEAD IS A naturally occurring element that has been used since the beginning of civilization. It has no biologic value. Therefore, the ideal blood level should be 0 mcg/dl (micrograms per deciliter—the unit used for blood lead levels). However, since it is a natural constituent of the earth's crust and has many industrial uses, lead is everywhere in the environment, so all humans have absorbed some lead into their bodies. As a matter of fact, the mean blood level in American preschool children is between 7 and 10 mcg/dl. The major sources of lead are paint, auto exhaust, food, water, and dust. For children, the most important pathways are ingestion of chips from lead-painted surfaces, inhalation of lead from car emissions, food from lead-soldered cans, and water drunk from lead-soldered plumbing. The lead in car emissions is inhaled directly or deposited in soil. Children playing near roads and freeways may not only breathe the exhaust fumes but may ingest contaminated dirt. Three to four million children in the United States are at risk of lead poisoning. It is especially toxic to children under six years of age, who are more likely to place objects with lead-contaminated dust in their mouths. Although lead poisoning occurs more commonly in inner city, underprivileged children, plumbism (lead poisoning) crosses all socioeconomic boundaries.

The lead content of paint was not regulated until 1977, and many older buildings have lead exterior and interior paint that is peeling, flaking, and chipping. Children ingest loose paint as a result of pica (compulsive eating of nonfood items). House dust has been found to have high levels of lead. Since farm vehicles are not required to use unleaded gasoline, lead may be deposited on crops and retained by leafy vegetables. Acidic foods leach lead from lead solder in cans and from lead glazes used in making some kinds of pottery and ceramics. Dishwashing may chip or wear off the protective glaze and expose the lead-containing pigments. Old water coolers with lead pipes are another source of lead exposure. If workers in lead-related industries do not shower and change clothes, they can bring lead dust home on their skin, shoes, clothing, and cars, thus endangering family members.

Children show a greater sensitivity to lead's effects than adults do. The lead enters the developing central nervous system, causing behavior disorders, lower intelligence, and delayed milestones. Lead also enters the kidneys, bone marrow, liver, bones, and teeth. As a result, the following complications can develop: anemia, short stature, low weight, kidney problems with high blood pressure, hearing loss, poor dentition, and infertility problems among men and women. Some children complain of fatigue, muscle aches, joint pains, stomachaches, headaches, vomiting, constipation, and difficulty in concentrating. Some have seizures. Many young children have iron and calcium deficiencies, which increase their gastrointestinal absorption of lead. Since lead readily crosses the placenta, the fetus is at risk for adverse neurological effects. Low birth weight and premature birth may result.

The exposure to lead need not be major for lead poisoning to develop. The body accumulates the lead a little at a time and releases it slowly. It is the total amount of lead in the body that relates to adverse effects, so a blood level determination is the most useful test for lead exposure. As expected, symptoms are dose-related. The higher the blood lead level, the worse the symptoms.

SAFETY TIPS: LEAD POISONING

At a blood level of 7 mcg/dl, transplacental transfer occurs.

At a blood level of 10, growth, hearing, and IQ are minimally affected.

At a blood level of 15, developmental milestones begin to be affected.

At a blood level of 40, anemia develops.

At a blood level of 60, abdominal pain may occur.

At a blood level of 80, kidney problems may develop.

At a blood level of 100, neurological problems often occur.

At a blood level of 130, death may occur.

The levels defining lead poisoning have been progressively declining. Currently, the official level of concern for children is 10 to 15 mcg/dl. In an adult, that amount of lead would weigh less than a paper clip. Recent estimates are that one out of six children in the United States fits into the "lead-poisoned" category. However, 93 percent of these have levels that are low enough to require little therapeutic action. Regardless, every child who has a developmental delay, behavior disorder, or speech problem and is at environmental risk should have a lead test.

TIPS:

1. The first rule of treatment is to separate the patient from the lead source. If the poisoning is caused by lead paint at home, the entire family should be rehoused while the home undergoes lead removal. Cover any cracked or flaking paint until it is removed. Hire only contractors licensed and experienced in lead removal. To find a qualified contractor, check the Yellow Pages under *Lead*, call the state health department, or contact the regional office of the U.S. Department of Housing and Urban Development.

A common danger is the improper removal of lead-based paint from older houses during renovation or, ironically, during cleaning to protect children. Torches, heat guns, and sanding machines are particularly dangerous because they blast the lead into a fine dust, whose small particles are more readily absorbed than paint chips. The contractor should remove all draperies, furniture, and rugs. He should turn off forced-air heating or cooling systems and seal all vents before he removes the lead. Be sure to cover floors with plastic, thoroughly vacuum all areas several times, and then seal floors with polyurethane. Sandblasting of exterior surfaces can also be a hazard. For outside paintwork, cover the ground with drop cloths and seal all windows and doors with plastic.

Covering lead paint with nonlead paint is not a solution, since the old paint will still chip, crack, and fall. An x-ray fluorescene analyzer, used by lead-detection experts, can quickly locate lead even under many layers of paint. A spoonful of chips or soil should be sent to a state lab for analysis, or homeowners can buy a home test kit for lead at a hardware store. If the child's blood level is between 15 and 25, these measures, plus removal of other sources, are usually enough. However, follow-up is always needed.

2. Chelation is a chemical reaction between the lead in the body and another agent (such as EDTA or BAL), in which the lead is leached out of the patient's body. The chelate has potentially serious side effects (e.g., kidney damage, fever) and is given as intramuscular injections in a hospital setting. If the child's blood level is 55 or higher, chelation should be started immediately. If the lead level is between 25 and 55, the response to a challenge test with one dose of a chelating agent will determine whether or not to continue the chelating process. Lead has a half-life, in blood, of 25 days; in internal organs, 40 days; in bone, more than 25 years. Therefore, it may take several chelation treatments until enough lead is leached from the body.

3. The child should be checked and treated for iron or calcium deficiency.

4. Limit the amount of dirt tracked into the home. If you work with lead-containing materials, wash your work clothes separately from the family clothes.

5. Run the tap water until it is very cold before using the water for cooking. Never cook with water from the hot tap, since lead leaches more quickly into hot water, and boiling concentrates this lead. Instead, boil the cold water.

6. Avoid putting acidic foods (such as tomato sauce or orange juice) in ceramic containers with lead glaze. Pregnant women should not drink coffee out of ceramic mugs.

7. Give children food that is high in calcium and iron to reduce lead absorption.

8. Wash children's hands before meals. Wash pacifiers, toys, and nipples before they are put into mouths.

9. Move cribs and playpens away from painted windowsills and doors. Replace or strip baby furniture that may be decorated with lead paint. Remember that antique toys may have a high lead content.

10. If exterior paint is a problem, plant thick shrubs and bushes near outside walls to discourage children from playing there.

11. Plant grass on contaminated soil to keep dust down.

12. Do not heat food in lead-soldered cans.

13. Be sure your contractor disposes of all lead waste and soil in a hazardous waste facility that has been approved by the U.S. Environmental Protection Agency. Do not burn newspapers or battery casings; their lead content requires that they be disposed of correctly.

In 1976 and 1984, the government drastically reduced the amount of lead in gasoline, but it remains a serious problem in other countries. Today, the average blood lead level in the United States has dropped from 16 down to 7 to 10, following the removal of lead from gasoline. In 1988, the use of lead solder and other lead-containing materials in connecting household plumbing to public water supplies was banned. Many older structures still have lead pipes or lead-soldered plumbing. The Environmental Protection Agency recommends that all families with young children obtain a professional analysis of their home's water supply. This service usually costs $30 to $60. In 1989, the lead content of drinking water coolers in schools was controlled by federal regulations. Some states offer a tax credit for homeowners who clean up the lead in their homes.

One last point: pencil "lead" is made of graphite carbon, not lead. It does not cause lead poisoning even if the child chews on the tip or "tattoos" himself by jabbing the pencil point into his skin. There is no lead in the paint that coats the outside of the pencil.

For more help, call the National Maternal and Child Health Clearinghouse at 1-703-821-8955, extension 254 or 265. Ask for a copy of *Childhood Lead Poisoning Prevention: A Resource Directory*. It is a state-by-state guide to sources for assistance. The Environmental Protection Agency hot line for lead is 1-800-LEAD-FYI.

SAFETY TIPS:

The Newborn: Crowds and Going Outside

ONE QUESTION most commonly asked of pediatricians is: "When can I take my newborn baby outside?" The answer demonstrates that pediatrics is an art, not a science; each pediatrician has his or her own rules of thumb. I always encourage parents to take their babies outside within a few days after they return home from the hospital. Babies love fresh air, and it is healthy for the mother to get outside too, as long as she feels well enough. A baby is discharged from the nursery when he can maintain his own temperature, so that is an indication to the parents that he can spend some time on a porch or a terrace and that he can be taken for a walk around the block or to the park. If it is not too cold (if it is over 20° F) or not too hot (if it is under 90° F), just dress him appropriately and notice how much he loves to sleep or to be taken for a walk outdoors.

Although we can't and don't isolate a baby from the bacteria and viruses that exist in his own home, there is no need to expose him to the microbes and potential colds and illnesses of others. I urge parents to have their baby avoid indoor crowds until he is a month old. This means that he should not go to stores, shopping centers, malls, churches, synagogues, restaurants, airplanes, etc., until he shows us that he is thriving and growing well at one month of age. If there is a party for his *bris* (ritual circumcision), christening, or just a family get-together, the baby should be kept in a separate room. He can come out for the ceremony but should return to relative solitude immediately afterward. Close family members, individually, can come to be with him as long as they are feeling fine and free of any infection. I find that this compromise—of allowing healthy friends and relatives, one at a time, to see and hold the baby for short periods but having the baby avoid indoor crowds —allays the fears and concerns of new parents while it allows others to share in the joy of a newborn. Uncle Joe who has a cold will get over the insult of not being allowed to hold the baby sooner than the baby would get over his cold.

If the baby is healthy, growing, and developing normally, and is free of infection himself, it is safe for him to go to indoor crowds after he is one month old.

SAFETY TIPS:

Playground and Backyard Safety

MORE THAN 150,000 playground injuries require hospital emergency room treatment yearly in the United States. Swings and swing sets account for the highest number of injuries.

Keep the following tips in mind before letting your child loose at the playground.

TIPS:

1. Be sure the child is wearing sneakers or shoes with nonslip soles.

2. Grass, asphalt, packed dirt, and concrete are poor buffers for a fall. Monkey bars and swings should be over rubber mats, wood chips, sawdust, shredded tires, or sand—nine to twelve inches in depth—to break a fall. A sandbox should be too shallow for a child to bury himself in. Cover the sandbox when it is not being used so that cats or other animals don't use it as a litter box.

3. Be sure the child sits in the center of the swing and does not stand on it. He should hold on with both hands and stop the swing before getting off. He should then walk around the swing—not too close to the front or back. Only one person should be on one swing at one time. Don't push empty swings and don't twist swing chains.

4. Swings should be surrounded by gates to keep other children from running in front of or behind chil-

dren already swinging. There should be at least two feet between swings and thirty inches between a swing and a support pole. Swing seats made of lightweight rubber or plastic are safer than metal or wooden seats.

5. Merry-go-rounds should have no sharp edges.

6. Slides should be smooth, without protruding nails or panels. They should be built over a tall mound of earth to break a fall. Don't allow your child to walk up the sliding surface. A slide takes one child at a time. He should slide down feet first, always sitting up. Be sure the front of the slide is clear. Be sure that a metal slide, placed in the sun, is not too hot.

7. Empty your portable wading pool as soon as you are finished using it. Store it upside down so that rain water does not collect in it.

8. If you have a swimming pool, have a telephone installed out near the pool, or bring a cordless phone outside with you. That way, you won't be tempted to leave the child unsupervised even for a minute to answer the phone. Remember, an inch of water is an ocean to a baby. A dangerous and potentially life-threatening old wives' tale is that newborns have a natural ability to swim. They may hold their breath briefly under water, but the vast majority will not swim. They will gag and drown.

9. Be sure pool ladders have skid-resistant steps that are at least three inches wide.

10. Remove your pool covers completely before swimming. Never allow your child to walk on the cover, as water may have accumulated on it, posing a threat for drowning. Your child could also fall through and become trapped underneath.

11. In a whirlpool, pin up your child's hair so that it will not get caught in the suction drain. Keep all protective drain covers in place. Choose a model of hot tub that automatically shuts off when anything is pulled into the drain. Be sure the "off" switch is within easy reach. Every pool, hot tub, and whirlpool should be surrounded by a five-foot-high fence.

12. Place deck furniture away from all railings. Cover the slats of the railings with a plastic shield or a net to prevent small children from squeezing through. Be sure the railings do not have protruding nails or splinters.

13. Put colorful decals on glass doors to remind children of the glass.

14. If you store appliances in the garage, remove doors from any discarded refrigerators, freezers, washers, or dryers so that children cannot trap themselves inside.

15. If you have an automatic garage door opener, make sure that the door reopens automatically if it hits any object as it is closing.

16. Never use a lawn mower with a child nearby. Flying debris could hit the child.

17. Avoid scented soaps, perfumes, or hairsprays, which are inviting to insects.

SAFETY TIPS:

Sunburns and Sunscreens

Sunburns:

A SUNBURN first develops two to four hours after exposure, with the worst symptoms occurring in twenty-four hours. Cloudy days do not stop the sun's ultraviolet rays from burning the skin. There is a higher risk of premature aging of the skin (wrinkling, sagging, brown spots) and of skin cancer in people who have sustained a serious sunburn or a series of less serious sunburns in their youth. Sunlight can be reflected off water, sand, snow, and concrete.

A minor sunburn is a first-degree burn that turns the

skin red. A more severe sunburn results in a second-degree burn and forms blisters. A sunburn does not cause a third-degree burn and does not result in scarring.

There are two types of rays that cause sunburns and tanning: ultraviolet A and ultraviolet B. Ultraviolet A plays a major role in long-term tanning of the skin but is only a minor cause of immediate sunburn reaction. Ultraviolet A radiation remains relatively consistent throughout the day. Ultraviolet B rays are called the "sunburn" rays, because they are the ones most responsible for immediate sunburns. Ultraviolet B radiation is greatest between 10 A.M. and 2 P.M. Although earlier sunscreens contained blockers only for ultraviolet B, there are several reasons that ultraviolet A exposure should not be ignored.

• Although ultraviolet A's ability to cause immediate sunburn is only a thousandth of ultraviolet B's, it nevertheless does have a cumulative effect.

• The amount of ultraviolet A reaching the earth is much greater (ten to fifteen times greater) than ultraviolet B.

• Ultraviolet A has a cumulative effect in causing skin cancer as well as sunburns.

• Effective ultraviolet B sunscreens have allowed users to stay in the sun longer, prolonging their exposure to ultraviolet A.

• Ultraviolet A is transmitted through window glass. Ultraviolet B is not.

• Sun exposure increases by 4 percent for each 1000 feet of elevation. Mountain climbers in particular should be aware of this problem.

TIPS:

1. Apply a cool compress to reddened and blistered areas. Cool baths with Aveeno can also be soothing. Showers may be too painful.

2. When inside, leave the affected area exposed to

the air. When outside, bandage any blistered areas. Loose-fitting cotton clothing will be less irritating to the sunburn than snug clothes.

3. Give acetaminophen or ibuprofen for relief of fever or pain. Over-the-counter moisturizing creams can also be soothing. They can be used again, a week later, when peeling starts.

4. Avoid direct sunlight to involved areas for two days.

5. Encourage the child to drink extra fluids to replace increased body needs after a sunburn.

6. Be sure the sheets on your child's bed are pulled tight so that wrinkles won't irritate the sunburn.

7. Don't forget to apply sunscreen on your child's scalp and the back of his neck. Have him wear a hat.

8. A blister is "nature's Band-Aid," so don't burst it. When the underlying skin is ready to be exposed, the blister will burst by itself. If it bursts prematurely, apply an antibiotic ointment (e.g., Neosporin) under a bandage. Consult your pediatrician if these second-degree burns develop, as an antibiotic may be needed.

9. Be sure tetanus immunizations are up-to-date.

10. If the sunburn itches, give an oral antihistamine (e.g., Benadryl or Tavist).

Sunscreens:

Zinc oxide is probably the most effective topical blocker. It is now available in brightly colored preparations popular with most kids. PABA (para-aminobenzoic acid) used to be popular, but actually has limited usefulness. The most dangerous wavelengths of ultraviolet B are not blocked by PABA. It is also highly water soluble, so it washes off too easily. Finally, PABA is responsible for more allergic reactions than any other sunscreen compound. However, some derivatives of PABA, like Padimate O, eliminate these problems and are very effective sunscreens.

The sun protection factor (SPF) measures sunscreen

effectiveness. It is the amount of ultraviolet B required to produce minimal redness in sunscreen-protected skin as compared with unprotected skin. The SPF of various products ranges from 2 to 45. Sunscreens with an SPF of 15 are considered sunblocks because they block more than 92 percent of ultraviolet B. SPF 30 blocks out 97 percent. The SPF is valid only if the sunscreen is applied liberally and as frequently as directed. A second measure of sunscreen effectiveness is the PPF— phototoxic protection factor—which rates how well the sunscreen protects against ultraviolet A. The maximum PPF of 4 is achieved by many commercially available products.

TIPS:

1. Although higher SPF sunscreens offer more protection, they also are more likely to cause a contact dermatitis. Try to determine the appropriate SPF for your child's skin coloring. It is usually safe to start with an SPF of 15.

2. Some drugs cause skin reactions when the skin is exposed to the sun. Common ones are tetracycline, sulfa drugs, Tegretol, Tofranil, and Retin-A. Sunscreens are important for these patients. Some moisturizers incorporate sunscreens.

3. Apply the sunscreen thirty minutes before sun exposure to give it time to penetrate the skin.

4. Apply sunscreens liberally and frequently. Use them for backyard play as well as at the beach. Don't forget to apply them to the scalp, especially along the part in your child's hair. Frequent applications are also needed behind the knees, where sweat and rubbing (from sitting) easily rinse away sunscreen. Use special lip protection with SPF 15 or 30. Lips don't tan, because they have no melanin, so they burn and blister easily and are prone to skin cancer. Remember that a "waterproof" sunscreen stays on for only thirty minutes in water. Don't hesitate to reapply.

5. The use of tanning salons should be discouraged,

as there is no evidence that the resulting tan is truly protective.

6. Sunglasses are rated according to their ultraviolet A and ultraviolet B filtering abilities.

7. Car window shades should be used on long drives to block the sun's rays in the car.

8. Start applying sunscreens when your child is one year old. Earlier than this, his sensitive skin may have allergic reactions to sunscreens. Simply keep him in the shade and protected from reflected light from nearby water, snow, or sand, and have him wear long clothing and a hat with a brim. I usually allow a maximum of ten to fifteen minutes per day in a pool or ocean for children under one year, as long as they are wearing a short-sleeved undershirt.

SUGGESTIONS:
> Water Babies (15, 30, 25)
> Pre-Sun (23, 30)
> Sundown (30+)
> Vaseline Intensive Care (15)

SAFETY TIPS:

Traveling with Children

TIPS:

1. Refer to the entry on "Motion Sickness" on page 230 and the "Safety Tips" on "Airplane Safety" on page 374 and "Car Safety" on page 378.

2. Be sure all immunizations are up-to-date. The Traveler's Hotline will supply up-to-date information on immunization needs for any country you plan to visit. This telephone number is 1-404-332-4559. I do not recommend giving the MMR (measles, mumps, rubella) vaccine within the week before travel, because any reaction would occur seven to ten days after the shot. It can be given on your return.

3. Bring your pediatrician's phone number with you. If the services of a local doctor are needed, it helps to know whether he is board-certified. This attests to a higher level of expertise and the doctor's ability to deal with common problems. It obviously does not tell you about the doctor's personality, office hours, or office staff. In case of an emergency, however, this little tip can make you feel more comfortable about seeing that doctor. Another suggestion is to call the pediatric department of a local hospital to obtain the name of a competent physician. Always carry your family health insurance cards and immunization records when traveling.

4. Pack the following first-aid kit: thermometer; acetaminophen and/or ibuprofen; antimotion sickness medicines, such as Dramamine Jr.; Benadryl or another antihistamine for allergic reactions; adhesive tape and Band-Aids; Neosporin or other topical antibiotic ointments; tweezers for splinters; topical medicine for teething; eardrops; calamine lotion; syrup of ipecac; scissors; sunscreen; and insect repellents.

5. When traveling with powdered formulas, use distilled water or boiled water. Bringing ready-to-use formula in throw-away bottles is expensive and heavy, but it does avoid the problems associated with contaminated water.

6. A small, plug-in night light may be indispensable in motels, hotels, or homes of friends and relatives.

7. Older children enjoy their own backpacks for carrying their personal supplies of goodies and necessities. Never forget a younger child's favorite blanket, toy, or doll.

8. Pack a few electric outlet covers if you have an exploring toddler.

9. Whether in a car, plane, or train, on a long trip you will sooner or later need discipline. Firmness without loss of temper is the operative phrase. Remember to praise good and cooperative behavior periodically. This goes a long way to keeping the trip a pleasant one.

10. Keep a change of clothes and plastic bibs readily available.

11. One cute trick is to take along a small inflatable pool to serve as a crib, playpen, and bathtub for smaller children.

12. It is wise *not* to make children's names very obvious on clothing, toys, etc., where strangers can see them. In places like air terminals, a child may respond to a stranger calling her name, and that could spell disaster. Names should be accessible but not obvious.

13. Fill prescriptions for children who regularly take medicine.

14. Mosquitoes can transmit diseases like malaria and yellow fever. Refer to Tip 2 (above) for the Traveler's Hotline to learn if these diseases are prevalent in your area of travel. Use insect repellents with DEET. Wear long sleeves and long pants at dusk, when malaria mosquitoes tend to bite. When traveling to areas that have malaria, use prophylactic medicines before, during, and after your trip. In some developing countries, it is advisable not to swim in fresh water unless a reliable source tells you that the water is not contaminated with parasites. Chlorinated pools and salt water are usually safe for swimming.

15. In areas of high altitude (over 10,000 feet), some children complain of headaches and shortness of breath due to the lowered oxygen in the air. It is advisable to rest for the first twelve to twenty-four hours when arriving at a place of high altitude.

16. When traveling abroad, you can take some measures to prevent traveler's diarrhea: avoid tap water, ice, uncooked vegetables, and dairy products. (Many countries do not routinely pasteurize milk.) In developing countries the poorer people defecate in ponds, streams, and fields. Since tap water is often collected from these contaminated sources, avoid all tap water use, even for brushing teeth. Even luxury hotels with "clean, filtered, or chlorinated" water only rarely check the water purity. Boiling the water for five to ten minutes is usually adequate. Bottled carbonated water is preferable because it assures you that the bottle was not filled with tap water. Bottled or canned soda and soft drinks are usually fine. In some countries it is advisable to eat only fruits and vegetables that have to be peeled. Avoid raw or rare meat or fish. All vegetables, meats, and fish should be thoroughly cooked.

Index

Abdomen
  newborn, 241–42
  pain in, 307. See also
    Stomachaches
  "surgical," 312
Abscess, 347
  brain, 288
  eyelid, 132
  peritonsillar, 305
  throat, 100
Abuse, 58–63
  emotional, 58
  physical, 58
  reporting, 61
  sexual, 58, 60, 61,
    223, 367
Accidents. See Safety
Achilles tendon, 134,
    214, 218
Acne, 1–3
  newborn, 1
Acquired
    immunodeficiency
    syndrome, 4–6, 168,
    197
  immunizations during,
    192
Acyclovir, 57, 58, 73
ADD. See Attention
    deficit disorder
Adenoids, 116, 119, 288
Adolescence
  acne in, 1
  cholesterol screening
    in, 67
  diabetes in, 108–9
  discipline in, 327

eating disorders in, 11–
    12
  migraine in, 157
  rebellion in, 332
  scoliosis in, 272
  sexual development in,
    282–84
  sleep in, 293–94
Adrenalin, 17
Aggression, 104, 326,
    331
AIDS. See Acquired
    immunodeficiency
    syndrome
Airplane safety, 374–75
Alice-in-Wonderland
    syndrome, 228–29
Allergies, 9, 42, 87
  "allergic salute," 78
  and antibiotics, 137
  to bites and stings, 28
  and colds, 78
  drug, 171
  and ear infection, 116
  and eczema, 126, 128
  food, 144, 147–50
  hives in, 148, 183, 184
  injections, 20, 28, 148
  milk, 7, 149, 150
  penicillin, 301
  "shiners" with, 78
  with sinusitis, 287
  testing for, 20, 21
Alopecia, 153–54
Amnesia, 163
Amniocentesis, 167
Amphetamines, 284

Anal fissures, 81
Analgesics, 28
  for broken bones, 33
  for burns, 45
  for chest pain, 51
  in chickenpox, 55
  for colds, 79
  for cold sores, 72
  and croup, 99
  for earaches, 121
  for ear infection, 117
  for fever, 135
  for frostbite, 151
  for headaches, 158
  for influenza, 199–200
  for migraine, 158
  in sickle cell anemia, 10
  for sinusitis, 288
  for sore throat, 300–1
  for teething, 323
  topical, 72
Anal ring, tight, 81
Anaphylactic shock, 148, 150
Anemia, 6–10, 391
  and crib death, 91
  fifth disease, 140
  iron deficiency, 7–9
  maternal, 91
  sickle cell, 9–10, 52, 197, 199, 200, 203, 228
Animal bites. See Bites and stings
Anorexia, 11–12, 123, 153
Antibiotics, 288
  for acne, 2
  for bronchitis, 40
  and colds, 80
  for cold sores, 73
  and diarrhea, 113
  for ear infection, 118, 119

  for fever, 137
  oral, 3, 85, 112, 198–99, 216
  problems with use of, 111, 137
  topical, 2, 44, 85
Antihistamines, 55, 79, 87, 271, 288
  for bites and stings, 28
  for ear infection, 118
  and eczema, 128
  for hives, 184
  for itching, 85
  for motion sickness, 230
  in pityriasis rosea, 260
Ants, fire. See Bites and stings
Anxiety, separation, 279–81, 327
Apgar scores, 12–14
Aphthous ulcers, 71
Appendicitis, 81, 308–9
Appetite
  decreased, 172, 308, 311
  picky, 122–26
Arrhythmias, cardiac, 53, 220, 303
Arthralgia, 215
Arthritis, 303
  juvenile rheumatoid, 54, 181, 182, 183, 196, 215–17
  with Lyme disease, 220
  septic, 182
Asthma, 14–21, 42, 52, 58, 77, 86, 87, 148, 197, 199, 200
  and eczema, 127
  with sinusitis, 287
Atopic dermatitis, 126

Attention deficit disorder, 148, 205, 207–9
Attention span, 8, 104, 208
  during meals, 125
Au pairs, 46

Baby sitters, 46–48
  and bedtime, 296
  and discipline, 327
  and separation anxiety, 280
Back
  curvature. See Scoliosis
  newborn, 243
Bacteria. See individual illnesses
  and antibiotics, 76
  in bronchitis, 40, 41
  and diphtheria, 115–16
  in epiglottitis, 100
  infection, 111, 138, 215, 216, 287–88, 299–303
  pneumococcal, 197
  stapholococcus, 198–99
  streptococcus, 198–99
  tetanus, 30
Bad breath, 21–22
Barotrauma, 287–88
Bathing
  newborn, 237
  "sitz," 367
  sponge, 135, 277
Batteries, button, 64
Bedbugs. See Bites and stings
Bedtime, 289–99
Bed-wetting, 22–25, 187, 345
  and abuse, 60
  and diabetes, 108
  secondary, 22
Bees. See Bites and stings

Behavior
  aggressive, 104, 284, 327, 331
  dieting, 12
  disorders, 148, 391
  modification, 24, 235, 341
  positive reinforcement, 235, 329, 332
  unacceptable, 326
Bell's palsy, 220, 228
Bellybutton, 241–42, 357–59
Bicycle safety, 375–77
Bilirubin, 9, 172, 201, 202, 203
Biofeedback, 158
Birthmarks, 25–26
  color, 25
  symmetry, 25
Bites and stings, 27–31
  animals, 29–30
  bedbugs, 29
  bees, 27–28
  cats, 30–31
  fire ants, 28
  fleas, 28
  hornets, 27–28
  human, 27, 59
  jellyfish, 31
  mosquito, 29
  rats, 31
  snakes, 31
  spiders, 28
  ticks, 29
  wasps, 27–28
Biting. See Temper tantrums
Bleeding
  disorders, 165–71
  intracranial, 159
  nose, 170, 179
  rectal, 81
  in skull, 163
Blisters

from burns, 44–45
chickenpox, 54, 55
in diaper rash, 111–12
fever, 71–73
in frostbite, 151
in impetigo, 198–99
in poison ivy, 84
Blocked tear ducts, 129
Blood
  bilirubin, 9, 172, 201,
    202, 203
  clotting, 166, 171
  group incompatibility,
    7
  hemoglobin, 6, 7, 9
  plasma, 6
  pressure, 141, 148,
    179–80, 245, 303,
    362, 391
  red cells, 6, 7, 10
  Rh factors, 7
  in stool, 148, 171, 307
  sugar, 160, 274, 275
  transfusions, 5, 10,
    202
Bones
  broken, 32–33, 50
  dislocated, 33–34,
    181–82
  infections, 215
  tumors, 218
Bottle feeding, 36–40
  bottle mouth syndrome
    in, 34–35
  discontinuing, 35
Bottle Mouth Syndrome,
    34–35
Botulism, 309
Bowel problems. See
    Constipation;
    Diarrhea;
    Stomachaches
Bowlegs, 134, 243–44
Brain
  abnormalities, 275

abscesses, 288
  pressure on, 266
  tumors, 160
Breast feeding, 35, 36–
    40, 203, 284
  advantages, 36–37
  and AIDS, 5–6
  and colic, 74
  and constipation, 112
  and crib death, 93
  and diarrhea, 112
  immunizations during,
    193, 194
  weaning, 39
Breasts
  development of, 281.
    See also Sexual
    development
  enlargement, 283–84
  masses in preadolescent
    males, 283–84
  newborn, 241
Breath
  bad, 21–22, 287
  holding, 92
  shortness of, 15
Breathing
  difficult, 100, 115, 148
  exercise, 103
  mouth-to-mouth, 65
  rapid, 41
  shallow, 52
Bris, 249, 396
Bronchiolitis, 15–16, 41–
    42, 77
Bronchitis, 40–43, 86,
    87, 199, 314. See
    also Asthma
  asthmatic, 40
  bacterial, 40, 41
  chronic, 16, 77, 200
  viral, 40, 41
Bronchodilators, 15, 16,
    41–42, 87, 88, 103
Bronchospasm, 14, 16

exercise-induced, 14, 20
Bruises, 59
  anal, 60
  and bleeding disorders, 169, 170
  genital, 60
Bruxism, 234–35
Bulimia, 11–12
Bumpers, 97
Burns, 43–45
  and abuse, 59
  chemical, 44, 45
  degrees, 43
  electrical, 44
  heat, 44
  sunburn, 399–401

Caffeine, 74, 158
Calamine lotion, 55
  for bites and stings, 28
  for poison ivy, 85
Calcium, 125, 150, 275, 320, 364, 391
Calluses, 217
Cancer, 7, 56, 57
  penile, 251, 253
  testicular, 333
Candida albicans, 111, 367
Canker sores, 71, 72
Car
  air bags, 379
  safety, 378–81
  seats, 378–79
Carbohydrates, 107
Carbon monoxide, 160, 262
Cardiac arrhythmias, 53, 220, 303
Cardiopulmonary resuscitation, 65
Carditis, 303
Caregivers. See Baby sitters; Day care

Carriages, 49–50
Cataracts, 239
Cat-scratch disease, 30–31
Celiac disease, 113, 309
Cellulitis, 131, 215
Cephalhematoma, 155, 238
Cereals, 141–43
Chest
  congestion, 15
  costochondritis, 50–51
  functional pain, 51
  musculoskeletal wall irritation, 50–51
  newborn, 241
  pain, 50–54, 69
  tsetse syndrome, 50
Chickenpox, 54–58, 76, 172, 198–99, 266, 368
Child abuse. See Abuse
Child care. See Babysitters; Day care
Choking, 64–65, 126
Cholesterol, 66–70
Cholybar, 69
Chordee, 253
Chorea, Sydenham, 303–4
Christmas disease, 168
Chromosomes, 166, 355
Chronic fatigue syndrome, 230
Circumcision, 167, 249–54, 362
  contraindications, 253
  and hemophilia, 167, 253
Cirrhosis, 174
Clavicle, fractured, 33
Clubfeet, 132, 218

Cold, common, 76–80, 87
  and bronchitis, 40
  cough in, 86
  and ear infection, 116
  and idiopathic thrombocytopenic purpura (ITP), 170
Cold sores, 71–73
Colic, 73–76
Colitis, 113, 311
Collarbone, fractured, 33
Colorado tick fever, 29
Conjunctivitis, 129–31, 223, 299
  allergic, 131
  with Lyme disease, 220
Consciousness, loss of
  in head trauma, 162
Constipation, 80–82, 143, 307. See also Toilet training
  causes, 81
  and cystic fibrosis, 103
  in eating disorders, 11
  and toilet training, 80, 81
Contact dermatitis, 83–86
Convulsion. See Seizures
Coronary artery disease, 66, 69
Costochondritis, 50–51
Coughing, 15, 50, 52
  antitussives, 42, 86, 87–88
  in asthma, 52
  bark-like, 98, 223
  in bronchiolitis, 41
  with cold, 77
  croupy, 115
  expectorants, 42, 79, 86, 88
  hoarse, 98
  medicines, 79, 86–88

  productive, 40, 87
  reflex, 138
  with sinusitis, 287
Counseling
  behavioral, 332
  genetic, 167, 257
Coxsackie virus, 52, 71, 72, 204–5
CPR, 65
Cradle cap, 89, 155
Crib Death, 90–95
Cribs, 96–98
Crohn's disease, 9, 311. See also Inflammatory bowel disease
Crossed eyes, 131–32, 239
Croup, 77, 98–100
Crowds, newborns in, 395–96
Crying, 100–2
  at bedtime, 290–91
  and head trauma, 163
  vomiting from, 291
Cuts. See Stitches
Cystic fibrosis, 16, 42, 58, 102–3, 197, 199, 200, 309
  and diarrhea, 113
  and sinusitis, 287
Cystitis, 359
Cytomegalovirus, 172

Day care, 47–48
  abuse in, 60
  and AIDS, 6
  hepatitis in, 176–77
  returning to after illness, 265
  and separation anxiety, 280
Deafness, 119, 231, 269
Decongestants, 87, 99,

117–18, 159, 224, 288
Dehydration, 42, 155, 229, 309, 314
  from burns, 45
  with colds, 79
  in diabetes, 107
  and diarrhea, 113, 115
Dental. See also Teeth
  bottle mouth syndrome, 34–35
  malocclusion, 34, 234, 339
Denver Developmental Screening Test, 104
Dermabrasion, 3
Dermatitis. See also Eczema; Rashes
  atopic, 126
  contact, 83–86
  seborrheic, 89
  shoe, 133
Dermatomyositis, 54, 219
Developmental
  disabilities, 156, 256
  milestones, 104–7
Diabetes, 22, 107–10, 197, 199, 367
  adult-onset, 108
  and coronary artery disease, 69
  in food poisoning, 309
  insipidis, 109–10
  juvenile-onset, 107–8
  paradoxical, 81
  Somogyi phenomenon in, 109
Diaper rash, 110–12
Diapers
  cloth, 111, 336
  disposable, 110, 112, 336
Diarrhea, 112–15. See also Constipation

and allergy, 144, 148
and antibiotics, 137
bloody, 311
causes, 112–13
in cystic fibrosis, 103
in food poisoning, 112
and formula change, 73
in hepatitis, 172
with influenza, 113, 199
paradoxical, 112–13
in poisoning, 260
in Reye's syndrome, 55
with stomachache, 309
traveler's 405–6
and urinary tract infection, 113
Diet
  and cholesterol, 67
  in cystic fibrosis, 103
  fat in, 67, 179
  in phenylketonuria, 256–57
  salt in, 179
  vegetarian, 146
Diphtheria, 76, 100, 115–16, 304
  complications of, 115
  immunizations, 190, 193–94
Discipline, 58, 62, 63, 210–11, 326–33
  grounding, 327, 328, 332
  time out, 211, 326–29
Diseases
  bacterial, 9
  cat-scratch, 30–31
  coronary artery, 66, 69
  fifth, 139–40
  heart, 67
  immunodeficiency, 56
  Kawasaki, 53, 204–5
  kidney, 77

Legg-Perthes, 218
liver, 77
Lyme, 219–21
Osgood-Schlatter, 246–47
psychological, 11
pulmonary, 14–21
reactive airway, 14–21
sexually transmitted, 60, 61, 172, 251, 362, 368
sixth, 268
Dislocations, 33–34, 181–82
hip, 356
Distractability, 208
Doctor, calling for, 377–78
Dog bites. See Bites and stings
Dosages, 225
Dreams, 109, 294–96
Drug use, 4
and crib death, 91
side effects, 153
Dyscalculia, 205
Dysgraphia, 205
Dyslexia, 205

Earache. See Ear(s), infection
Eardrops, 117, 120, 383
Eardrum, 118–19
Ear(s), 116–22
bleeding from, 163
drops, 117, 120, 383
infection, 79, 86, 106, 116–22, 157, 199, 224, 305, 314
newborn, 240
otitis externa, 120–21
otitis media, 116–20
wax in, 121–22
Eating
disorders, 11–12

finger-feeding, 124
habits, 122–26
Eczema, 14, 89, 126–28, 153, 267
infant, 148
with PKU, 256
Electrolyte solutions, 113, 135
Embolism, pulmonary, 52
Encephalitis, 56, 224, 228, 231, 269
Encopresis, 81
Enemas, 82
Enuresis. See Bed-wetting
Epiglottitis, 100, 196
Epilepsy, 159, 274–75
grand mal, 274
petit mal, 275
Epinephrine, 28, 109, 150, 184
Epiphysis, slipped capital femoral, 218
Epistaxis, 244–46
Epstein-Barr virus, 172, 228, 229, 300
Erythema infectiosum, 139–40
Erythema toxicum, 128
Esophagitis, 9, 51
Esophagus, 51, 310–11
Ethnicity
and crib death, 90–91
and eating disorders, 11
and sickle cell anemia, 10
Exanthem subitum, 268
Exercise, 126
breathing, 103
and cholesterol, 67, 69–70
and hypertension, 179
Eyedrops, 130, 131, 383
Eyelids, 131

and head trauma, 163
Eye(s), 129–32
  blocked tear ducts, 129
  bulging, 342
  conjunctivitis, 129–31
  crossed, 131–32, 239
  and diabetes, 109
  drops, 130, 131, 383
  foreign bodies in, 130
  infections, 288
  inflammation, 216
  lazy, 239
  newborn, 238–39
  pupils in head trauma,
    162
  reddening, 204
  "shiners," 163
  strain, 159
  styes, 132
  watery, 77

Failure to thrive, 103,
    123
Febrile convulsions. See
    Seizures
Feeding
  bottle, 36–40
  breast, 36–40
  burping after, 38, 74
  equipment, 338
  in phenylketonuria,
    256–57
  solid foods, 141–47
Feet, 132–34
  choosing shoes, 133
  clubfeet, 132
  flat, 133–34
  in-toeing, 132
  pigeon toe, 132, 244
  shoe problems, 217
  toe-walking, 134, 218
Fever, 52, 134–39
  with appendicitis, 308
  blisters, 71–73
  in bronchitis, 41

with colds, 77, 78
with croup, 98, 99
and fifth disease, 140
hay, 148
in hepatitis, 172
with influenza, 199
in Kawasaki disease,
    204
low-grade, 120, 134,
    140
with Lyme disease, 220
with measles, 223
in meningitis, 226, 227
with mononucleosis,
    228
with mumps, 231
with polio, 264
postoperative, 138
rheumatic, 53, 198–99,
    215–16, 302, 303
in roseola, 268
with rubella, 269
scarlet, 139, 302, 368
and seizures, 137, 275–
    76
with sinusitis, 287
with sore throat, 299
with teething, 120
in tetanus, 334
with tuberculosis, 353
Fifth disease, 139–40
Filetov-Dukes disease,
    139
First-aid, 27
Fits. See Seizures
Flatfeet, 133–34
Flatulence, 307, 313
Flea bites. See Bites and
    stings
Flu. See Influenza
Fluoride, 34, 35, 318,
    319
Fontanelle, 154–55, 342
Food
  additives, 150

allergies, 144, 147–50
cereal, 141–43
choking on, 126
cholesterol-containing, 67
dairy products, 146–47
and eczema, 127
eggs, 146–47, 148
fads, 123
fruits, 143–45
and headaches, 158
and hives, 183
intolerances, 147
introducing new, 144
juices, 145
meats, 146
poisoning, 112, 260, 309–10, 314
preservatives, 19
starting solid, 141–47
vegetables, 145–46
Foreign objects
in the ear, 120
in the eye, 130
inhalation of, 16, 40, 64, 100, 287
in nose, 21
swallowed, 51
in vagina, 367
Formula feeding, 36–40, 73
Fractures, 32–33
clavicle, 33
greenstick, 32
rib, 50
skull, 33, 155, 163
Friends, imaginary, 188–89
Frostbite, 151–52
Fruits, 143–45
Fungus, 111, 153, 188, 267, 367

Gangrene, 31, 151
Gastroenteritis, 112, 309
Gastroesophageal reflux, 94, 310–11
Genes, 166
German measles. See Rubella
Glands, 102
lymph, 30, 204, 212, 353
parotid, 231
pituitary, 110, 342, 343
salivary, 231
sweat, 164
swollen, 115, 198–99, 204, 212, 216, 220, 228, 231, 268, 269, 299, 353
thyroid, 341
Glaucoma, 159, 239
Glomerulonephritis, 179, 303, 364
Goiter, 342
Growing pains, 152, 217
Gums, infected, 22
Gynecomastia, pubertal, 283

Haemophilus influenzae B, 100, 191, 196, 227
Hair
loss, 59, 153–54, 267
pubic, 281, 282
pulling, 153
twisting, 153, 235
underarm, 283
Halloween precautions, 385–86
Hand, foot, and mouth disease, 71, 205
Hay fever, 14, 127, 148
Head
aches, 157–61
banging, 235, 292–93
"battle" sign in trauma, 162

cephalhematoma, 155
fontanelle, 154–55, 342
hydrocephalus, 155–56
lice, 212–13
microcephaly, 156
newborn, 238
postconcussion
syndrome, 159, 162
"raccoon sign" in
trauma, 163
rolling, 292–93
soft spot, 154–55
trauma, 159, 161–63,
314
Headaches, 77, 157–61
and bruxism, 235
cluster, 157
in head trauma, 162
in hepatitis, 172
and hypertension, 179
with influenza, 199
with Lyme disease, 220
in meningitis, 226
migraine, 157–58, 274
with mumps, 231
with polio, 264
in roseola, 269
sinus, 159, 287
with sore throat, 299
tension, 158
with tuberculosis, 353
Hearing loss, 106, 120,
122, 227, 391
Heart
arrhythmia, 53, 220,
303
attack, 53, 66, 69,
179, 204
and chickenpox, 56
disease, 53, 67, 77,
197
failure, 109, 115
infections, 52
mitral valve prolapse,
53

murmurs, 164
problems, 53
rheumatic disease,
302–3
Heartburn, 11, 50, 51
Heat rash, 164–65
Heimlich maneuver, 65
Hematoma, subdural,
163
Hematuria, 363–64
Hemophilia, 165–69
Henoch-Schönlein
purpura, 171
Hepatitis, 76, 168, 172–
77, 183, 363–64
immunizations, 10,
169, 190, 196
infectious, 173
neonatal, 173, 203
serum, 173
vaccine, 174, 177, 190,
196
Hereditary factors
in allergies, 148
in asthma, 14
in attention deficit
disorder, 207
in bed-wetting, 22, 345
and cholesterol, 68
in cystic fibrosis, 102
in diabetes, 107
in eczema, 126
in epilepsy, 274
in hemophilia, 166–67
in microcephaly, 156
in migraine, 157
in motion sickness, 230
in scoliosis, 272
in sickle cell anemia,
10
in sleepwalking, 298
tooth decay, 34
Hernias
inguinal, 241–42, 312,
334, 359

scrotal, 243
umbilical, 241–42, 358–59
Herpangina, 71
Herpes virus, 54, 57, 71–73, 172, 198–99
Hib. See Haemophilus influenzae B
Hiccups, 178
High blood pressure, 141, 179–80, 245, 303, 362, 391
Highchairs, 180
Hips, 181–82
  dislocated, 181–82
  toxic synovitis, 182
Hirschprung's disease, 81
HIV. See Human immunodeficiency virus
Hives, 183–84
  and allergy, 148, 183, 184
  and arthritis, 183
  and cold, 183–84
  and food, 183
  and Henoch-Schönlein purpura, 171
  and hepatitis, 172, 183
  and hyperthyroidism, 183
  and infectious mononucleosis, 183
  and lupus, 183
Home monitors, 92–93
Homosexuality, 4, 5
Honey, 309
Hormones, 11, 222, 367
  in adolescence, 283
  antidiuretic, 24, 110
  cortisol, 109
  estrogen, 3
  growth, 109
  insulin, 107, 108, 110
  in puberty, 1

sex, 333
thyroid, 341, 342
vasopressin, 110
Hospitalization, 185–87
Human bites. See Bites and stings
Human immunodeficiency virus, 4, 251
Humidifiers, 42, 79, 98, 128, 187–88, 288, 304
Hydrocele, 243, 334
Hydrocephalus, 155–56
Hyperactivity, 17, 205, 208, 256
Hypercholesterolemia, 68–69, 70
Hyperlipidemia, 53. See also Cholesterol
Hypertension, 141, 179–80, 245, 303, 362, 391
Hyperthyroidism, 179, 183, 342, 343
Hypoglycemia. See Blood sugar
Hypospadias, 253
Hypothyroidism, 81, 342, 343

Idiopathic thrombocytopenic purpura, 170–71
Imaginary friends, 188–89
Immune disorders, 287
Immune system, 190–91
  and allergies, 147
Immunizations, 10, 189–98
  diphtheria, 116, 190, 193–94
  haemophilus influenza B, 196

hepatitis, 169, 174, 190, 196
influenza, 197, 200
measles, 190, 195–96
misconceptions about, 192–93
mumps, 190, 195–96
pertussis, 190, 193–94, 256
pneumonia, 197
polio, 190, 194–95, 264
rubella, 190, 195–96
schedule, 189–91
tetanus, 27, 45, 151, 190, 193–94, 334
typhoid, 197
whooping cough, 256
Immunodeficiency disease, 56
Impetigo, 153, 198–99
secondary, 271
Impulsivity, 208–9
Incubation period
chickenpox, 54
cold sores, 72
diphtheria, 115
fifth disease, 140
hepatitis, 173, 175
herpes, 72
influenza, 199
measles, 223
meningitis, 227
mononucleosis, 228
mumps, 231
pertussis, 255–56
polio, 264
rabies, 30
roseola, 268, 269
warts, 372
whooping cough, 255–56
Indigestion, 51
Infancy
acne in, 1
bowleggedness, 134
choking in, 65
crowds in, 395–96
eczema in, 148
going outside, 395–96
jaundice in, 201–4
seizures in, 275
vitamins in, 369
Infections
in anemia, 7
bacterial, 100, 111, 115, 131, 138, 171, 215, 216, 287–88, 299–303
bites and stings, 27
bone, 215
delayed, 139
and diabetes, 107
ear, 79, 86, 106, 120–21, 157, 199, 224, 305, 314
fungal, 111, 153, 267
gum, 22
Haemophilus influenzae B, 10
heart, 52
herpes in, 72
joint, 215
kidney, 303
liver, 172–77
lower respiratory, 86
lung, 52, 138
meningitis, 225–26
oral, 21
rashes in, 128
respiratory, 265
and seizures, 274
sexually transmitted, 60, 61
strep, 138, 299–303
throat, 120
tonsil, 299–300
upper respiratory, 55, 86
urinary tract, 22, 60,

138, 250, 307, 359–63

viral, 139, 171, 182, 216

yeast, 111

Inflammatory bowel disease, 307, 309, 311

Influenza, 76, 199–200, 266, 309, 314. See also Fever

and arthritis, 216

diarrhea in, 113

and idiopathic thrombocytopenic purpura, 170

immunizations, 10, 190, 197, 200

Ingrown nails, 233

Inhalers, 384

Injury, 386. See also Safety

prevention, 386

Insect bites. See Bites and stings

Insulin, 107, 108, 109, 110

Intercourse, sexual, 4, 5, 60

In-toeing, 132

Intussusception, 112, 311–12

Ipecac, 261, 262, 263

Iron, 7–9, 81, 143, 146, 391

Irritable bowel syndrome, 81, 312

Itching

in chickenpox, 56

in eczema, 126

and fifth disease, 140

in impetigo, 198–99

in poison ivy, 83–84

rectal, 258, 367

with ringworm, 153, 267

Jaundice

in anemia, 9

in hepatitis, 172

newborn, 201–4, 236–37

phototherapy for, 202

Jealousy, 284–86

Jellyfish bites. See Bites and stings

Jet lag, 375

Jock itch, 267

Joint

pain, 171, 172, 220, 231

problems, 213–19

swollen, 214

tenderness, 215, 269

Juices, 145

Kawasaki disease, 53, 204–5

Kernicterus, 202

Kicking. See Temper tantrums

Kidney, 11, 141, 171

disease, 7, 77, 197

failure, 109, 362

infection, 303

tumors, 179

Kissing disease. See Mononucleosis

Kitchen safety, 387–89

Knees. See Joint problems; Limping

Knock-knees, 134

Koplik's spots, 223

Lactase deficiency, 7

Lactose intolerance, 113, 147, 307, 309, 312–13

Language, delayed, 104

Lanugo, 237
Laxatives, 3, 11, 82, 229, 308
Lazy eyes, 239
Lead, 96, 97
    poisoning, 262, 390–95
Learning disabilities, 156, 205–7, 227, 269
Legg-Perthes disease, 218
Legs
    bow-legs, 134, 243–44
    growing pains in, 152
Lethargy
    and diabetes, 108
    in meningitis, 226–27
    in Reye's syndrome, 55
Lice, 212–13
Ligaments, 214
    torn, 32
Limping, 213–19
Lipoproteins, 66, 67, 68, 69
Liver
    cancer, 174
    cirrhosis, 174
    disease, 77
    enlargement of, 216
    infections, 172–77
    in Reye's syndrome, 266
Lockjaw, 334–35. See also Tetanus
Lumbar puncture, 226
Lung
    collapsed, 52
    infections, 52, 138
    pneumothorax, 52
Lupus, 7, 54, 153, 183, 219
Lyme disease, 219–21

Malabsorption illness, 113
Mantoux test, 353

Masturbation, 3, 222–23, 367
Mattresses, 96
Measles, 76, 100, 139, 223–24
    and arthritis, 216
    complications, 224
    German. See Rubella
    immunizations, 190, 195–96
    infant, 268
Meats, 146
Medic Alert bracelets
    for allergies, 150
    for diabetes, 109
    for hemophilia, 169
    for seizure activity, 277
Medications. See also specific names
    acyclovir, 57, 58, 73
    adrenalin, 17
    albuterol, 16
    antiasthmatic, 88
    antibacterial, 2, 198–99, 284
    antibiotic, 2, 10, 30, 40, 73, 76, 80, 85, 100, 103, 111, 112, 113, 118, 119, 137, 198–99, 216, 220, 288
    anticancer, 154
    anticonvulsant, 159, 277
    antidepressant, 12, 24
    antidiuretic, 24, 110
    antifungal, 111, 267, 367
    antihistamine, 28, 55, 79, 85, 87, 88, 118, 128, 184, 230, 260, 271, 288
    antihypertensive, 179, 303

anti-inflammatory, 55–56
antiparasitic, 259
antipyretic, 135
antispasmodic, 75, 312
antivenom, 31
for burns, 44
cholesterol-lowering, 69
cholestyramine, 69
colestipol, 69
cough, 42, 79, 86–88
cromolyn sodium, 17
decongestant, 87, 88, 99, 117–18, 159, 224, 288
desmopressin, 24
dosages, 225
eardrops, 117, 120, 383
and eczema, 127
eyedrops, 130, 131, 383
giving and taking, 381–85
hydrocortisone, 85
imipramine, 24
immunosuppressive, 57
measurements, 225
mebendazole, 258–59
metaproterenol, 16
migraine, 158
nosedrops, 79, 245, 383
penicillin, 10, 301, 302
side effects, 17
steroid, 17, 58, 72, 85, 89, 103, 127, 171, 184, 260, 271, 284, 288
theophylline, 17
Memory disability, 207
Meningitis, 90, 157, 196, 197, 220, 225–28, 231, 276, 288, 314
bacterial, 226, 227
partially treated, 227
vital, 226, 227
Menstruation
and acne, 1
and anemia, 8
delayed, 282
in eating disorders, 11–12
false, 242
and migraine, 157
onset, 282
Mental retardation, 202, 256, 342, 343. See also Developmental disabilities
and chickenpox, 56
and microcephaly, 156
Microcephaly, 156
Migraine headaches, 157–58, 274
Milk, 42
breast, 7, 36–40
cholesterol in, 70
cow's, 7, 146, 147, 148, 150
and diarrhea, 113, 114, 115
formula, 36–40
freezing, 38
lactose intolerance, 113, 147, 307, 309, 313
pneumonia, 38
warming, 38–39
witch's, 241
Minerals, 7, 37, 143
Mites, 270, 271, 272
Mitral valve prolapse, 53
Mobiles, 96
Mongolian spots, 26
Monilia infection, 111
Monitors, home, 92–93
Mononucleosis, 228–30
chronic, 229–30

complications, 228–29
infectious, 172, 183,
  299, 300, 304
Monosodium glutamate,
  19, 158
Mosquitoes. See Bites
  and stings
Motion sickness, 160,
  230–31, 314, 374
Motor development,
  105–6
Mouth
  Epstein's pearls, 240
  natal teeth, 240–41
  newborn, 240–41
MSG. See Monosodium
  glutamate
Mucocutaneous lymph
  node syndrome,
  204–5
Mumps, 76, 231–32
  complications, 231
  immunizations, 190,
  195–96

Nails, 232–34
  biting, 234
  cutting, 232–33
  ingrown, 233
Nannies, 46
Naps, 293–94
Nebulizers, 15, 16, 384–
  85
Neglect, 58, 59
Nevi. See Birthmarks
Newborn appearance,
  236–44. See also
  specific areas
Night
  lights, 290
  sweats, 109, 353
  terrors, 274, 294–96
  tremor, 109
Nightmares, 294–96
Nose

discharge from, 287
drops, 79, 245, 383
injuries, 33
newborn, 239–40
runny, 77, 148, 199
Nosebleeds, 163, 170,
  244–46

Obesity, 68, 69
  and hypertension, 179
  and television
  watching, 325
Organization disability,
  207
Osgood-Schlatter disease,
  246–47
Osteomyelitis, 215
Otitis, 116–21
Outside, going with
  newborn, 395–96

Pacifiers, 34, 35, 178,
  247–48, 320, 341
  See also Bottle mouth
  syndrome
Pain
  abdominal, 171, 172,
  307
  bone, 9
  chest, 50–54, 69
  functional, 51
  growing, 152, 217
  intestinal, 9
  joint, 171, 172, 220,
  231
  referred, 120, 182,
  321–22
  teething, 321–22
Paleness
  in anemia, 9
  in bites and stings, 28
  in frostbite, 151
  and head trauma, 163
Pancreas, 102, 103, 107
Pancreatitis, 231

INDEX

Paralysis, 115, 264

Parasites, 183, 212–13, 257–59, 309

Paronychia, 233

Peer pressure, 51, 332

Penis, 282, 364
  bleeding, 167
  circumcision, 167, 249–54
  ejaculation, 283
  foreskin, 248, 249–54
  newborn, 243, 248–49
  zipper entrapment, 254

Periods. See Menstruation

Peritonitis, 308

Pertussis, 255–56
  immunizations, 190, 193–94, 256

Pharyngitis, 77, 299–305

Phenylketonuria, 256–57

Phimosis, 249, 250, 253

Phlebitis, 139

Phobias, school, 51

Photophobia, 223, 224

Phototherapy, 202

Pica, 390–91

Pillows, 97

Pink eye, 129–31, 220, 223, 299

Pinworms, 22, 223, 235, 257–59, 367

Pituitary gland, 110

Pityriasis rosea, 259–60

PKU. See Phenylketonuria

Plantar warts, 217, 372–73

Playground safety, 397–99

Pleurodynia, 52

Pneumonia, 40, 42, 76, 86, 90, 196, 197, 199, 224
  and chickenpox, 56
  and cystic fibrosis, 103
  and diphtheria, 115
  immunizations, 197
  milk, 38
  recurrent, 353

Pneumothorax, 52

Poisoning, 260–63
  carbon monoxide, 262
  food, 112, 260, 309–10, 314
  lead, 262, 390–95

Poison ivy, 83–84

Polio, 76, 264
  immunizations, 190, 194–95, 264

Pools, swimming, 398

Postconcussion syndrome, 159, 162

Postnasal drip, 86, 159

Postural drainage, 103

Precordial catch syndrome, 54

Pregnancy
  and antibiotic use, 3
  asthma, 18–21
  and crib death, 91
  immunizations during, 192, 195, 200
  informing other children, 285
  iron in, 7–8
  rubella during, 269

Prematurity, 13, 193, 356

Preparing for the baby, 335–39

Prevention
  AIDS, 4, 5
  of choking, 64–65
  contact dermatitis, 84–86
  head trauma, 161
  heat rash, 165
  hepatitis, 176

of high cholesterol, 69–70
of injuries, 386
lead poisoning, 392–95
Lyme disease, 220–21
speech problems, 106–7
Prickly heat, 164–65
Pseudomenses, 242
Pseudostrabismus, 131
Psoriasis, 267
Psychotherapy, 12
and abuse, 61
Puberty, 1
breast enlargement in. See Sexual development
delayed, 342
onset, 283
Pulmonary embolism, 52
Purpura
Henoch-Schönlein, 171
idiopathic thrombocytopenic, 170–71
Pyelonephritis, 359
Pyloric stenosis, 313–14

Rabies, 29–30, 76
Race. See Ethnicity
Rape, 60
Rashes
allergic, 144, 148
in chickenpox, 55
in contact dermatitis, 83
diaper, 110–12
with fifth disease, 139
heat, 164–65
in Kawasaki disease, 204
with Lyme disease, 219–20
with measles, 223

with mononucleosis, 228
newborn, 128
in pityriasis rosea, 259
in roseola, 268, 269
with scabies, 271
Reflux
gastroesophageal, 94, 310–11
vesicoureteral, 361, 362
Relaxation therapy, 158
Respirators, 264
Respiratory problems, 14–21, 55, 86, 98–100
Reye's syndrome, 55, 56, 135, 266
Rheumatic fever, 53, 198–99, 215–16, 302, 303
Rheumatic heart disease, 302–3
Rheumatoid arthritis, 54
Rhinitis
medicamentosum, 245
Ribs, 50, 51
Ringworm, 153, 267
Rocking, 235, 292–93
Rocky Mountain spotted fever, 29
Roseola, 268, 269
Rubella, 139, 172, 269–70
and arthritis, 216
and birth defects, 269–70
immunizations, 190, 195–96
Rubeola. See Measles

Sacral dimple, 243
Safety
on airplanes, 374–75

backyard, 397–99
bicycle, 375–77
car, 378–81
Halloween, 385–86
kitchen, 387–89
party, 285–86
playground, 397–99
in toys, 349
travel, 374–75, 403–6
Salmonella, 309
Salmon patches, 26
Salt, 141
Scabies, 270–72
Scarlet fever, 139, 302, 368
Scarring
from acne, 1
in chickenpox, 55
in ear infection, 119
surgical, 138–39
School, returning to after illness, 265
Scoliosis, 272–73
Scrotum, 282, 307, 333, 334
newborn, 243
Scurvy, 166
Seizures, 160, 274–77, 391
febrile, 137, 139, 275–76
and head trauma, 163
and immunizations, 194
in meningitis, 227
newborn, 275
with PKU, 256
Sensitive topics, 277–78
Separation anxiety, 279–81, 327
Sequencing disability, 206
Sexual
abuse, 58, 60, 61, 223
characteristics, 283

development, 281–84
intercourse, 4, 5, 60
Sexually transmitted disease, 172, 251, 362, 368
Shigella, 309
Shingles, 54, 57
Shin splints, 214
Shoes, 133
Short attention span. See Attention deficit disorder; Attention span
Sibling rivalry, 284–86
Sickle cell anemia, 9–10, 52, 197, 199, 200, 203, 228
Side effects
asthma medications, 17
immunizations, 195
SIDS. See Sudden infant death syndrome
Sinusitis, 77, 79, 86, 131, 159, 199, 287–88
complications of, 288
Sixth disease, 268
Skin. See also Acne; Birthmarks; Rashes
birthmarks, 25–26
eczema, 126–28, 153
in frostbite, 151
impetigo, 153, 198–99
newborn, 236–37
photosensitivity, 2
Skull fractures, 33, 155, 163. See also Head Trauma
Sleep
apnea, 305
naps, 293–94
with parents, 296–98
position and crib death, 93–94
problems, 187, 289–99
and use of pillows, 97

vomiting during, 94
walking in, 298–99
Slipped capital femoral
    epiphysis, 218
Smallpox, 190, 197
Smoking
    and coronary artery
        disease, 69
    and ear infection, 117
    and hypertension, 179
Snake bites. See Bites and
    stings
Sneakers, 133
Snoring, 305
Sodium, 141
Somogyi phenomenon,
    109
Sore throat, 157, 299–
    305
    and bad breath, 21
    in bronchitis, 40
    with colds, 77
    and diphtheria, 115
    and idiopathic
        thrombocytopenic
        purpura, 170
    with influenza, 199
    in Kawasaki disease,
        204
    with mononucleosis,
        228
    with polio, 264
Spanking, 291, 326, 328,
    329
Speech
    delayed, 106
    developmental
        milestones, 105–6
    dysfluency, 316–17
    problems, 35, 104–5,
        160, 316–17
    and toilet training, 344
Spiders. See Bites and
    stings
Spinal

problems, 272–73
    tap, 226
Spleen, 9, 171, 197, 216,
    228, 229
Splinters, 213–14
Sprains, 32, 214
Stenosis, pyloric, 313–14
Sternum, 51
Still disease, 216
Stings. See Bites and
    stings
Stitches, 306
Stomachaches, 9, 307–15
    and antibiotics, 137
Stool
    black, 8
    blood in, 80, 148, 171,
        307, 311, 312
    bulky, 103
    color, 315–16
    "currant jelly," 312
    foul smelling, 103
    light, 172
    with mucus, 312
    transitional, 112
Storkbites, 26
Strabismus, 131–32, 239
Strains, 214
Strawberry nevi, 26
Strep
    complications of, 302–
        3
    infection, 138, 299–
        303
Stress
    and asthma, 14
    and bed-wetting, 22
    and cold sores, 71
    and colitis, 311
    and diarrhea, 112
    and eczema, 127
    and headaches, 158
    and hypertension, 179
    management, 179
    parental, 59

and stomachache, 309
and tics, 234, 235
and viruses, 57
Stroke, 9, 179
Strollers, 49–50
Stuttering, 316–17
Styes, 132
Sudden infant death
    syndrome, 90–95
Suffocation, 96
Sugar, 125. See also
    Blood sugar;
    Diabetes
  blood, 160, 274, 275
Sunburn, 43, 83, 399–
    401
Sunscreen, 2, 401–2
Suppositories, 82
Sweating
  adolescent onset, 283
  and cystic fibrosis, 103
  feet, 133
  and heat rash, 164
  night, 109
Swelling
  and allergy, 148
  in bites and stings, 28,
    30
  lymph gland, 30
Swimmer's ear, 120–21
Sydenham chorea, 303–4
Symptoms
  asthma, 15
  attention deficit
    syndrome, 209–10
  cold, 77–78
  diabetes, 107–8
  food allergies, 148
  hepatitis, 172, 175
  inflammatory bowel
    disease, 311
  influenza, 199
  iron deficiency anemia,
    8

learning disabilities,
    209–10
  meningitis, 226–27
  mononucleosis, 228
  mumps, 231
  poisoning, 260
  polio, 264
  rabies, 30
  roseola, 269
  sinusitis, 287
  tuberculosis, 353
  urinary tract infection,
    359–60
Synovitis, toxic, 182, 216
Systemic lupus
    erythematosis, 219

Tanner scale, 281–83
Tear ducts, 129
Teeth, 317–23
  brushing, 21, 319
  buck, 339
  decay in, 22, 34, 35,
    318
  enamel, 35, 235
  fluoride use, 34, 35
  grinding, 234–35
  and headaches, 159
  malocclusion, 34, 234
  natal, 240, 321
  permanent, 35, 317,
    319–20
  wisdom, 318
Teething, 321–23
  and diarrhea, 113
  and earache, 120
  and fever, 120
Television, 323–25, 330–
    31
Temperature. See also
    Fever
  in chickenpox, 55
  normal, 134
  taking, 136–37
Temper tantrums, 325–33

at bedtime, 290–91
Temporomandibular
    joint, 159–60, 235
Tendonitis, 214
Tendons, 214, 218
Testes, 333–34
    torsion in, 312, 334
    undescended, 333–34
Tetanus, 27, 30, 334–35
    immunizations, 45,
        190, 193–94, 334
Thalassemia, 7, 197
Thermometers, 136–37
    broken, 139
Thirst, 108
Throat infections, 120
Thrush, 111, 367
Thumb sucking, 187,
    339–41
Thyroid, 341–43
    abnormalities, 275
    deficiency, 81
    disorders, 153, 179
Ticks, 29, 219–21
Tics, 274
    nervous, 234–36
    repetitive, 235–36
Tine test, 353
Toilet training, 285–86,
    344–46. See also
    Bed-wetting
    and constipation, 80,
        81
Tongue
    black, 346
    geographic, 346
    thrust habit, 247
    tied, 347
Tonsils, 228, 288, 299–
    300, 304–5
Torticollis, 347–48
Tourette syndrome, 236
Tourniquets, 31
Toxic synovitis, 182, 216
Toxoplasmosis, 172

Toys, 349–52
Treatment
    acne, 2–3
    asthma, 16–18
    bed-wetting, 23–25
    broken bones, 32–33
    bronchitis, 40–41, 42–
        43
    burns, 44–45
    of colic, 74–76
    conjunctivitis, 130–31
    constipation, 82
    contact dermatitis, 84–
        86
    cystic fibrosis, 103
    diabetes, 108–9
    diarrhea, 113–15
    diphtheria, 116
    dislocations, 181
    eczema, 127–28
    fever, 135–38
    food allergies, 149–50
    hair loss, 154
    hepatitis, 176
    hypertension, 179
    idiopathic
        thrombocytopenic
        purpura, 171
    influenza, 199–200
    iron deficiency anemia,
        8
    jaundice, 203–4
    juvenile rheumatoid
        arthritis, 216–17
    lead poisoning, 392–95
    Lyme disease, 220
    measles, 224
    middle ear infection,
        117–20
    migraine, 158
    mononucleosis, 229
    mumps, 231–32
    nosebleed, 244–46
    osteomyelitis, 215
    pertussis, 255–56

pinworms, 258–59
pityriasis rosea, 260
poisoning, 260–63
Reye's syndrome, 266
rubella, 270
seizure, 276–77
sibling rivalry, 284–86
sinusitis, 159, 288
Sydenham chorea, 304
teething, 322–23
torticollis, 348
toxic synovitis, 182
tuberculosis, 354
urinary tract infection, 361
whooping cough, 255–56
Trichotillomania, 153
Triglycerides, 66, 68
Tsetse syndrome, 50
Tuberculosis, 42, 76, 284, 352–55
Tumors
bone, 218
brain, 160
and headaches, 160–61
kidney, 179
and seizures, 274
and sinusitis, 287
testicular, 333
thyroid, 342, 343
Twins, 355–57
Typhoid immunizations, 197

Ulcerative colitis, 311
Umbilical cord, 242, 357–59
Urinary problems
frequent urination, 364–65
painful urination, 366
Urinary tract infection, 22, 60, 113, 138, 250, 307, 359–63

Urine
blood in, 363–64
color change, 365
dark, 113, 172, 303
odor, 365
Urticaria, 183–84

Vaccine. See also Immunizations
adverse effects, 192
chickenpox, 56, 198
diphtheria, 193–94
haemophilus influenza B, 196
hepatitis, 174, 177, 190, 196
inactivated, 192, 194
influenza, 197, 200
live, 192, 194
measles, 190, 195–96
mumps, 190, 195–96
pertussis, 193–94
pneumococcal, 197
polio, 190, 194–95
rubella, 190, 195–96
smallpox, 197
tetanus, 193–94
typhoid, 197
Vagina, 281, 359, 366–68
discharge from, 367
injury to, 61
newborn, 242
Vaginitis, 3, 22, 137, 359, 366
Vaporizers, 79, 98, 187–88, 224, 232, 245, 256
Varicella. See Chickenpox
Vernix, 236
Vertigo, 157
Video games, 324
Viruses, 76–77, 137, 199, 226, 259–60, 264, 268, 372–73

and antibiotics, 76–77
in bronchitis, 40, 41
chickenpox, 54
Coxsackie, 52, 71, 72, 204–5
and croup, 98
Epstein-Barr, 172, 228, 229, 300
and fifth disease, 139
in hepatitis, 172
herpes, 54, 57, 71–73, 172
infection, 182, 216
rabies, 29–30
respiratory syncytial, 15–16, 41–42
stomach, 309
Vision, 163
Visual perception disabilities, 206
Vitamins, 3, 37, 126, 143, 146, 154, 167, 369–70
in anemia, 7
and colds, 80
in cystic fibrosis, 103
deficiency, 166
in infancy, 369
Volvulus, 312
Vomiting
and allergy, 148
with appendicitis, 308
in bronchitis, 40
from crying, 291
and formula change, 73
in head trauma, 162, 163
in hepatitis, 172
and hypertension, 179
with influenza, 199

in meningitis, 227
with motion sickness, 230
in poisoning, 260, 309
projectile, 160, 314
recurrent, 162, 163
with Reye's syndrome, 55, 266
during sleep, 94
with stomachache, 307, 314–15

Walkers, 371
Walking, toe, 134
Warts, 372–73
plantar, 217, 372–73
Weaning, 39, 124
Weight
and asthma, 20
and failure to thrive, 103
inadequate, 123–24
loss, 12, 108, 179, 307, 311
low at birth, 90
Wheezing, 14, 15, 87
allergic, 144, 148
in asthma, 52
in bites and stings, 28
in bronchiolitis, 41
in bronchitis, 40
Whiteheads, 1
Whooping cough, 255–56
immunizations, 190, 193–94
Withdrawal, 104
Wounds, head, 29–30

Xiphoid process, 241